SCHOOL·BASED HEALTH CARE
ADVANCING EDUCATIONAL SUCCESS AND PUBLIC HEALTH

D1212605

SCHOOL·BASED HEALTH CARE

ADVANCING EDUCATIONAL SUCCESS AND PUBLIC HEALTH

Editors

Terri D. Wright, MPH and
Jeanita W. Richardson, PhD, MEd

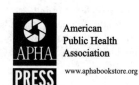

American
Public Health
Association

APHA
PRESS

www.aphabookstore.org

WASHINGTON, D.C. • 2012

American Public Health Association
800 I Street, NW
Washington, DC 20001-3710
www.apha.org

Georges C. Benjamin, M.D., F.A.C.P., F.A.C.E.P. (Emeritus), Executive Director
Howard Spivak, M.D., Publications Board Liaison
Printed and bound in the United States of America
Interior Design and Typesetting: Manila Typesetting Company
Cover Design: Alan Giarcanella
Printing and Binding: Victor Graphics, Inc.

Library of Congress Cataloging-in-Publication Data

School-based health care : advancing educational success and public health / edited by Terri D. Wright and Jeanita W. Richardson.
   p. ; cm.
Includes bibliographical references.
ISBN-13: 978-0-87553-006-2
ISBN-10: 0-87553-006-2
I. Wright, Terri D. II. Richardson, Jeanita W., 1957– III. American Public Health Association.
[DNLM: 1. School Health Services--organization & administration. 2. Health Policy. 3. Public Health Practice. 4. Students. WA 350]
  362.1—dc23
              2011038456

Table of Contents

Section IV. School-Based Health Care: Looking to the Future   **321**

List of Tables

List of Figures

Foreword

S *chool-Based Health Care: Advancing Educational Success and Public Health* is a revelation about a little known resource for closing the achievement gap and improving life outcomes for millions of children in the United States. In an age of countless articles and books about access to health care, health care reform, and an equal or greater amount of literature on education reform, this book offers a remarkable story of success against great odds. The success can be defined as the exponential growth of a movement that meets the concrete needs of vulnerable children and adolescents. Every year, about four million school-age youth receive care through school-based health centers (SBHCs). More than 70% are children of color. Almost all are in low-income neighborhoods, both rural and urban. SBHCs have not replaced the school nurses that many "baby boomers" may recall. No, SBHCs have boldly expanded access to care by providing more services, on a regular basis, in the form of a "medical home" to young people at times when that care may be pivotal to their continued school success and to school engagement.

Story is a powerful medium for change. This book is a "story" culled from many stories about nearly 2,000 SBHCs in 44 states and the District of Columbia. The stories of these SBHCs are the narratives of real communities who managed to put children's needs above politics of fear and division to provide, figuratively speaking, "open arms and safe embraces," or literally safe, accessible places for healing.

And as impressive as the rapid expansion of SBHCs in the 1990s was (from less than 100 in the 1980s to almost 2,000 in 44 states by 2000), this growth has slowed to an almost snail's pace since that time. The growth has decreased by a conservative estimate of 50%. According to the 2010 census from the National Assembly on School-Based Health Care, today less than 10% of this nation's 50 million school-age children have access to the fundamental resource, a center for health care—a medical home—in the place where they spend the bulk of their waking and learning hours.

SBHCs provide needed access to primary care and behavioral health, as well as preventive health care, to the most vulnerable community members, children. A disproportionate number of these children are children of color, who might otherwise have no source of primary health care. In addition to improving student chances for better school attendance, achievement, and outcomes, SBHCs are also an important resource for reducing health disparities. The American Academy of Pediatrics reminds us that extensive, pervasive, and persistent racial and ethnic health disparities in health and health care exist. By providing quality, timely care, SBHCs offer an important lever for change. In addition to care, however, the school-based health care movement (with funding from the W. K. Kellogg Foundation) has developed an intentional and sustained focus on multicultural and racial equity skills development.

Persistent inequitable health outcomes, or disparities, can be viewed as symptoms of deeper protracted social dynamics embedded in historical systems of racial discrimination and limited opportunity. The prevalence of residential segregation and the subsequent over-representation of children of color within low-income neighborhoods and schools is the clearest illustration of this phenomenon.

Incorporating an intentional racial equity and multicultural lens in this school-based health care movement as it looked to engage more policymakers and elected officials helped to prepare community advocates, parents, and students with needed strategies for effective engagement and cross-cultural communication. The challenges of identifying community-level barriers, building multisector alliances, and engaging diverse constituencies were handled more efficiently as a result of this added dimension. Readers of this book will benefit from the multicultural and racial equity conceptual framework, theories of action, and tools that are so clearly delineated. Latino, Native American, African American, and many immigrant children and families have reported significant benefit from these resources.

The World Health Organization's Commission on Social Determinants of Health reminds us of the forces that truly shape health and well-being. "Inequities in health, avoidable health inequalities, arise because of the circumstances in which people grow, live, work, and age, and the systems put in place to deal with illness. The conditions in which people live and die are, in turn, shaped by political, social, and economic forces."[a]

SBHCs should be the hallmark of the "system" put in place to deal with illness and prevention of illness in every school district in America. A recent victory for this movement, "authorization as a federal program" in the nation's health

---

[a] World Health Organization, Commission on the Social Determinants of Health. *Closing the Gap in a Generation: Health Equity Through Action on the Social Determinants of Health. Final Report of the Commission on Social Determinants of Health.* Geneva, Switzerland: World Health Organization; 2008.

care law, the Patient Protection and Affordable Care Act (PPACA) makes it more possible, if not probable, that this vision will become reality. Authorization as a federal program is an empty pot without an appropriation. Certainly in a climate of shrinking state revenues and deficit-based budgeting, the odds for accelerating the expansion of this movement are stacked against hope.

But odds have never stopped the proponents of school-based health care. They have had help, however. The W. K. Kellogg Foundation has been a strategic friend and generous ally to this important work for many decades. Since 2004 alone, the W. K. Kellogg Foundation has invested more than $39 million in support of communities that organized to implement and sustain school-based health care, as well as in support of the national infrastructure for the expanding movement.

This comprehensive book is the first of its kind. It captures the on-the-ground-realities of building the movement for school-based health care with explicit detail and lessons learned the hard way, through both failure and success. By addressing practical professional practice, advocacy, and sustainability strategies unique to school-based health care, this book offers contemporary knowledge and resources that are needed for the continued expansion of the work in communities across America. As important, it provides insight and strategies that are transferable to major social change endeavors. Readers will learn in the most credible way—within context—about designing and launching successful messaging and media campaigns when opponents have more money and more power. They will also be taken by the hand into the halls of Congress and shown the nuanced steps to educating and influencing champions that "at a heart" level share common values for the well-being of children. The rhetoric of cross-disciplinary collaboration moves from concept to form in the stories of communities that decided to move young people out of the "dropout danger zone," once they were helped to see the school dropout crisis as a public health crisis. This is probably the most salient message of this comprehensive volume—"public education and public health are inextricably linked."

It is impossible to return to education or health "business as usual" after reading this book. The public health system and the public education system are literally bookends—the lives and future well-being of the nation shelved between them.

These two pillars of vibrant democracy, public health and public education, must work together in complementary ways on many fronts, from disaster preparedness and response to education about climate change and environmental stewardship. Yet, as important as these curriculums are, the most fundamental vehicle for collaboration between these two disciplines is in the form of providing school-based health care for the 50 million young people in our nation's schools.

This book shows readers how others are bridging the disciplinary divides of language, culture, turf protection, and budget silos to truly work together on behalf of vulnerable children. This work is perfectly aligned with the original vision of Will Keith Kellogg, and it is at the heart of the Foundation's mission as it is expressed today—81 years later:

> The W. K. Kellogg Foundation supports children, families, and communities as they strengthen and create conditions that propel vulnerable children to achieve success as individuals and as contributors to the larger community and society.

Will Keith Kellogg created the Foundation after attending President Hoover's White House Conference on Child Health and Protection. The conference produced "The Children's Charter," which recognized the rights of the child. The Charter contains an impressive set of 19 fundamental rights for every child, regardless of race, or color, or situation, wherever he/she may live under the protection of the American flag. Among these rights are:

V: For every child health protection from birth through adolescence, including periodic health examination and, where needed, care of specialists and hospital treatment; regular dental examination and care for the teeth; protective and preventive measures against communicable diseases; the insuring of pure food, pure milk, and pure water.

VI: For every child from birth through adolescence, promotion of health, including health instruction and a health program, wholesome physical and mental recreation, with teachers and leaders adequately trained.

VII: For every child a dwelling place safe, sanitary, and wholesome, with reasonable provisions for privacy, free from conditions which tend to thwart his development; and a home environment harmonious and enriching.

VIII: For every child a school which is safe from hazards, sanitary, properly equipped, lighted, and ventilated. For younger children nursery schools and kindergartens to supplement home care.

Many of the earliest investments of the W. K. Kellogg Foundation during its first 11 years were in providing health care and nutrition in local schools in Michigan. These grants were a prelude to the school-based health care movement, and subsequent support of SBHCs was a natural outgrowth of donor intent.

That said, the progress of that support was the direct result of leadership, skill, tenacity, and brilliance of the Foundation staff who shepherded the work through its most vital period. Terri Wright, MPH, brought amazing talent to her role as Program Director throughout the 1990s through 2009. It was during this period that the school-based health care movement experienced its most significant expansion in scale and impact.

Terri Wright and her coeditor of this volume, Jeanita W. Richardson, PhD, MEd, have compiled an impressive set of articles in this book that collectively make the most compelling case for the primacy of school-based health care to the well-being of the nation's children and, as such, to this nation's future. The true power of their "case" grows from authentic engagement in the work, on the ground and in communities.

Practitioners will return to this work time and time again for its jewels of wisdom about how to and how *not* to move a program from, just that, a program to an organization; then to a coalition, to a movement, and ultimately, to a system (that works well with other systems) for lasting social change. Such is the story and the case that is made eloquently in this important book.

Timing is also critical. Most Americans have been hoodwinked into believing media "spin" and sound bites about the PPACA. The general public knows far too little about the hard-fought victories embedded in this long-awaited, although first of many, steps toward universal access to health care. As this landmark legislation winds its way through state courts, legislatures, and governors cabinets for implementation, its potential for changing lives, immediately, is underestimated. Budget debates at all levels of government threaten the realization of that potential. But the authorization of school-based health care (along with an appropriation), coupled with the health care reform law's emphasis on public health prevention, health-in-all policies, and community transformation, combine to create an unprecedented opportunity for improving the health and life trajectories of our nation's most vulnerable young people. Between now and 2014, when most of health care reform change takes effect, there is a unique moment in history for reshaping understanding of health, health care, disease prevention, and the role of communities and schools. This truly informative and wise book will help to deepen conversations about adult, student, and community engagement in both education and public health.

It is an urgent, must read for policymakers, public health practitioners, educators, and parents, but most importantly for the students whose future is being determined now.

Gail C. Christopher, DN
Vice President for Program Strategy
W. K. Kellogg Foundation
Battle Creek, MI

Acknowledgements

"You can't educate people that are not healthy. But you certainly can't keep them healthy if they're not educated."

—*Jocelyn Elders*

The editors are grateful to all of the authors who by virtue of their submissions and their commitment to the well-being of children and youth demonstrate the power of linking the just causes of educational and health equity. The patience, commitment, and professionalism of Brian Selzer and his colleagues were indispensable. We deeply appreciate your grace.

This book is dedicated to the practitioners, advocates, researchers and educators who struggle daily to understand and remedy the complex issues faced by America's youth.

Jeanita W. Richardson
Terri D. Wright

Introduction

Debate rages about the strengths and weaknesses of the national health care delivery system and the attendant legislative interventions designed to provide access to health care for millions of uninsured and underinsured Americans in general. Of particular concern in this volume are the millions of children who find themselves unable to access health care for several reasons, including being uninsured or under insured. Children and youth are particularly vulnerable because they are fiscally and politically dependent upon adults and social systems for support. Further complicating the optimal development of childhood and youth potential are the reciprocal influences of health and learning readiness and success.[1] Given the calls for fiscal conservatism, accountability, efficiency, and high quality of care, it seems rational to consider programs and practices that successfully meet the needs of children where they spend significant time: their schools.

Support for supplying health services in and near schools comes from both the health and educational sectors. The persistent challenge has been to bring both disciplines together as advocacy partners in support of children and youth. As one example, American Public Health Association's policy #20101, as well as its Center for School, Health, and Education, supports the value of breaking down the silos between health and education professionals, particularly in the case of children and youth, because health and education are inextricably linked. Schools are one of the last institutions central to every community and have proven themselves to be a logical location to provide all manner of support services for children, youth, and their families. Furthermore, 90% of the nation's children attend public schools, and educators and health professionals have practical knowledge of the relationships between health and attendance.[2] For example, children with fair to poor health status are six times more likely to have learning disabilities as their healthy counterparts and are apt to be absent

11 or more days of school per year.[1,3-6] Graduation rates, in addition to being a predictor of economic status, are now identified as a way to derail health disparities.[7,8]

While numerous books and articles concern themselves with dimensions of health and school-aged children and youth, there does not appear to be one volume addressing practice, policy, and applied research on outcomes and impacts particular to school-based health care. This edited book attempts to address that need by capturing the current knowledge on school-based health care from the field of practitioners, researchers, and policy advocates. Their voices demonstrate the wide array of those committed to advancing the school-based health care movement. Collectively they share their experiences and wisdom on strategies that not only improve access to comprehensive health care, services, and programs but favorably impact health and educational equity as well. In addition, they share insight into the components of a national policy initiative designed to secure favorable local, state, and national policies.

Contributors to this book reflect the levels of engagement needed to advance the health and wellness of America's children and youth through the school-based health care movement. Borrowing from the public health ecological model, practitioners intimately acquainted with youth and their families and schools represent the power of interventions focusing on relationships and communities. Hands-on involvement at these levels typically leaves little time for authorship, which speaks to the value of inclusion of these school building– and community-level "voices." Propelling a health care model into mainstream consciousness also requires attention to a systems-level view of successful practices. As a result, attention is also given to placing school-based health centers (SBHCs) in a national and state political context. These "voices" advance lessons learned and strategies helpful in positioning SBHCs for the future. Given the diversity of contributors, it is our hope that every reader will identify with at least one "voice" and feel empowered to replicate, augment, and advance strategies and policies supportive of school-based health care for the nation's children and youth.

WHY SCHOOL-BASED HEALTH CARE AND WHY NOW?

SBHCs are unsung heroes of preventative and medical care for children and youth. There are over 1,900 school-based and school-linked health centers throughout the country, at least 41% of which are located in Title I schools, a designation given to schools with high numbers of economically disadvantaged and otherwise at-risk students.[9,10] As per the most recent SBHC census conducted by the National Assembly on School-Based Health Care, 80% of survey respondent centers serve at least one grade of adolescents. SBHCs primarily serve school populations with significant numbers of ethnic and racial minorities who historically experience poverty, inadequate access to health care, health care disparities, and health inequities.[11] Most SBHCs are located in urban communities (57%), however, their presence is increasing in rural schools (27%).[12,13] The scope of services is community specific and determined through consensus between service providers, the schools in which they are located, and the communities served. The range of services most consistently offered include comprehensive primary care and; of particular importance to the public health community, have as a primary focus health promotion and disease prevention, early intervention and risk reduction, and mental health services.[9,10,14]

SBHC interventions can mitigate the impact of health disparities that are a function of poverty and, in partnership with schools, have a profound effect on children and youth. Health and education disciplines have their own lexicons with terms that overlap in meaning. For example, many of the social determinants of health are also educational risk factors, i.e., poverty, linguistic minority status, being a racial and ethnic minority, rurality, and inadequate housing. SBHC interventions can promote early diagnoses of preventable or treatable health conditions, thereby theoretically improving the quality of academic experiences. As a result of the interaction among and between income, health, and cognitive development, introducing health facilities in schools holds the potential of high returns on investment.[1]

In his article on school health policies and programs, Kolbe writes, "Today, more than ever, school health programs could become one of the most efficient means available to improve the health of our children and their educational achievement."[15(p226)] Similarly, in an article concerned with school–community partnerships, Lee-Bayha and Harrison posit, "The best of teaching cannot always compete successfully with the challenges many students face outside of school."[16(p1)] As these quotes and research would suggest, bridging the two disciplines and providing preventative and acute care in schools has been proven as a rational, efficient, and effective means of supporting the health and educational success of young people.

Studies of the impact of SBHCs affirm their positive influence on reducing absenteeism, improved management of chronic diseases such as asthma, and early identification of risk behaviors because of their ecological approach to child and youth health.[12,14,17] Evidence substantiating the cost-benefit and improved health care access associated with school-based and school-linked health centers has finally begun to mitigate the significant barrier to securing long-term, sustainable funding streams in the form of statutory acknowledgment of SBHCs as valued contributors to the continuum of medical care.[12,13,18,19] More recent studies are revealing the relationship between health and educational success. For example, users of SBHCs for mental health services had an increased grade point average over nonusers, African American male users were three times more likely to stay in school than were nonusers, and SBHCs positively impacted the school learning environment.[20,21]

The favorable evidence of school-based health care has successfully propelled it into the national policy arena. The profile and value of SBHCs has risen significantly in the last five years among federal and state legislators, as well as in the educational and health sectors. As examples, SBHCs became an authorized federal program in Section 4101(b) of the Patient Protection and Affordability Care Act of 2010, and in 2009 became recognized providers in the Child Health Insurance Program Reauthorization Act. Both of these policies will contribute to the long-term viability of school-based health care.

Equally important are advances that have been made between health and educational policy. Early in 2010, Secretary of Health and Human Services Kathleen Sebelius spoke at the Coalition for Community Schools' biannual convention where she affirmed that she and the Secretary of Education (Arne Duncan) are actively seeking ways to increase the footprint of SBHCs in both educational and health policy reform.

All evidence points to the need for a cadre of advocates and practitioners who understand the inextricable connections between the health and educational potential of children and youth, possess strategic political intervention skills, and knowledge of successful health care delivery practices if SBHCs are to take advantage of the current momentum, such as in the process of the reauthorization of the Elementary and Secondary Education Act (ESEA).

SBHCs are well positioned to build on what has been learned from almost 40 years of serving school-age youth, and major strides have been made in public policy to support this model of health care delivery. Now it is time to optimize the inherent potential of SBHCs by expanding their impact beyond their clinic walls and enrolled patients into the broader school population regardless of enrollment status. The chapters of this book capture what is now known and can provide the impetus to mobilize on behalf of the future well-being of school-age youth.

School-Based Health Care: Advancing Educational Success and Public Health is divided into four sections: (1) "School-Based Health Care Practice, Interventions, Outcomes, and Impacts From the Field"; (2) "Propelling the

School-Based Health Care Movement: The W. K. Kellogg Foundations School-Based Health Care Policy Program"; (3) "Strategic Partnerships for Fiscal and Policy Advocacy"; and (4) "School-Based Health Care: Looking to the Future."

The first section entitled "School-Based Health Care Practice, Interventions, Outcomes, and Impacts From the Field" includes eight chapters providing an array of empirical research, analytical essays, commentaries, and descriptions of evidence-based interventions. It offers insight into the breadth of clinical interventions and public health approaches unique to SBHCs.

"Propelling the School-Based Health Care Movement" deconstructs the W. K. Kellogg Foundation's six-year national School-Based Health Care Policy Program investment. Lessons relative to the various program elements and the need to nurture organizations, advocates, and policy decision-makers are central to this section. We believe the focus on how policy advocacy at the local, state, and federal levels takes shape over time is instructive to organizations and individuals interested in propelling the school-based health care movement forward.

As was noted earlier, sustainability has always been tenuous for school-based health care. "Strategic Partnerships for Fiscal and Policy Advocacy" provides practical examples of how to engage partners of different types to advance the work of SBHCs. Likewise, diversified resources are described that allow SBHCs to lessen their vulnerability to shifts in the legislative appropriations process through revenue generation and strategic partnerships.

Finally, "School-Based Health Care: Looking to the Future" includes chapters that place SBHCs in the contemporary educational, health, and political context. The opportunities for school-based health care are examined in light of educational partnerships for resiliency, impacting the school climate, and health care reform.

This book is the first of its type in over 20 years. Educational attainment is widely acknowledged as the most reliable means of decimating the impact of poverty. Health fuels the resilience of otherwise at-risk children and youth, enabling them to actualize their innate potential. With hindsight and research as our evidence, SBHCs now more than ever are positioned to take their rightful place in the health and educational reform movements on behalf of the populations they most often care for: economically disadvantaged youth. The clarion call to advance the strategies in this volume and encourage those who read it to advocate for the educational success and health of the nation's youth is perhaps summed up best by the words of Nelson Mandela and Graca Machel: "We cannot waste our precious children. Not another one, not another day. It is long past time for us to act on their behalf."[22]

REFERENCES

1. Richardson JW, Juszczak LJ. Schools as sites for health-care delivery. *Public Health Rep.* 2008;123(6):692–694.

2. Richardson JW. From risk to resilience: promoting school–health partnerships for children. *Int J Educ Reform.* 2008;17(1):19–36.

3. Federal Interagency Forum on Child and Family Statistics. *America's Children: Key National Indicators of Well-Being 2007.* Washington, DC: Federal Interagency Forum on Child and Family Statistics, US Government Printing Office; 2007.

4. National Center for Children in Poverty. *United States Early Childhood Profile.* New York, NY: Columbia University Mailman School of Public Health; 2007.

5. US Department of Education—National Center for Education Statistics. *The Condition of Education 2006.* Washington, DC: US Government Printing Office; 2006.

6. Taras H, Potts-Datema W. Chronic health conditions and student performance at school. *J Sch Health.* 2005;75(7):255–266.

7. Alliance for Excellent Education. *The High Cost of High School Dropouts: What the Nation Pays for Inadequate High Schools.* Issue Brief. Washington, DC: Alliance for Excellent Education; 2008.

8. Freudenberg N, Ruglis J. Reframing school dropout as a public health issue. *Prev Chronic Dis.* 2007;4(4):A107.

9. National Assembly on School-Based Health Care. *School-Based Health Centers: A National Definition.* Washington DC: National Assembly on School-Based Health Care; 2002.

10. Richardson JW, Wright TD. Advancing school-based health care policy and practice. *Am J Public Health.* 2010;100(9):1561.

11. Strozer J, Juszczak L, Ammerman A. *2007–2008 School-Based Health Center Census.* Washington, DC: National Assembly on School-Based Health Care; 2010.

12. Geierstanger SP, Amaral G, Mansour M, Walters SR. School-based health centers and academic performance: research, challenges, and recommendations. *J Sch Health.* 2004;74(9):347–352.

13. Schlitt JJ, Juszczak LJ, Eichner NH. Current status of state policies that support school-based health centers. *Public Health Rep.* 2008;123(6):731–738.

14. Juszczak L, Schlitt J, Odum M, Barangan C, Washington D. School-based health centers: a blueprint for healthy learners—data from the 2001–2002 School-Based Health Center Census. In: Lear JG, Isaacs SL, Knickman JR, eds. *School Health Services and Programs.* San Francisco, CA: Jossey-Bass; 2006:294–307.

15. Kolbe LJ, Kann L, Brener ND. School health policies and programs study 2000: overview and summary of findings. In: Lear JG, Isaacs SL, Knickman JR, eds. *School Health Services and Programs*. San Francisco, CA: Jossey-Bass; 2006:163–181.

16. Lee-Bayha J, Harrison T. *Using School–Community Partnerships to Bolster Student Learning*. Policy Brief. San Francisco, CA: WestEd; 2002.

17. Guo G, Harris KM. The mechanisms mediating the effects of poverty on children's intellectual development. *Demography*. 2000;37(4):431–447.

18. Richardson JW. Building bridges between school-based health clinics and schools. *J Sch Health*. 2007;77(7):337–343.

19. Wade TJ, Mansour ME, Guo JJ, Huentelman T, Line K, Keller KN. Access and utilization patterns of school-based health centers at urban and rural elementary and middle schools. *Public Health Rep*. 2008;123(6):739–750.

20. Basch CE. *Healthier Students Are Better Learners: A Missing Link in School Reforms to Close the Achievement Gap*. New York, NY: The Campaign for Educational Equity, Teachers College Columbia University; 2010.

21. Bireda S. Healthy students are better students: health reform bill gives a boost to school-based health centers. Center for American Progress. May 19, 2010.

22. UNICEF. United Nations Special Session on Children. May 8–10, 2002.

SECTION I

School-Based Health Care Practice Interventions, Outcomes, and Impacts From the Field

OVERVIEW

The delivery of health care in schools dates back to the days of public health efforts to eradicate poliomyelitis by ensuring that every child received the newly created vaccine against this preventable infectious disease.[1] School nurses were also an essential ally of the public school system to care for the sudden onset of illness, provide first aid, follow up on compliance issues, and ensure that infections were contained. School-based health centers (SBHCs) are the next generation of this tradition and provide a broader array of services that constitute primary care, often including mental health services that supplement the school counselor's or social worker's interventions. A critical mass of SBHCs appeared in the 1980s[2] and today there are over 2,000 SBHCs in 47 states that serve the K–12 student population with an array of primary health and mental health services including, in some cases, oral health services as well.[3] The rationale for this model of care has been predicated on improving access to much needed care for children and adolescents where they spend the majority of their hours. As such, almost 2 million racially and ethnically diverse students receive their health care in schools largely located in urban and rural communities.[3] These young people tend to be underserved, uninsured or underinsured, and are often most in need of support and care to complete the school day.

This section uncovers the role and impact of school-based health care when responding to the numerous health and social issues faced by students. Its content includes the promising results of both empirical research as well as the descriptive results of evidence- or practice-based interventions.

In Chapter 1, Clayton and colleagues provide several descriptive and promising examples of a range of programs and services offered by SBHCs in California that have integrated clinical care and services with public health concepts. Centers are providing primary and public health programs that focus on obesity prevention and improved access to healthy food in schools, for example. They are providing mental health services while changing the school climate for improved race relations between students and faculty and implementing antibullying campaigns. Asthma management offers a special opportunity to integrate public health with clinical care. While clinicians and health educators work with students to manage their asthma and keep them in school, other school personnel conduct indoor air assessments to identify possible triggers within the school building. In fact, from the school bus drivers to cafeteria workers to teachers, faculty and staff throughout the school milieu are trained to be the eyes and ears into the lives and experiences of students. They become the pathway for students to engage with the SBHC for assistance and intervention.

The remaining chapters in this section will explore a variety of evidence- or practice-based approaches that SBHCs employ to impact the health and well-being of young people in schools. Schools offer a safe and convenient location for students to access an array of services needed to be well and stay in school ready to learn.

In Chapter 2, Soleimanpour et al. reveals how young people at risk for not receiving much needed physical and mental health care find their SBHCs a safe and confidential medical home. The researchers share their findings about SBHCs improving access and having favorable outcomes particularly in reproductive health and health care and utilization of mental health services.

Exciting results of a cohort prospective study are explored by McNall et al. in Chapter 3, who examined the health and health behaviors of users and nonusers of SBHCs in middle and high schools at two points in time. The findings shed light on the impact of the SBHC on health promoting behaviors.

SBHCs have increasingly been shown to have a favorable impact on the utilization of mental health services by particularly vulnerable children and adolescents.[4] Postdisaster poses a time of increased need for mental health services by those affected. In Chapter 4, Broussard and colleagues share the experience of post-Katrina New Orleans and how the capacity of school nurses was developed to recognize and refer students in need of behavioral health services. The impact is extensive and includes not only tens of thousands of traumatized students but the school nurses as well.

Mandel and Kulig offer a provocative perspective on the rationale for gender specific prevention of substance use in SBHCs in Chapter 5. This longitudinal demonstration project reveals the unique role of the SBHC on girls and substance use prevention.

At its core SBHCs respond to the need to have middle and high school students fully immunized. Achieving full compliance with immunization requirements is particularly challenging as the scientific community releases new vaccines and updated guidelines.[1] Schools hold a historically unique position beyond the physician's office to reach large numbers of young people in one venue.[1] Chapter 6, by Salerno, shares a project to achieve full compliance with the state health department's priorities for childhood and adolescent immunizations. Salerno discusses a successful, comprehensive approach that included students, parents, and school personnel.

Floodwaters damaged or destroyed all of the SBHCs in the greater New Orleans area after Hurricane Katrina in 2005. An infusion of philanthropic resources aided in the rapid rebuilding and restoration of vital school-based health care, particularly behavioral health services. In Chapter 7, Broussard and colleagues describe the impact of SBHCs on access to quality health care and in the reduction of high-risk behaviors in a post-trauma environment.

Childhood obesity represents another prevalent societal reality. The Centers for Disease Control and Prevention reports that approximately 17% (or 12.5 million) of children and adolescents aged two to 19 years old are obese, a condition that has almost tripled since 1980.[5] In Chapter 8, van Helden demonstrates how a public health nutritionist in an SHBC impacted the health of adolescents through the design and implementation of a weight management program. This comprehensive approach for middle and high school students included nutrition education and intervention based on the Nutrition and Physical Activity Program. Increased physical activity was incorporated through a Walking Club and Fitness Club that included information and education as well as counseling. The results of this program are discussed, as is the transformation of one young man who at the program's beginning weighed 385 pounds.

This collection of chapters substantiate the breadth of the impact that school-based health care can have not only on the physical and mental health needs of school-age youth but also on the social and environmental challenges that can sabotage a student's ability to learn and succeed in school.

REFERENCES

1. Mazyck D. School-located vaccination clinics; then and now. *J Sch Nurs*. 2010; 26(4 Suppl):3S–6S.

2. Brindis CD, Klein J, Schlitt J, Santelli J, Juszczak L, Nystrom RJ. School-based health centers: accessibility and accountability. *J Adolesc Health*. 2003;32(6 Suppl):98–107.

3. Strozer J, Juszczak L, Ammerman A. *2007–2008 National School-Based Health Care Census*. Washington, DC: National Assembly on School-Based Health Care; 2010. Available at: http://www.nasbhc.org/atf/cf/%7Bcd9949f2-2761-42fb-bc7a-cee165c701d9%7D/NASBHC%202007-08%20CENSUS%20REPORT%20FINAL.PDF. Accessed December 6, 2010.

4. Soleimanpour S, Geierstanger SP, Kaller S, McCarter V, Brindis CD. The role of school health centers in health care access and client outcomes. *Am J Public Health*. 2010;100(9):1597–1603.

5. Ogden C, Carroll M. *Prevalence of obesity among children and adolescents: United States, Trends 1963–1965 through 2007–2008*. Atlanta, GA: National Center for Health Statistics Health E-Stat, Centers for Disease Control and Prevention; 2010.

Different Setting, Different Care: Integrating Prevention and Clinical Care in School-Based Health Centers[*]

Serena Clayton, Teresa Chin,
Samantha Blackburn, and
Cecilia Echeverría

Although insuring the 8.1 million uninsured children in the United States is a critical first step, improving children's and adolescents' health requires going beyond insurance coverage and providing better access and preventive services. Obesity, adolescent pregnancy, dental disease, uncontrolled asthma, and many mental health conditions are serious child and adolescent health concerns whose amelioration requires a combination of clinical services and preventive strategies. The pediatric health care system falls far short in the delivery of preventive care.[1,2] A recent study examined pediatric medical records for 175 indicators of quality care defined by an expert panel of physicians. Adherence to these quality standards was 67.6% for acute care but only 40.7% for preventive care, dropping to 34.5% when only adolescents were considered.[3]

Many authors have highlighted the need to tackle the multiple determinants of children's health. The resiliency paradigm emphasizes the importance of supportive environments and psychosocial skill development as protective factors mediating both adolescent risk behaviors and health outcomes.[4] The life course health development framework points to the importance of biological, behavioral, social, and economic determinants of health status that require integrated health interventions.[5] Most recently, with the growing obesity epidemic, we are seeing increasing attention to environmental determinants of health such as opportunities for

---

* This chapter previously appeared in the September 2010 issue of the *American Journal of Public Health* and is reprinted with permission in its entirety. Clayton S, Chin T, Blackburn S, Echeverría C. Different setting, different care: integrating prevention and clinical care in school-based health centers. *Am J Public Health*. 2010;100(9):1592–1595.

SCHOOL-BASED HEALTH CARE   15

physical activity and access to produce. A successful system for children's health requires a multisector approach that integrates medical, public health, educational, and social services, sectors that today remain an uncoordinated patchwork of categorical programs.[6]

The ability of school-based health centers (SBHCs) to increase access to health care has been well documented.[7-9] SBHCs, which deliver primary medical and mental health care, increase access and utilization by providing health care in a location that is convenient for students and their families. Less well recognized, however, is that health care services can be qualitatively different in an SBHC than they are in a community provider's office. Because of their unique location, SBHCs have the potential to implement health care models for children and adolescents that fully integrate prevention—primary, secondary, and tertiary—into clinical care and that address biological, behavioral, social, and economic determinants of health. We describe 4 school-based programs that exemplify this integration of clinical and preventive care and discuss opportunities for expanding these innovative models.

PROFILES OF 4 INNOVATIVE SCHOOL-BASED PROGRAMS

The school setting is a crucial factor in the ability of SBHCs to integrate multiple levels of prevention into clinical care. We chose 4 programs in California as examples of SBHCs that have maximized the value of their location in a school. The care they provide is not simply better access to the same care a community pediatrician would provide, it is health care that reaches outside the exam room to better address the myriad determinants of children's and adolescents' health.

Obesity Prevention

Edison High School in Stockton serves 2500 students, 57% of whom qualify for free or reduced lunch. The student population is ethnically diverse: 50% Hispanic, 30% Asian, and 14% African American. In 2003, a survey conducted by the University of the Pacific, Stockton, of physical fitness scores in high school physical education classes, which included a sample of 304 Hispanic ninth graders, found that 1 in 4 high school freshmen were obese or at risk for obesity. Furthermore, obese children in the survey had significantly lower school attendance and lower test scores compared with their nonobese peers. These findings prompted Edison's SBHC to start an obesity prevention and reduction program in 2004 called Healthy Hearts.

To recruit students for the program without creating a sense of stigma, the SBHC began with broader school-based screenings of height, weight, and blood pressure. Health center staff conducted presentations in classes, encouraging all students to come in for a physical. As an incentive, each student who complied received a T-shirt conforming to the school's physical education dress code, which normally would have to be purchased by the family. In addition, students who wished to participate in a popular salsa dance club were required to enroll in the health center and record their height, weight, and blood pressure.

Through these outreach efforts, the SBHC identified students who had a body mass index at or above the 85th percentile or blood pressure at or above the 90th percentile (in 3 consecutive readings) and approached them individually about Healthy Hearts. Fifty-five students were recruited to the program. Before beginning the intervention, each student received a baseline health assessment; the students considered to be at highest risk also had blood drawn for lipid panels. An innovative component of the program was the inclusion of mental health screenings that identified underlying issues that may not have been picked up in a traditional clinical setting. Counselors assessed for depression, safety issues, and substance abuse. Approximately 10% of the participants needed additional mental health services, which were integrated seamlessly into the other services the students received in the program.

All participants met with a clinician to create a plan for their personal nutrition and physical activity. Physical activities such as yoga, salsa dancing, and conditioning were provided after school. Because of their proximity to the students, SBHC staff were able to monitor the students to keep them engaged in the program and to resolve obstacles to continued participation. For example, health center staff called students out of class if they missed an appointment, and students could easily check in regularly to talk about why they were not able to attend exercise classes or what foods they had available at home. Free Lunch Fridays were weekly workshops in which participants came to the clinic during the lunch hour, were provided with healthy foods, and learned how to prepare nutritious meals.

The program reached families through workshops held after popular school events such as student performances. A registered dietician provided Spanish-language instruction on healthy eating, cooking, and reading nutrition labels. Family members of all ages were encouraged to attend, and Healthy Hearts provided food for everyone. As an incentive, the SBHC partnered with teachers to offer students extra credit in 1 of their core classes if their parents attended the workshops. Approximately 50% of participants had at least 1 parent participate. At the end of 1 year, program coordinators conducted an internal evaluation and found that 60% of the students who participated in Healthy Hearts for the entirety of the 2004 to 2005 school year (51 of the original 55) had lowered their body mass index score, with a mean reduction of 0.9 points.

Mental Health Care and Social Change

In 1999, the James Morehouse Project (JMP) was founded to provide health services, mental health care, and youth development opportunities at El Cerrito High School in El Cerrito, California. JMP was initiated by a history teacher, who observed that her ability to teach was severely challenged by the many health and psychosocial issues of her students. The majority of the school's 1400 students are from low-income communities in Northern California with high rates of violence and trauma.

In 2006, a social work intern alerted her supervisor that 6 of the students she was counseling individually, all of whom were African American, were raising issues related to race at the high school. The supervisor suggested that the intern invite her clients with these concerns to take part in a group conversation on racial issues at school. This approach was feasible because the therapy sessions took place on the same school campus where the problems occurred and needed to be addressed. The social justice orientation of the mental health program at the JMP encourages clinicians to see clients as change agents and to focus on social and environmental conditions rather than individual pathology.

All of the 6 students agreed to participate and were joined by 3 others. The majority had a history of low academic achievement, and many had been disciplined or suspended in the previous year. The group decided to conduct research into attitudes and behaviors related to race—particularly with respect to classroom learning and teaching. Guided by the intern, the students conducted focus groups and surveyed more than 300 of their peers.

When the students presented their findings to school staff, these young people who had felt marginalized for years found themselves offering data and critiques of teaching practices and attitudes they identified as contributing to low expectations and unfair disciplinary treatment. For some of the group members, defiant behavior that led to disciplinary actions in the past found a positive outlet as they became advocates and felt that, for the first time, people were listening to their opinions.

In both written evaluations of student presentations and informal oral feedback, teachers reported that they were more aware of the ways that they unknowingly treated students differently because of race. One teacher commented that the students' insights affected her teaching practice more than anything she learned in her master's degree program. In written evaluations after the presentations, students reported that teachers were more willing to have difficult classroom conversations about issues of racism. Through this innovative extension of clinical mental health services, the JMP created a campus-wide dialogue about race that contributed to an improved school environment.

Managing Asthma

Roosevelt Health Center was started in 1999 at Roosevelt Middle School in Oakland in response to a community needs assessment calling for increased access to adolescent health and support services. This SBHC annually serves more than 800 middle school students, including many immigrants and children of immigrants. In 2001, the SBHC implemented a comprehensive asthma prevention and management program in partnership with Oakland Unified School District called Oakland Kicks Asthma. The program was funded by the Centers for Disease Control and Prevention and led by the American Lung Association of the East Bay.

The SBHC providers collaborated with the school district's facilities department on an indoor air quality assessment. Poor air quality measurements in classrooms resulted in changes to reduce exposure to allergens and improve ventilation. Most problems were minor (e.g., blocked ventilation ducts, chemicals stored improperly, windows not opened for ventilation), so many solutions were quick and cost little or nothing. The SBHC screened students' families smoking histories to determine the level of secondhand smoke exposure or other allergens in the home. When they identified concerns, they contacted public health nurses to conduct home evaluations and help families reduce triggers.

A second component of the program was early identification of students with asthma. This required support from the school principal and staff. The SBHC organized a presentation at a faculty meeting which opened a dialogue among school personnel about student absences and problems at school caused by poorly controlled asthma. The SBHC then worked closely with the sixth-grade language arts teachers to screen all incoming students for asthma symptoms with an in-class survey.[10] Students with asthma were also identified at registration and by referrals from teachers, office staff, parents, and administrators.

With the SBHC just down the hall from the main office, students and families had easy access to medical providers when any asthma-related conditions arose. Sometimes the clinician went to a classroom or to the school yard to see a student, another way to ensure timely intervention. Many students elected to keep an inhaler in the SBHC and came in to use it at critical times during the day, such as right before they went to physical education class. The SBHC also furnished families with asthma action plans and permission forms for students to carry so that they could self-administer their medications.

All students with asthma were invited to participate in education and management classes at lunchtime, with lunch provided. High school peer educators performed skits to make these classes fun. Evaluation of the classes across the school district found that participating students had fewer activity limitations and emergency room visits than they did before the Oakland Kicks Asthma classes began.[11]

Oral Health Access

California children miss an estimated 847 000 days of school each year because of dental problems.[12] This statistic impelled the Santa Barbara County Office of Education to take a leading role in improving children's oral health. Their Health Linkages Program coordinated and provided dental services that emphasized preventive care to children from infancy to age 6 years. Health Linkages identified students from preschools and elementary schools by conducting parent workshops on the benefits of oral health assessment and fluoride varnish and distributing fact sheets and service consent forms. Health advocates, who were trained paraprofessionals, worked with schools and preschools to deliver oral health education. The Health Linkages staff assisted teachers in preschool programs in doing dry toothbrushing with the children and educated both students and parents about oral health. Outreach efforts resulted in more than 5000 children receiving fluoride varnish at multiple school sites in 2008 and 2009; these varnishes were applied by the health advocates under the supervision and direction of the project director.

Health Linkages recruited volunteer dentists to treat, at reduced fees, the many students who needed restorative work. A critical component of this effort was cooperation between the county office of education and public health department, working through the Dental Access Resource Team and the Oral Health Executive Committee. These groups brought together dental providers, community organizations, stakeholders, and leaders in the field of children's oral health to develop the community resources and school and community partnerships necessary to prevent dental disease in elementary and preschool settings, improve access to oral care services for children, and keep students in class.

ADVANTAGES OF THE SCHOOL SETTING

SBHCs provide a place-based form of health care. Rather than serving individual patients who are united by nothing more than their selection of a particular medical practice, SBHCs serve a population of children and families united by a common institution and by the relationships they have with each other and with school staff. As the profiles illustrate, the location of clinical services in a school setting creates unique opportunities to integrate care with primary, secondary, and tertiary prevention.

Primary Prevention

Because children spend a large portion of their waking hours in school, their health can be substantially affected by school policies and environments, both social and physical. Antibullying campaigns, recreation opportunities, sun protection, and health education are all examples of primary prevention strategies that are often successful in schools. The impact of these strategies can be strengthened when clinical care is also provided on the school campus. The Healthy Hearts program demonstrated how a clinical strategy can be used to identify students at greatest risk and provide supportive services that allow them to derive greater benefit from broader environmental and educational strategies, such as opportunities for physical education.

When patients share a connection to a place, it is easier to develop public health approaches that involve education campaigns, group interventions, social action, or environmental change. The Roosevelt asthma program demonstrated how clinicians can raise awareness of a health issue and galvanize support for primary prevention, such as indoor air quality assessment. The James Morehouse Project illustrated how experiences in the clinical setting (identification of racial issues) can lead to a focus on the school's social environment. Another clinic in California identified anemia among students as a common clinical problem and responded by providing nutrition education in the classroom and at parent meetings as well as making iron-rich foods more available at school.

Secondary Prevention

Schools are ideal locations for early detection and intervention. The Health Linkages program identified oral health needs by conducting systematic screenings. The Healthy Hearts program used incentives related to the school (T-shirts for physical education) to encourage students to get screened. Moreover, integrating clinical staff into the school can greatly expand the number of people who contribute to the effectiveness of the health care system. Because school staff have regular contact with students, they are well positioned to identify health concerns such as changes in students' motor skills, affect, class attendance, and behavior that may be early signs of physical or mental health issues. For example:

- A teacher's observation that a student was sleeping in class led to a diagnosis of uncontrolled diabetes.
- An English teacher's attention to a student writing assignment resulted in identification of depression.
- A bus driver's concern about a student stumbling on and off the bus led to the diagnosis of a brain tumor.
- A student's concern about her friend's behavior resulted in detection of sexual abuse.
- Cafeteria workers' observation that the arms of students in the lunch line were marked with cuts and burns led to greater awareness of the extent of self-mutilation and mental health issues.

Training school staff to identify medical and psychosocial issues increases the likelihood that these issues will be detected early. Implementing standardized protocols within the school for referring students to the health center, protecting student privacy, and conducting routine screenings all further maximize the effectiveness of secondary prevention as part of an SBHC.

Tertiary Prevention

Proximity of clinical care to the patient population allows for effective follow-up and case management. The school provides a setting in which a clinician can be deployed promptly and provide immediate intervention. School-based clinicians also have more frequent opportunities to educate students and parents about how to manage health conditions. For example, it is easy for a school-based clinician to call a child back for a brief follow-up to determine if an ear infection has cleared or to ask a diabetic high school student to come back every day for a week to check whether a lesson on how to count carbohydrates has been fully understood.

In a school setting, both patients and clinicians can initiate contact with each other to ask questions, provide updated information, or recheck symptoms. This type of access is extremely difficult to achieve through a community practice, where layers of recorded messages, front office staff, and voice mail boxes often separate patients and providers. Even with today's advanced communications technology, there is no substitute for the ability to talk face to face. This is particularly important for populations such as adolescents, immigrants, low-wage working families, and non–English speakers, who all experience numerous barriers to accessing care.

OPPORTUNITIES FOR INNOVATIVE SCHOOL-BASED HEALTH SERVICES

Public health advocates have long fought for an expanded focus on prevention in health care delivery and policy. Recently, the obesity epidemic has heightened awareness that clinical care alone cannot address what, at one time, was considered a personal health issue. The related increase in type 2 diabetes prevalence calls for improved strategies for chronic disease management. New opportunities for prevention, including new funding for SBHCs, are provided by the 2010 health care reform legislation. All these developments provide new impetus to consider schools, the one institution to which virtually all children are connected, for the delivery of primary, secondary, and tertiary prevention.

Comprehensive preventive care is also integral to the growing efforts to establish a medical "home" for all children. Once this concept connoted merely a physical location where medical records are housed and care is centered, but it has expanded, with support from the American Academy of Pediatrics, to focus on patient-centered coordination of care across a network of community based services.[13,14] SBHCs can be a valuable asset to a pediatric medical home by working with community-based providers to deliver the components of preventive care that are more efficiently and effectively delivered in a place-based setting that is part of families' daily lives. Furthermore, as technologies to facilitate health information exchange go to scale, it will become more feasible to coordinate services provided on a school site with those provided in community facilities, thereby enhancing the medical home with school-based approaches to prevention.

The potential for SBHCs to provide preventive care can only be realized if schools themselves are receptive partners. The unique ability of SBHCs to link health care providers with school staff, students, and families represents a value not only to public health but to education as well. From a public health lens, it is easy to see schools as a useful delivery site for health interventions and forget that for educators, SBHCs are an educational intervention. The climate for health and support services in schools may be improving as federal policymakers embrace a broader view of education than that set forward in No Child Left Behind. This change provides an opening for public health professionals who see the benefit of school-based health services to work more closely with colleagues in education.

SBHCs engage teachers, peers, parents, school staff, and clinicians in preventive health care as well as treatment for underserved children and adolescents. By drawing on the strengths of the health care and educational systems, expansion of this unique model for accessible and comprehensive health services has the potential to effect substantive improvements in health, educational, and life outcomes for American students and their families.

REFERENCES

1. Leatherman S, McCarthy D. *Quality of Health Care for Children and Adolescents: A Chartbook*. New York, NY: Commonwealth Fund; 2004.

2. Chung PJ, Schuster MA. Access and quality in child health services: voltage drops. *Health Aff (Millwood)*. 2004;23(5):77–87.

3. Mangione-Smith R, DeCristofaro AH, Setodji CM, et al. The quality of ambulatory care delivered to children in the United States. *N Engl J Med*. 2007;357(15):1515–1523.

4. Irwin CE Jr, Igra V, Eyre S, Millstein S. Risk-taking behavior in adolescents: the paradigm. *Ann N Y Acad Sci*. 1997;817:1–35.

5. Halfon N, Hochstein M. Life course health development: an integrated framework for developing health, policy, and research. *Milbank Q.* 2002;80(3):433–479.

6. Inkelas M, Halfon N, Wood DL, Schuster MA. Health reform for children and families. In: Andersen RM, Rice TH, Kominski GF, eds. *Changing the U.S. Health Care System: Key Issues in Health Services Policy and Management.* 3rd ed. San Francisco, CA: Jossey-Bass; 2007:405–438.

7. Juszczak L, Melinkovich P, Kaplan D. Use of health and mental health services by adolescents across multiple delivery sites. *J Adolesc Health.* 2003;32(6 Suppl):108–118.

8. Kaplan DW, Calonge BN, Guernsey BP, Hanrahan MB. Managed care and SBHCs. Use of health services. *Arch Pediatr Adolesc Med.* 1998;152(1):25–33.

9. Kisker EE, Brown RS. Do school-based health centers improve adolescents' access to health care, health status, and risk-taking behavior? *J Adolesc Health.* 1996;18(5):335–343.

10. Davis A, Savage Brown A, Edelstein J, Tager I. Identification and education of adolescents with asthma in an urban school district: results from a large scale intervention. *J Urban Health.* 2008;85(3):361–374.

11. Magzamen S, Patel B, Davis A, Edelstein J, Tager IB. Kickin' Asthma: school-based asthma education in an urban community. *J Sch Health.* 2008;78(12):655–665.

12. Pourat , Nicholson G. *Unaffordable Dental Care Is Linked to Frequent School Absences.* Los Angeles, CA: UCLA Center for Health Policy Research; 2009.

13. American Academy of Family Physicians, American Academy of Pediatrics, American College of Physicians, American Osteopathic Association. Joint principles of the patient-centered medical home. March 2007. Available at: http://www.medicalhomeinfo.org. Accessed January 13, 2010.

14. American Academy of Pediatrics. Policy statement: organizational principles to guide and define the child health care system and/or improve the health of all children. *Pediatrics.* 2004;113(5 Suppl):1545–1547.

About the Authors

Serena Clayton, PhD – is the Executive Director of the California School Health Centers Association, which improves the health and academic success of underserved children and youth by increasing access to health services in schools. Dr. Clayton has been a leading advocate for adolescent and school health in California since 1998. Her expertise also includes evaluation and planning in teen pregnancy prevention, early childhood, and youth development. Her prior experience includes international development, and she continues to support health and educational projects in Haiti. Dr. Clayton received her Doctorate in Public Health and her Master's in Educational Psychology from UCLA.

Teresa Chin – is a graduate student at the UC Berkeley School of Journalism. She also completed a Bachelor's in Biology and a Master's degree in Public Health at Berkeley. She has produced pieces on education and health for Bay Area news outlets Oakland North and North Gate Radio. Prior to her current degree, Chin taught high school math and chemistry and worked as the technical assistance coordinator at the California School Health Centers Association. Chin was also a columnist at *The Daily Californian*, where her work garnered national attention and has been featured in national publications including *Cosmopolitan*, *Esquire*, and *Playboy* magazines.

Samantha Blackburn – is the Technical Assistance Director at the California School Health Centers Association, where she leads development and implementation of school health center trainings, technical assistance, toolkits, and practice guidelines. She has worked in school health for 20 years, initially as a health educator and then as a credentialed school nurse and pediatric nurse practitioner starting and managing a school-based health center. Ms. Blackburn has also developed statewide after-school health training programs and conducted strategic planning for school health services at the local, regional, and statewide level.

Cecilia Echeverría – is a Program Officer for the Blue Shield of California Foundation's Health Care and Coverage team, managing grants focused on strengthening California's health care safety net. Previously, Ms. Echeverría served as a senior program officer with The California Endowment where she provided strategic direction on school health, insurance coverage, and the health care safety net. She also worked for California HealthCare Foundation as a policy analyst and as a legislative analyst for the Congressional Research Service in Washington, DC. Ms. Echeverría has a Bachelor's in Social Welfare and Master's degrees in Public Policy and Public Health from University of California, Berkeley.

The Role of School Health Centers in Health Care Access and Client Outcomes [*]

Samira Soleimanpour, Sara P. Geierstanger,
Shelly Kaller, Virginia McCarter, and
Claire D. Brindis

School-based and school-linked health centers (hereafter "school health centers") represent a model of care that responds to the unique physical and mental health issues of adolescents by offering care in an accessible, youth-friendly environment. Studies have found that access to school health centers increases use of primary care, reduces use of emergency rooms, and results in fewer hospitalizations.[1-3] School health centers also expand access to and quality of care for underserved adolescents; one study found that school health center users were more likely than were traditional outpatient clients to have received primary and preventive care services despite the fact that they were less likely to be insured.[4] Furthermore, adolescents with alternate forms of health care report high degrees of comfort-seeking care at school health centers.[5]

Adolescent mental health outcomes have also improved because of school health centers. Studies have shown a significant decline in depression among students who received school health center mental health services[6] and a reduced likelihood of suicide ideation among students attending schools with school health centers.[7] Studies have also documented the positive impact of school health centers on reproductive health outcomes,[8] including improved contraceptive use.[9]

Although research has demonstrated how the school health center model of care can affect health access and outcomes, many studies have been limited by relatively

---

[*] This chapter previously appeared in the September 2010 issue of the *American Journal of Public Health* and is reprinted with permission in its entirety. Soleimanpour S, Geierstanger SP, Kaller S, McCarter V, Brindis CD. The role of school health centers in health care access and client outcomes. *Am J Public Health*. 2010;100(9):1597–1603.

small sample sizes. Collecting uniform outcome data from larger coalitions of school health centers is challenging, given the obstacles of different school districts, community health providers, service structures, and data confidentiality regulations. Our aim was to demonstrate the impact of 12 school health centers on clients' access to care, satisfaction, and reproductive and mental health outcomes. We incorporated data collection from both client and provider perspectives through a standardized evaluation process that documents services provided, as well as provider assessments of 2 outcome measures that school health centers have been known to affect: reproductive health and mental health.

METHODS

Established in 1996 by the Alameda County (California) Health Care Services Agency, the Alameda County School Health Services Coalition seeks to improve adolescent health by providing base funding and building the capacity of 12 comprehensive school health centers located on 1 middle school and 11 high school campuses, operating in 6 school districts.

The school health centers offer 16 to 40 hours of medical, mental health, and health education services per week, as well as a variety of development programs for youths. School health center staff include physicians, midlevel practitioners, and medical assistants, and mental health providers include clinical supervisors, therapists, and substance abuse cessation staff. All practitioners provide internal referrals to onsite services, as well as external referrals to community health services. School health center enrollment requires active parental or guardian consent; however, California law allows adolescents to access "sensitive services," including reproductive health services and alcohol and drug counseling, without parental consent.[10] As a condition of funding, coalition members must provide a minimum level of services at their site and participate in a standardized evaluation.

Since 1997, the University of California, San Francisco, has worked closely with the coalition's school health centers to develop a set of evaluation indicators, establish common evaluation tools, and collect and analyze data. Results have been used to refine program outcomes and to make programmatic modifications.

Our evaluation study used both qualitative and quantitative methods. First, all school health center providers completed standardized Medical and Health Education Encounter Forms and Mental Health Encounter Forms to document clients' demographics, the services provided, and clients' outcomes. School health center staff entered this information into Clinical Fusion[11] (2001/02–2007/08) or Efforts to Outcomes[12] (2008/09) software. Data were provided to us in a de-identified format and reported in the aggregate. We analyzed provider-reported clinic data from 7410 clients who made 39 754 visits in 2008–2009.

To track impact data, mental health providers recorded the status of clients' presenting concerns and resiliency factors on Mental Health Encounter Forms at every visit. This list of presenting concerns and resiliency factors was based on a review of the adolescent mental health and resiliency literature and on feedback from mental health providers at the 12 school health centers. Providers were asked to rate the client on each of these factors, based on their clinical expertise. We examined only the data of clients with at least 3 mental health visits by comparing their "baseline visit" (first mental health visit between July 2008 and March 2009) and their "follow-up visit" (last visit, at least 3 months after the baseline visit). If clients were missing provider-reported data at baseline or follow-up, they were excluded from the analysis. Youths qualifying for inclusion in the sample made an average of 17 visits each (range = 4–184; SD = 16.2).

During each family planning visit, medical and health education providers used Medical and Health Education Encounter Forms to record data related to clients' reproductive health behaviors. We examined only the data of female clients with at least 3 family planning visits by comparing their "baseline visit" (first visit between July 2008 and March 2009) and their "follow-up visit" (last visit, which occurred at least 3 months after the baseline visit). If clients were missing provider-reported data at baseline or follow-up or if gender was not documented, their data were excluded from the analysis. The average number of visits for clients included in this analysis was 6 (range = 2–24 visits; SD = 3.2). We also calculated a mean score for these questions by assigning the following values to the response options: never = 1, rarely = 2, sometimes = 3, most times = 4, always = 5.

A second data collection method was a pre–post client survey, which clients completed at the first visit of the year and at follow-up (2.5 to 4 months later) to assess satisfaction and health outcomes from their perspective. Clients received a $10 gift card for the follow-up survey. The analysis included 286 matched surveys administered during a 3-year period (n = 89 in 2006–2007, n = 97 in 2007–2008, and n = 100 in 2008–2009). A 3-year data collection period was used to increase the power of the study sample.

We analyzed clinic and client survey data with SAS version 9.2 (SAS Institute, Cary, NC), using descriptive statistics and the χ^2 test or the t test for significance. Missing data were excluded from all analyses, unless noted otherwise.

Lastly, focus groups were used to obtain qualitative data. Twelve focus groups were conducted with 105 students. Two gender-specific focus groups, consisting of both school health center users and nonusers, were held at 6 school health centers in May and June 2009. Group sizes ranged from 7 to 12 participants. To recruit participants, school health center staff posted flyers at the school and school health center and made announcements in various group settings. To participate, students were required to submit a consent form signed by both themselves and their parents or guardians. S.S., S.K., and 4 research assistants moderated the groups and took notes. At the completion of each focus group, students received $20 for their participation. Participants in all groups consented to having the discussions audio-recorded, and the recordings were used to supplement notes taken during the discussions.

During data analysis, notes were reviewed for consistency and clarity, with use of recordings as needed. Data were analyzed by content to identify themes and salient points and to explore relationships among themes.[13] Themes were summarized and reported based on the number of participants within and across groups that mentioned the topic and how much discussion the topic generated.

RESULTS

The following is a summary of the results from the 3 evaluation data sources: provider-reported clinical data, pre–post client survey data, and focus group data.

Provider-Reported Clinic Data Findings

The majority of school health center clients were female, and the client population was racially diverse. Insurance status was known and documented for 62% of clients (n = 4561), with government and private sources being most common (Table 2.1).

SCHOOL HEALTH CENTER VISITS

From the 2006–2007 school year to the 2008–2009 school year, the number of clients increased from 6624 to 7410 and visits increased from 27078 to 39754. On average, clients made 5.4 visits each in the 2008–2009 school year.

In the 2008–2009 school year, 33% of client visits were for medical care (n = 13060), 27% (n = 10650) for mental health, 25% (n = 9904) for first aid, and 15% (n = 6107) for group visits. Medical services were defined as triage, comprehensive health assessments, screenings, treatment and management, and referrals to other school health center services and primary care physicians. Mental health services were defined as primary prevention; individual, family, and group therapy; crisis intervention; clinical case management; psychiatric consultation; and linkages to external providers. Group visits primarily consisted of group health education, support groups, peer educator trainings, and ongoing youth leadership and development programs.

TABLE 2.1—DEMOGRAPHICS OF STUDENT CLIENTS USING SCHOOL HEALTH CENTERS, BY DATA SOURCE: ALAMEDA COUNTY, CA, 2008–2009

	Provider-Reported Clinic Clients, No. or No. (%)	Pre–Post Client Survey Respondents, No. or No. (%)	Focus Group Participants, No. or No. (%)
Sex			
Male	2764 (37)	50 (17)	54 (51)
Female	4636 (63)	236 (83)	51 (49)
Missing data	10 (0)	0 (0)	0 (0)
Total	7410	286	105
Race			
Non-Hispanic African American	2480 (33)	98 (34)	38 (36)
Hispanic	1883 (25)	86 (30)	30 (29)
Asian/Asian Pacific Islander	1152 (16)	47 (16)	21 (20)
Non-Hispanic White	748 (10)	18 (6)	3 (3)
Biracial or multiracial	387 (5)	22 (8)	11 (10)
Other	285 (4)	15 (5)	2 (2)
Missing data	475 (6)	0 (0)	0 (0)
Total	7410	286	105
Client insurance			
Private	1591 (21)	83 (29)	...
Medi-Cal[a] or other government insurance	2141 (29)	54 (19)	...
No insurance	735 (10)	13 (5)	...
Other	95 (1)	...	...
Not sure or unknown	2811 (38)	76 (27)	...
Missing data	37 (0)	60 (21)	...
Total	7410	286	...

Note. All data are from 2008/09, except for pre–post client survey data, which are from 2006 through 2009. Ellipses indicate that data are not available.

[a]Medi-Cal is California's Medicaid program.

MEDICAL SERVICES

Of the services received during medical visits in the 2008–2009 school year, 55% (n = 11 310) were for family planning, 24% (n = 4928) were for other medical services (e.g., sports physicals and chronic disease management), and 20% (n = 4147) were for health education. During their first medical and health education visits, the vast majority of clients were screened for sexual activity (90%; n = 4155), tobacco use (85%; n = 3910), marijuana use (80%; n = 3716), and feeling unsafe in the school, home, or community (83%; n = 3817).

MENTAL HEALTH SERVICES

The most common reasons for referrals to mental health services for new or returning clients (n = 1239) were for academic performance (33%; n = 415), family conflicts (33%; n = 403), depression or suicide ideation or attempt (31%; n = 378), peer relationships (30%; n = 367), anxiety or adjustment (i.e., maladaptive reaction to an identifiable stressful life event [23%; n = 279]), and anger management (21%; n = 260). The most common mental health service provided was individual therapy (38%; n = 4393). Other types included intake or assessment (16%; n = 1790), collateral contacts with clients' significant support persons (12%; n = 1440), and case management or brokerage (11%, n = 1256). More than 1 service could be provided per visit, and the type of service was not documented for 499 visits.

REFERRALS TO OTHER NEEDED SERVICES AFTER INITIAL SERVICE

Of the 1528 clients who received mental health services, 42% (n = 643) also received school health center medical services. Of clients whose initial school health center visit was for first aid, 22% (n = 487) subsequently returned for a medical, mental health, or group visit. Of the clients who returned, 50% (n = 243) returned for a medical visit, 21% (n = 104) for a mental health visit, and 7% (n = 34) for a group visit. An additional 22% (n = 106) returned for more than 1 type of visit.

IMPACT ON MENTAL HEALTH OUTCOMES

Mental health providers reported significant improvements ($P < .05$) from baseline to follow-up in 9 of 12 documented presenting concerns: anxiety or nervousness; depression or sadness; eating disorders; grief, loss, or bereavement; oppositional, defiant behavior, or anger management problems; relationship issues or conflict; self-injury; substance abuse; and suicidal ideation or attempt. The presenting concerns that did not improve significantly over time were identity issues, school behavior or academic performance issues, and posttraumatic stress disorder (Table 2.2).

TABLE 2.2—PROVIDER ASSESSMENTS OF BASELINE AND FOLLOW-UP MENTAL HEALTH STATUS OF STUDENT CLIENTS USING SCHOOL HEALTH CENTERS: ALAMEDA COUNTY, CA, 2008–2009

	No.	Baseline Score	Follow-Up Score	P^a
Presenting concerns[b]				
Anxiety or nervousness	376	1.03	0.79	<.001
Depression or sadness	378	1.32	0.99	<.001
Eating disorders	357	0.15	0.07	.002
Grief, loss, or bereavement	374	0.72	0.45	<.001
Identity issues	364	0.29	0.26	.334
Oppositional, defiant behavior, or anger management problems	374	0.75	0.58	<.001
Relationship issues or conflict (family, peers, partners)	383	1.50	1.19	<.001
Posttraumatic stress disorder	363	0.25	0.21	.266
School behavior or academic performance issues	386	1.07	1.04	.638
Self-injury (cutting, pulling out hair, gouging, and so on)	362	0.12	0.04	.003
Substance abuse (alcohol or drugs)	363	0.26	0.19	.046
Suicidal ideation or attempt	361	0.18	0.08	.003
Resiliency factors[c]				
Attending school regularly and applying self at school	355	1.55	1.45	.051
Expressing feelings and emotions (sadness, anger, and so on) in healthy ways	356	1.26	1.40	.003
Expressing a sense of hope for his or her life or future	349	1.50	1.62	.008
Involved in organized recreational or vocational activities	349	1.01	1.17	.004
Motivated to participate in counseling for himself or herself	355	1.86	1.83	.447

[a]P for difference between baseline and follow-up score (significant at < .05).

[b]Client was asked on the day of the visit if he or she had any of the given problems or concerns. Scoring was as follows: no longer a problem or not available = 0, somewhat a problem = 1, a problem = 2, very much a problem = 3.

[c]Client was asked on the day of the visit if each of the given statements regarding resiliency was true. Scoring was as follows: not true = 0, somewhat true = 1, true = 2, very true = 3.

Providers also reported significant improvements ($P < .05$) from baseline to follow-up in 3 of 5 documented resiliency factors: expressing feelings and emotions in healthy ways, expressing a sense of hope for one's life or future, and involvement in organized recreational or vocational activities. There were no significant changes in reports of clients being motivated to participate in counseling or of clients attending school regularly and applying themselves (Table 2.2).

IMPACT ON REPRODUCTIVE HEALTH BEHAVIORS

Medical and health education providers reported a significant improvement ($P < .001$) from baseline to follow-up in the use of birth control other than condoms (from 14% [n = 55] to 40% [n = 153] "always" using) among female clients. The mean score for this behavior increased from 1.72 to 2.87 (from "rarely" to "sometimes"). There was also a significant improvement ($P < .001$) from baseline to follow-up in the use of condoms with another form of birth control (from 5% [n = 18] to 10% [n = 38] "always" using). The mean score for this behavior increased from 1.41 to 1.93 (from approximately "never" to approximately "rarely"). There was a significant decrease ($P < .001$) reported in condom use in the past month (from 35% [n = 138] to 25% [n = 98] "always" using). The mean score for this behavior declined from 3.5 to 3.08 (from approximately "most times" to approximately "sometimes"; Table 2.3).

Pre–Post Client Survey Findings

The majority of respondents were female (83%; n = 236), which represented a larger percentage than in the overall clinic population (63%; n = 4636). Respondents' ethnic backgrounds reflected the general clinic population; however, Hispanics were slightly overrepresented and Whites slightly underrepresented in the survey sample (Table 2.1).

USUAL SOURCES OF CARE

The school health center was the most commonly reported source for medical care (30%; n = 84), family planning services (63%; n = 177), and counseling (31%; n = 85). Other "usual" sources of medical care included Kaiser Permanente, a local health maintenance organization (21%; n = 60); doctor's office or community clinic (10%; n = 27); and another hospital (10%, n = 27). Very few clients (2%; n = 7) reported that they did not get medical care when they needed it and few (2%; n = 5) reported using an emergency room for medical care. However, approximately 1 in 10 clients (11%; n = 30) reported that they did not get needed mental health services through any source (Table 2.4).

TABLE 2.3—PERCENTAGE OF FEMALE STUDENT CLIENTS OF SCHOOL HEALTH CENTERS USING BIRTH CONTROL AT BASELINE AND FOLLOW-UP, BY TYPE OF BIRTH CONTROL USED: ALAMEDA COUNTY, CA, 2008–2009

Past-Month Frequency of Birth Control Use (% of Time)	% Condom Use at Baseline (n=398)	% Condom Use at Follow-Up[a] (n=398)	% Birth Control Other Than Condoms Used at Baseline (n=384)	% Birth Control Other Than Condoms Used at Follow-Up[a] (n=384)	% Both Condoms and Other Form of Birth Control Used at Baseline (n=380)	% Both Condoms and Other Form of Birth Control Used at Follow-Up[a] (n=380)
Always (100%)	35	25	14	40	5	10
Most times (75%)	25	20	1	6	3	8
Sometimes (50%)	16	19	4	4	6	11
Rarely (25%)	5	10	2	3	2	9
Never (0%)	20	26	78	47	85	63

[a]Significant change from baseline to follow-up (P <.001).

TABLE 2.4—USUAL SOURCES OF MEDICAL CARE, FAMILY PLANNING CARE, AND COUNSELING CARE SELF-REPORTED BY STUDENT CLIENTS OF SCHOOL HEALTH CENTERS: ALAMEDA COUNTY, CA, 2006–2009

Usual Source of Care	Clients Reporting Use of Medical Care, No. (%)	Clients Reporting Use of Family Planning, No. (%)	Clients Reporting Use of Counseling, No. (%)
School health center or school nurse	84 (30)	177 (63)	85 (31)
Did not need care	54 (19)	59 (21)	119 (43)
Kaiser Permanente	60 (21)	13 (5)	8 (3)
Doctor's office or community clinic	27 (10)	4 (1)	6 (2)
Another hospital	27 (10)	0 (0)	2 (<1)
Did not know	18 (6)	18 (6)	27 (10)
Did not get the care he/she needed	7 (2)	6 (2)	30 (11)
Emergency room	5 (2)	0 (0)	0 (0)
Planned Parenthood	0 (0)	3 (1)	1 (<1)

IMPACT ON REPRODUCTIVE HEALTH BEHAVIORS

Most respondents had previously had sexual intercourse at both presurvey (70%; n = 193) and postsurvey (74%; n = 204). The most commonly reported birth control method by sexually active females at last sexual encounter was condoms, and use of this method increased significantly ($P < .001$) from presurvey (48%; n = 78) to postsurvey (65%; n = 105). Reported birth control use by females also increased significantly ($P < .001$), from 7% (n = 11) to 23% (n = 37). Use of other methods, including "no method," did not change significantly.

CLIENTS' REPORT OF OTHER IMPACTS

Most postsurvey respondents "agreed" or "strongly agreed" that the school health center helped them get information and resources they needed (94%; n = 264), get help sooner than they would have otherwise (88%; n = 251), and get access to services they would not have received otherwise (80%; n = 225). Respondents also reported that the school health center helped them to improve a variety of health behaviors and academic indicators, including using protection more often when they had sex (81%; n = 230), eating better or exercising more (60%; n = 168), staying in school (59%; n = 167), and dealing with stress or anxiety better (59%; n = 166; Table 2.5).

REASONS CLIENTS LIKED SCHOOL HEALTH CENTERS

Respondents reported in the postsurvey that they chose to use the school health center for the following reasons: privacy or confidentiality (62%; n = 177), convenient location (56%; n = 159), they liked the staff (45%; n = 130), free services (45%; n = 130), convenient hours (43%; n = 122), it was the only place they knew of (10%; n = 29), teacher or school staff referrals (7%; n = 21), and other reasons, such as proximity or comfort (6%; n = 16). Nearly all postsurvey respondents "agreed" or "strongly agreed" that the school health center staff were people they could go to for advice or information (94%; n = 264) and that they were easier to talk to than were other doctors or nurses (89%; n = 249).

Student Focus Group Findings

Compared with the ratio in the clinic population, there were more males in the focus group population. Clients' ethnic backgrounds were similar to those of the school health center clients (Table 2.1).

REASONS STUDENTS LIKED SCHOOL HEALTH CENTER SERVICES

Participants reported liking the school health center because it was free, confidential, convenient, and youth-friendly. They appreciated the staff because of their

TABLE 2.5 — IMPACT OF USE OF SCHOOL HEALTH CENTERS AS SELF-REPORTED BY STUDENT CLIENTS: ALAMEDA COUNTY, CA, 2006–2009

Survey Statement[a]	Agree or Strongly Agree With Statement, No. (%)	Disagree or Strongly Disagree With Statement, No. (%)	Do Not Know Agreement or Statement Does Not Apply, No. (%)
Get information and resources I need	264 (94)	8 (3)	8 (3)
Get help sooner than I would otherwise	251 (90)	17 (6)	12 (4)
Use protection (like condoms, birth control) more often when I have sex	230 (81)	14 (5)	39 (14)
Get services I would not get otherwise	225 (80)	39 (14)	19 (7)
Feel safe talking about my problems	212 (75)	26 (9)	43 (15)
Eat better or exercise more	168 (60)	43 (15)	68 (24)
Stay in school	167 (59)	29 (10)	85 (30)
Deal with stress or anxiety better	166 (59)	47 (17)	69 (24)
Improve my grades	131 (47)	63 (22)	87 (31)
Get involved in leadership programs	114 (41)	70 (25)	96 (34)
Use tobacco, alcohol, or drugs less	108 (39)	72 (26)	98 (35)

[a]Clients were presented with the statement "The school health center has helped me. . . ." and asked to rate their agreement with the given student health center services.

nonjudgmental care, ability to listen, and friendly dispositions. Many participants explained that because the school health center staff members were integrated in the school and were familiar, students might be more comfortable seeking care from the school health center than from another health facility. They felt strongly that school health center services were helpful and facilitated better health care for students.

SUGGESTIONS TO IMPROVE STUDENT ACCESS

Participants explained that students who did not use the school health center (1) might not think they needed care, (2) received care elsewhere, or (3) did not know about the school health center and the services it offered. Many expressed concern about what other students would think if they saw them going to the school health center. To counter these barriers, participants suggested increased outreach to spread the word about the clinic, and use of more peer-provided services, youth development, and after-school activities to normalize involvement by youths with the school health center.

SUGGESTIONS TO IMPROVE CLIENTS' SATISFACTION

Although participants said that wait times were longer at other clinics and that being able to seek care at school took less time out of their day, they still reported disliking waiting for appointments at the school health center. Additionally, they felt that larger waiting rooms and expanded clinic spaces would increase confidentiality and keep their health concerns more private. Students also wanted longer hours of school health center operation and increased provider availability.

DISCUSSION

Consistent with previous research,[5,14-16] the Alameda County school health centers were able to overcome traditional barriers to care and serve ethnically and racially diverse clients, groups who experience the greatest likelihood of being uninsured or underinsured and who face the greatest barriers to care. Moreover, the majority of clients were screened for risk factors and received comprehensive primary care, consistent with medical guidelines.[17] Research has shown that most youths generally do not receive screening or preventive counseling at rates consistent with clinical guidelines.[18-20] Our findings demonstrate that school health centers can provide this necessary care. Additionally, adolescents are best served with improved and coordinated health systems that meet criteria highlighted by the National Academy of Sciences: accessibility, acceptability, appropriateness, effectiveness, and equity.[21] This study points to the importance of developing systems of care, whether at school or nonschool settings, to improve adolescent health, including integrated health promotion, disease prevention and management, physical and mental health services, and coordination as a means of eliminating health disparities.

Integration of Medical and Mental Health Services

The integration of physical health and mental health services, as well as overall convenience of location and services provided, enabled students to seek and receive a wide variety of on-site services. The staff's commitment to screen and refer students to available services also ensured that clients' diverse health needs were met.

For students who might initially have come for a first-aid visit, school health center staff had the opportunity to actively engage and encourage them to return for subsequent medical, mental health, or group visits.

Meeting Mental Health Needs

We showed that approximately 1 in 10 clients (11%) did not get needed mental health services from any source, despite being registered school health center clients. Although this identifies a need for improvement, national data demonstrate an even higher unmet need. In 2007, among all adolescents with emotional, developmental, or behavior problems who needed mental health services, more than one third (34%) did not receive these services.[22] Thus, the Alameda County school health centers were able to fill an important gap in access to mental health services.

Improving Reproductive Health Behaviors

As with previous research showing that school health centers can improve contraceptive use,[9] the providers in this study reported a significant improvement in the use of birth control other than condoms and in the dual use of condoms and another form of birth control. The significant decrease in provider-reported past-month condom use after the adoption of hormonal methods has also been documented in other research.[23,24] Additionally, the majority of clients (81%) reported in the client survey that the school health center helped them to use protection more often when they had sexual intercourse, which supports findings from another study that showed that adolescents who used a school health center were more likely to have received preventive counseling on pregnancy and sexually transmitted infections and were also more likely to report that the care they received was helpful.[25]

Conflicting Findings on Condom Use

There were conflicting results between the provider- and client-reported condom use data, pointing to the importance of collecting data through a variety of methods to untangle diverse perceptions. These conflicting perceptions may be due to the different time frames that were referenced ("last month" vs "last sexual encounter") or to the client survey's smaller sample size. Linking data from specific clients and providers may also be useful in ensuring that providers and clients are in greater concordance as a symbol of provider–client communication, although this process can be complicated because of confidentiality concerns and consent requirements.

Clients' Perceptions of Confidentiality

Overall, client survey and focus group participants cited confidentiality as a main reason they liked the school health center, which indicates that assurance of confidentiality is a major factor in their decision to pursue school health center services. However, focus group participants also said that they felt that larger waiting rooms and expanded clinic spaces would increase confidentiality. Although most existing clinics face space and funding restrictions, upcoming school health centers should consider this feedback in their planning and design.

Limitations

Our multisite, multimethod, outcomes-based evaluation faced several methodological challenges. First, although we regularly trained providers, not all data fields were consistently completed in the clinic data collection. For example, insurance status was documented for only 62% of clients. In addition, the matched pre–post client surveys represented only a small percentage of the clients served from 2006 to 2009, reflecting the challenges of instituting a client pre–post survey in this setting. Furthermore, 3 years of client survey data were combined to obtain a larger sample for statistical analysis. Although the respondent demographic profile between years was similar, potential biases exist when 3 years of client survey data are compared with only 1 year of clinic and focus group data.

Moreover, the research study did not have longitudinal data or a comparison group because of a lack of resources; this would have allowed us to better document how school health centers differ from traditional health services for this population. A final limitation was the lack of examination of dosage effects on client outcomes, as well as other potential mitigating or contributing factors. Because of confidentiality policies, the design was not able to link the client survey to the clinic database.

Despite these limitations, we showed that school health centers can provide a variety of health and wellness services to a racially diverse population in a safe, accessible environment where young people spend a great deal of their time. The school health center provider- and client-reported outcome data provide important evidence of the value and impact of school health center services. Furthermore, the use of multiple methods to collect evaluation data allowed us to answer more comprehensively how the school health centers affect youths' access to care and health outcomes.

Conclusions

This study contributes to the field by demonstrating that a multimethod, multisite evaluation can document the impact of school health centers on utilization and self-reported health outcomes, despite variations in sites. Such information can be vital for counties and school districts seeking to understand the value of such services to the system as a whole.

The field of school health center evaluation needs to establish a more standardized set of health services indicators, with a stronger emphasis on health outcomes, to better document the value of this model of care. Although future evaluations will benefit from additional comparison and longitudinal methodological designs, this study contributes to the increasing understanding of the characteristics of effective health care programs that meet the diverse needs of adolescents as a means of diminishing barriers that contribute to health disparities.

REFERENCES

1. Morone JA, Kilbreth EH, Langwell KM. Back to school: a health care strategy for youth. *Health Aff.* 2001;20(1):122–136.

2. Kaplan DW, Calonge BN, Guernsey BP, Hanrahan MB. Managed care and school-based health centers: use of health services. *Arch Pediatr Adolesc Med.* 1998;152(1):25–33.

3. Santelli J, Kouzis A, Newcomer S. School-based health centers and adolescent use of primary care and hospital care. *J Adolesc Health.* 1996;19(4):267–275.

4. Allison MA, Crane LA, Beaty BL, Davidson AJ, Melinkovich P, Kempe A. School-based health centers: improving access for low-income adolescents. *Pediatrics.* 2007;120(4):e887–e894.

5. Brindis C, Kapphahn C, McCarter V, Wolfe AL. The impact of health insurance status on adolescents' utilization of school-based clinic services: implications for health care reform. *J Adolesc Health.* 1995;16(1):18–25.

6. Weist MD, Paskewitz DA, Warner BS, Flaherty LT. Treatment outcomes of school-based mental health services for urban adolescents. *Community Ment Health J.* 1996;32(2):149–157.

7. Kisker EE, Brown RS. Do school-based health centers improve adolescents' access to health care, health status, and risk-taking behavior? *J Adolesc Health.* 1996;18(5):335–343.

8. Peak GL, McKinney DL. Reproductive and sexual health at the school-based/school-linked heath center: an analysis of services provided by 180 clinics. *J Adolesc Health.* 1996;19(4):276–281.

9. Galavotti C, Lovick SR. School-based clinic use and other factors affecting adolescent contraceptive behavior. *J Adolesc Health Care.* 1989;10(6):506–512.

10. Gudeman R. *Minor Consent, Confidentiality and Child Abuse Reporting in California.* Oakland, CA: National Center for Youth Law; 2006:3–4.

11. Clinical Fusion software. Denver, CO: National Center for School-Based Health Information Systems, University of Colorado. Available at: http://www.clinicalfusion.com. Accessed October 28, 2009.

12. Efforts to Outcomes software. Baltimore, MD: Social Solutions Inc. Available at: http://www.socialsolutions.com. Accessed October 28, 2009.

13. Ryan GW, Bernard HR. Techniques to identify themes. *Field Methods.* 2003;15(1):85–109.

14. Juszczak L, Melinkovich P, Kaplan D. Use of health and mental health services in a large, urban school district. *J Adolesc Health.* 2003;32(6):108–118.

15. Kaplan DW, Brindis CD, Naylor KE, Phibbs SL, Ahlstrand KR, Melinkovich P. Elementary school-based health center use. *Pediatrics.* 1998;101(6):e12.

16. Wade TJ, Mansour ME, Guo JJ, Huentelman T, Line K, Keller KN. Access and utilization patterns of school-based health centers at urban and rural elementary and middle schools. *Public Health Rep.* 2008;123(6):739–750.

17. *Guidelines for Adolescent Preventive Services (GAPS): Recommendations Monograph.* Chicago, IL: Dept of Adolescent Health, American Medical Association; 1997. Available at: http://www.ama-assn.org/ama/upload/mm/39/gapsmono.pdf. Accessed February 26, 2009.

18. Halpern-Felsher BL, Ozer EM, Millstein SG, et al. Preventive services in a health maintenance organization: how well do pediatricians screen and educate adolescent patients? *Arch Pediatr Adolesc Med.* 2000;154(2):173–179.

19. Fleming M, Elster AB, Klein JD, Anderson SM. *Lessons Learned: National Development to Local Implementation, Guidelines for Adolescent Preventive Services (GAPS).* Chicago, IL: American Medical Association; 2001.

20. Klein JD, Wilson KM. Delivering quality care: adolescents' discussion of health risks with their providers. *J Adolesc Health.* 2002;30(3):190–195.

21. Committee on Adolescent Health Care Services and Models of Care for Treatment, Prevention, and Healthy Development. *Adolescent Health Services: Missing Opportunities. Report Brief.* Washington, DC: National Academy of Sciences; 2008. Available at: http://www.bocyf.org/ahc_brief.pdf. Accessed October 28, 2009.

22. *The Health and Well-Being of Children: A Portrait of States and the Nation 2007.* Rockville, MD: US Dept of Health and Human Services, Health Resources and Services Administration, Maternal and Child Health Bureau; 2009. Available at: http://mchb.hrsa.gov/nsch07/national/1child/2healthcare/pages/07mhc.html. Accessed October 28, 2009.

23. Ott MA, Adler NE, Millstein SG, et al. The trade-off between hormonal contraceptives and condoms among adolescents. *Perspect Sex Reprod Health.* 2002;34(1):6–14.

24. Woods JL, Shew ML, Tu W, et al. Patterns of oral contraceptive pill-taking and condom use among adolescent contraceptive pill users. *J Adolesc Health.* 2006;39(3):381–387.

25. Klein JD, Handwerker L, Sesselbeg TS, Sutter E, Flanagan E, Gawronski B. Measuring quality of adolescent preventive services of health plan enrollees and school-based health center users. *J Adolesc Health.* 2007;41(2):153–160.

About the Authors

Samira Soleimanpour, MPH – is a Senior Researcher with the Philip R. Lee Institute for Health Policy Studies (PRL-IHPS) at the University of California, San Francisco (UCSF). Since joining UCSF in 2000, her work has focused on child and adolescent health research and program evaluation. She has extensive experience designing and conducting youth-led participatory research projects and evaluations of school health programs, including school-based health centers and mental health services, and pregnant and parenting teen programs. She received her Master's in Public Health from the George Washington University and is currently pursing doctoral studies at the Johns Hopkins University.

Sara P. Geierstanger, MPH – is a Senior Researcher at UCSF's PRL-IHPS, where she has worked since 1994 designing and directing multisite program evaluation research projects on adolescent, school health, and community health services to inform local, state, and national programs and policies. She received her Master's in Public Health from the University of California, Berkeley, in 1994 and served as both a US Peace Corps Volunteer (Guinea, West Africa) and a US Fulbright Scholar (Norway). A Yoga Alliance Registered Yoga Teacher, she has also recently started teaching yoga to children in schools as part of her commitment to school and community health.

Shelly Kaller, MPH – is a Senior Researcher at UCSF's PRL-IHPS, where she has worked since 2005 conducting and evaluating adolescent health programs. Her expertise in school health includes substance abuse prevention, teen pregnancy prevention, school-based health centers, and nutrition and physical activity programs. Currently, she is directing multimethod evaluations of school-based health centers in Alameda County, California, and in Colorado. She is also part of an assessment team planning for the development of new school health services in Oakland, California, and coordinating youth-led participatory research projects. She received her Master's in Public Health from Columbia University's Mailman School of Public Health.

Virginia McCarter, PhD – is a Statistician at UCSF's PRL-IHPS. She has been involved in adolescent health care research at UCSF for over 21 years, where she specializes in database management and statistical analysis. She has over 25 years experience as an SAS programmer and research analyst. She received a PhD in Sociology from Texas A&M University in 1987.

Claire D. Brindis, DrPH, MPH–is a professor in UCSF's Department of Pediatrics, Division of Adolescent Medicine, and the Department of Obstetrics, Gynecology and Reproductive Sciences. She is Director of the Bixby Center for Global Reproductive Health and Director of UCSF's PRL-IHPS. She is also Executive Director of UCSF's National Adolescent Health Information and Innovation Center and the Policy Information and Analysis Center for Middle Childhood and Adolescence. Dr. Brindis's research focuses on program evaluation and the translation of research into policy, particularly in the areas of women's health, reproductive health, and teen pregnancy prevention.

The Impact of School-Based Health Centers on the Health Outcomes of Middle School and High School Students[*]

Miles A. McNall,
Lauren F. Lichty, and Brian Mavis

At school-based health centers (SBHCs), multidisciplinary teams of providers, including physicians, nurse practitioners, registered nurses, physician assistants, and social workers provide a comprehensive range of primary care, preventive care, and early intervention services to children from elementary school through high school. SBHCs located in medically underserved areas have helped increase access to and utilization of primary care services among a wide variety of students, including low-income,[1] urban,[1-3] rural,[2,4,5] female,[5] and African American[5] students. SBHC utilization rates are highest among children with public insurance or no insurance.[5] Thus, SBHCs serve as an important health care safety net for disadvantaged and medically underserved youth.

Most students who use SBHCs do so infrequently, averaging slightly more than 1 visit per year. An analysis of the diagnostic categories associated with SBHC visits paints a portrait of the typical SBHC user as a student who occasionally visits the SBHC for the treatment of an acute illness or to receive a physical examination.[6] In addition to providing direct health care services, SBHC staff members engage in a wide range of other activities to promote student health. A recent study found that 20% of all clinical activity in a sample of SBHCs was devoted to patient, classroom, and group education activities and to contacts with parents and school staff.[7] Such activities hold the promise of spreading the effects of SBHCs to students who do not directly receive SBHC health care services.

[*] This chapter previously appeared in the September 2010 issue of the *American Journal of Public Health* and is reprinted with permission in its entirety. McNall MA, Lichty LF, Mavis B. The impact of school-based health centers on the health outcomes of middle school and high school students. *Am J Public Health*. 2010;100(9):1604–1610.

The strongest evidence for the impact of SBHCs on the health of the children they serve is found among children with chronic diseases. For children with asthma, SBHC use is associated with fewer hospitalizations,[8,9] fewer visits to emergency rooms,[8,10] and better school attendance.[9] The evidence for the health benefits of SBHCs for children in the general population is less compelling. A study sponsored by the Robert Wood Johnson Foundation's School-Based Adolescent Health Care Program[11] compared the health status and health outcomes of 9th- and 10th-grade students in schools with SBHCs to a national random sample of 9th- and 10th-grade students attending schools without SBHCs. The presence of SBHCs in schools had no significant effect on the overall health status or health outcomes of students. A second study,[2,5] funded by the Health Foundation of Greater Cincinnati, compared the health-related quality of life of students in 4 elementary schools with SBHCs to students in 4 comparison schools without SBHCs. SBHC users reported significant improvement in student-reported quality of life over 3 years when compared with students in non-SBHC schools.

It is worth noting that, whereas the Robert Wood Johnson Foundation–funded study compared *all* students in schools with SBHCs to a national random sample of students in schools without SBHCs, the Health Foundation of Greater Cincinnati–funded study involved a comparison among 3 groups of students: students in schools without SBHCs, students in schools with SBHCs who used their school's SBHC, and students in schools with SBHCs who did not use their school's SBHC. Distinguishing between SBHC users and nonusers within the same school is critical because it allows for analysis of the direct effects of SBHC services on users.

The purpose of this study was to extend understanding of the effects of SBHCs on the general population of school-aged children by analyzing the impact of SBHCs on a range of health and health behavior outcomes among middle and high school students over a 2-year period. In particular, we sought to answer the following research questions: (1) What is the direct impact of SBHC use on middle and high school students' health and health behaviors? (2) What is the indirect impact of having an SBHC in a school on the health and health behaviors of students in that school, regardless of whether students use SBHC services? To answer these questions we used multilevel modeling to model school-level (i.e., SBHC status) and individual-level (i.e., student use of SBHCs) predictors of health separately.

METHODS

We used a prospective cohort design, surveying cohorts of middle school and high school students over 2 consecutive school years (2006–2007 and 2007–2008). Seven middle schools and 9 high schools in Michigan were recruited to participate in the study. Five sites contained well-established SBHCs (i.e., centers that had been in operation for at least 6 years at time 1); 6 sites contained newly implemented SBHCs (i.e., centers that had been in operation for less than 1 year at time 1, here called "implementation" sites); and 5 comparison sites did not have SBHCs. Comparison sites were matched with established sites on the basis of the percentage of students receiving free and reduced-price lunches, the racial/ethnic composition of the student body, and school size (implementation sites were not included in the matching process because the original study design did not include data from those sites in the outcomes study). The 16 schools constituted a geographically dispersed sample, varying by region of the state, urban and suburban communities, and predominant race/ethnicity. Whereas the established sites were located in urban settings with large populations of low-income residents, the implementation sites represented a mix of urban and rural settings.

In middle schools, we recruited students in grades 6 or 7, depending on what the first grade of the middle school was. In high schools, we recruited students in grade 9. Parental consent was obtained through a variety of means, including mailings to the homes of all children in grades 6 or 7 (in the selected middle schools) and 9 (in the selected high schools); having research staff attend back-to-school events or parent-teacher conferences; and sponsoring in-school competitions between classrooms for the most returned consent forms, regardless of whether consent to participate was granted.

Sample

In year 1, parental consent was obtained for 1134 students, representing 26% of eligible students across all schools. Of these students, 969 (85%) provided written assent to participate and completed a survey. Of the 969 completed surveys, 959 were usable. In year 2, we surveyed 833 (73%) of the 1134 students who provided assent in year 1: 317 middle school students (38%) and 516 high school students (62%). Only participants who completed surveys in both years were included in our study sample (n = 744, 89% of the year 2 participants).

Tests of baseline differences in demographics by SBHC type (Table 3.1) revealed that middle school students at implementation schools were older than their counterparts at established or comparison schools ($F_{2, 282} = 8.67$; $P < .01$), which is an expected result given that 1 implementation middle school begins at seventh grade. Implementation schools also had more White students and fewer minority students than established or comparison schools ($\chi^2_6 = 50.84$; $P < .01$). Given that SBHCs were first established in largely urban, minority communities and that newly implemented SBHCs are more frequently located in rural, predominantly White communities, this finding is not surprising.

TABLE 3.1—DEMOGRAPHIC CHARACTERISTICS OF STUDENTS WHO COMPLETED STUDY QUESTIONNAIRES AT BOTH TIME 1 AND TIME 2: MIDDLE SCHOOL AND HIGH SCHOOL STUDENTS, MICHIGAN, 2006–2008

	Entire Sample: 16 Schools (n=744), Mean (SD) or %	Comparison Sites: 5 Schools (n=229), Mean (SD) or %	Established Sites: 5 Schools (n=267), Mean (SD) or %	Implementation Sites: 6 Schools (n=248), Mean (SD) or %	Tests of Differences Across School Types	P
Age, y, at time 2						
Middle school	7 schools: 12.8 (0.68)	2 schools: 12.7 (0.62)	2 schools: 12.6 (0.61)	3 schools: 12.9 (0.74)	$F_{2,282}=8.67$	<.01
High school	9 schools: 15.6 (0.65)	3 schools: 15.5 (0.58)	3 schools: 15.6 (0.61)	3 schools: 15.7 (0.61)	$F_{2,456}=2.69$	.07
Gender					$\chi^2_2=2.99$	.22
Male	45%	45%	41%	48%		
Female	55%	55%	59%	52%		
Race/ethnicity					$\chi^2_6=50.84$	<.01
White	45%	41%	35%	59%		
African American	29%	26%	35%	25%		
Hispanic	12%	14%	19%	4%		
Native American	3%	<1%	2%	8%		
Asian/Pacific Islander	2%	3%	1%	1%		
Other[a]	9%	15%	9%	4%		
Free or reduced-cost lunches at time 1	56%	55%	67%	46%	$F_{2,741}=0.07^b$	.93

[a]Typically self-reported multiracial ethnicity.

[b]Analysis of variance–tested scores on the socioeconomic status scale.

Data Collection

MEASURES

Participants completed the self-administered Child Health and Illness Profile–Adolescent Edition (CHIP-AE) survey annually for both of the 2 study years. The CHIP-AE contains 107 items reflecting 6 domains and 20 subdomains that measure the physical, mental, and social aspects of health of youth aged 11–18 years.[12] It has been used and found both valid and reliable with racially and economically diverse middle and high school student samples in urban, rural, clinical, and community settings.[12–14]

DEPENDENT VARIABLES

We examined 5 health outcomes: satisfaction with health, physical discomfort, emotional discomfort, physical activity, and nutrition. Nutrition was divided into 2 subscales: healthy eating and unhealthy eating. All scales were constructed following the instructions provided by the measure authors, with higher scores indicating better health. We reverse-scored some scales so that higher scores reflected more of the construct (e.g., higher physical discomfort scores reflected higher levels of discomfort). We computed all scales by taking the average response across scale items; scale characteristics are shown in Table 3.2.

INDEPENDENT VARIABLES

The focal predictors in this study included 1 student-level variable, SBHC use, and 1 school-level variable, SBHC type. At the student level, participants were asked whether they had ever used the SBHC in their school, where nonusers were coded zero and those who had used the SBHC at least once were coded 1. Analyses focusing on this predictor used only the subsample of students with access to an SBHC. Approximately 72% of participants at implementation sites and 76% of participants at established sites reported that they were SBHC users. At the school level, analyses compared the impact of attending a school with no SBHC, a newly implemented SBHC, or an established SBHC. SBHC type was dummy-coded with comparison sites as the reference group.

COVARIATES

A single school-level covariate—grade level—was included in all models. Five student-level covariates were included: age, gender, race/ethnicity, socioeconomic status (SES), and the outcome at time 1. Time 1 means and standard deviations for the outcome variables across SBHC types and user statuses are presented in Table 3.3. We detected significant time 1 differences by SBHC type for healthy eating and by user status for physical discomfort and physical activity. At time 1, students at

TABLE 3.2—DESCRIPTIONS OF SURVEY OUTCOME MEASURES: MIDDLE SCHOOL AND HIGH SCHOOL STUDENTS, MICHIGAN, 2006–2008

Scale	Description	No. of Items	Internal Consistency[a]	Mean (SD)
Satisfaction with health	Measures perceptions of and beliefs about one's health; includes questions about the extent to which one feels full of energy, resists illness well, or is physically fit.	7	0.77	3.12 (0.57)
Physical discomfort	Measures both positive and negative somatic feelings and symptoms, asking individuals to identify how many days in the past 4 weeks they experienced various types of physical discomfort, such as cough, headache, or stomachache.	24	0.85	1.63 (0.42)
Emotional discomfort	Measures both positive and negative emotional feelings and symptoms, asking respondents how many days in the past 4 weeks they experienced various types of emotional discomfort, such as trouble sleeping, feeling depressed, or feeling nervous.	14	0.84	1.72 (0.57)
Physical activity	Measures participation in activities that promote physical fitness, such as walking or running.	5	0.69	3.07 (0.98)
Nutrition: healthy eating	Measures the frequency with which students drink milk and eat healthy foods such as fruits and vegetables.	4	0.64	3.44 (0.83)
Nutrition: unhealthy eating	Measures the frequency with which students eat unhealthy foods, such as fast food, salty foods, and sweets (this scale was reverse-coded so that higher scores reflected better nutrition).	3	0.72	3.38 (0.80)

[a]Calculated using the Cronbach α.

TABLE 3.3—TIME 1 OUTCOMES ACROSS SBHC TYPE AND USER STATUS: MIDDLE SCHOOL AND HIGH SCHOOL STUDENTS, MICHIGAN, 2006

	Comparison Sites, Mean (SD)	Implementation Sites		Established Sites		ANOVA; P^a	t Test; P^b
		SBHC User, Mean (SD)	SBHC Nonuser, Mean (SD)	SBHC User, Mean (SD)	SBHC Nonuser, Mean (SD)		
Satisfaction with health	3.14 (0.56)	3.12 (0.63)	3.16 (0.62)	3.04 (0.61)	2.99 (0.64)	$F_{2,736}=2.53$; $P=.08$	$t=0.02$; $P=.99$
Physical discomfort	1.65 (0.43)	1.76 (0.51)	1.58 (0.43)	1.69 (0.46)	1.62 (0.39)	$F_{2,728}=1.31$; $P=.27$	$t=-2.78$; $P<.01$
Emotional discomfort	1.75 (0.57)	1.81 (0.63)	1.77 (0.69)	1.83 (0.64)	1.70 (0.71)	$F_{2,728}=0.43$; $P=.65$	$t=-1.27$; $P=.21$
Physical activity	3.09 (0.91)	3.18 (1.00)	2.92 (0.89)	3.02 (0.95)	2.65 (0.88)	$F_{2,725}=2.62$; $P=.07$	$t=-3.07$; $P<.01$
Healthy eating	3.29 (0.85)	3.37 (0.93)	3.42 (0.86)	3.12 (0.92)	3.07 (0.90)	$F_{2,724}=6.35$; $P<.01$	$t=0.18$; $P=.86$
Unhealthy eating	3.27 (0.88)	3.09 (0.93)	3.19 (0.92)	3.23 (0.93)	3.28 (0.89)	$F_{2,726}=2.02$; $P=.13$	$t=0.73$; $P=.47$

Note. ANOVA = analysis of variance; SBHC = school-based health center. Comparison sites did not have SBHCs. Implementation sites had SBHCs that had been in operation for less than 1 year at time 1, and established sites had SBHCs that had been in operation for at least 6 years at time 1.

^{a}ANOVA compared time 1 means across comparison, implementation, and established sites, with implementation and established means collapsed across SBHC users and SBHC nonusers.

^{b}The t test compared mean differences across SBHC users and SBHC nonusers, collapsed across site type.

implementation sites reported eating more healthy food than students at established sites, and SBHC users reported *significantly* more physical discomfort and physical activity than SBHC nonusers. Race/ethnicity and SES were included as covariates to account for the well-documented health disparities that exist across different social locations.[15-18]

AGE AND GRADE LEVEL

Age and grade level were entered into all models as separate age-related constructs. Grade level was coded zero for middle school and 1 for high school. Age was group-mean-centered, resulting in a variable that reflected variation from the typical age of one's classmates.

Gender. Participants reported whether they identified as male or female. Male was coded zero; female was coded 1.

RACE/ETHNICITY

Survey instructions allowed participants to select 1 racial/ethnic group: White, African American, Latino, Native American, Asian/Pacific Islander, or "other." Race/ethnicity was dummy-coded, with White participants (the largest racial/ethnic group in the sample) as the reference group. The Native American, Asian/Pacific Islander, and "other" categories were combined into "Other" because of the small number of individuals who endorsed each category. Ultimately, there were 3 dummy categories that permitted comparison of African American students, Latino students, and "other" students to White students.

SES

The composite family SES scale combined measures of financial capital, human capital, and social capital; it was constructed following the CHIP-AE developers' instructions.[19] This mean composite measure included the following items: mother's or female guardian's education level and employment status, father's or male guardian's employment status, family structure, whether the participant or any sibling received a free or reduced-cost lunch at school, and whether the family received food stamps. Father's or male guardian's education level and family welfare status were excluded because much of these data were missing.

Data Analysis

We used 2-level hierarchical linear modeling to account for a design in which students were clustered within schools. This approach also allowed us to separately model the effect of the presence or absence of SBHCs on student health at the school level and the effect of SBHC use or nonuse at the student level. We also examined whether there were differences in the effects of SBHC use at the student level depending on gender (i.e., an SBHC user by gender interaction effect) and type of SBHC (i.e., an SBHC user by SBHC type interaction). All analyses examining SBHC user effects were performed on data from the subsample of participants (n = 515) who had access to an SBHC in their schools. We used HLM version 6.0[20] to analyze the data, making use of full information maximization likelihood methods. For each outcome, nested models were built beginning with the covariates, which were entered 1 at a time; nonsignificant covariates were excluded from subsequent models so as to generate the most parsimonious final model possible. Hedge g effect sizes were computed for each significant SBHC-related predictor.[21]

RESULTS

For each section of results below, we report only those covariates that were significantly related to the outcome, followed by our findings regarding the influence of SBHC type and SBHC use on the outcome. Full results from the final models of each outcome, including effect sizes for all significant predictors, are presented in Table 3.4.

Satisfaction With Health

Being male ($\gamma = -0.27$; $P < .05$), being in middle school ($\gamma = -0.13$; $P < .05$), and having higher satisfaction with health at time 1 ($\gamma = 0.47$; $P < .05$) were significantly related to higher levels of satisfaction with health at time 2. No significant differences were found between students at schools with SBHCs and students at schools without SBHCs.

Among students who had access to an SBHC in their school, health center users reported significantly greater satisfaction with health at time 2 than did nonusers ($\gamma = 0.12$; $P < .05$). Interaction effects for user by gender and user by SBHC type were not significant, suggesting that gender and SBHC type had no effect on the relationship between being a user and satisfaction with health.

Physical Discomfort

Being female ($\gamma = 0.11$; $P < .05$), being White compared with "other" race/ethnicity ($\gamma = -0.10$; $P < .05$), being in high school ($\gamma = 0.07$; $P < .05$), and higher levels of physical discomfort at time 1 ($\gamma = 0.51$; $P < .05$) were all related to greater

TABLE 3.4—FINAL MODEL COEFFICIENTS, STANDARD ERRORS, AND EFFECT SIZES FOR SBHC-RELATED EFFECTS FOR EACH OUTCOME: MIDDLE SCHOOL AND HIGH SCHOOL STUDENTS, MICHIGAN, 2006–2008

Variables	Satisfaction With Health b (SE)	ES	Physical Discomfort b (SE)	ES	Emotional Discomfort b (SE)	ES	Physical Activity b (SE)	ES	Healthy Eating b (SE)	ES	Unhealthy Eating[a] b (SE)	ES
Covariates												
Gender[b]	−0.27** (0.03)	…	0.11** (0.03)	…	0.14** (0.03)	…	−0.25** (0.06)	…	…	…	…	…
SES[c]	…	…	…	…	…	…	…	…	…	…	…	…
African American[d]	…	…	−0.06* (0.03)	…	…	…	…	…	−0.23** (0.06)	…	−0.29** (0.06)	…
Latino[d]	…	…	0.06 (0.04)	…	…	…	…	…	−0.03 (0.09)	…	−0.14 (0.09)	…
Other[d]	…	…	−0.10** (0.04)	…	…	…	…	…	−0.04 (0.09)	…	−0.10 (0.08)	…
Age[c]	…	…	…	…	…	…	…	…	…	…	…	…
Middle school or high school[e]	−0.13** (0.05)	…	0.07** (0.03)	…	0.17** (0.03)	…	…	…	…	…	…	…
Time 1 outcome	0.47** (0.03)	…	0.51** (0.03)	…	0.50** (0.03)	…	0.57** (0.03)	…	0.42** (0.03)	…	0.35** (0.03)	…
Predictors												

Implementation SBHC[f]	0.0006 (0.06)	...	−0.02 (0.03)	...	−0.08* (0.04)	−0.13	0.16 (0.12)	...	−0.002 (0.07)	...	−0.07 (0.07)	...
Established SBHC[g]	−0.02 (0.06)	...	−0.05 (0.03)	...	−0.08* (0.04)	−0.14	0.05 (0.12)	...	0.04 (0.07)	...	0.04 (0.06)	...
SBHC user[h]	0.12** (0.05)	0.21	−0.04 (0.03)	...	−0.08* (0.05)	−0.14	0.20** (0.08)	0.20	0.18** (0.07)	0.22	−0.06 (0.07)	...
User×gender interaction	−0.10 (0.09)	...	−0.14** (0.07)	−0.22[i]	−0.15 (0.09)	...	−0.04 (0.16)	...	−0.01 (0.14)	...	0.18 (0.15)	...
User×SBHC type interaction	0.01 (0.09)	...	0.06 (0.07)	...	0.08 (0.09)	...	0.02 (0.16)	...	0.14 (0.14)	...	0.14 (0.15)	...

Note. SBHC = school-based health center; b = parameter estimate; ES = effect size; SES = socioeconomic status. We computed Hedge g effect sizes following the recommendations by the Institute for Educational Sciences (available at http://ies.ed.gov/ncee/wwc/help/idocviewer/Doc.aspx?docId=19&tocId=8#hm) from the What Works Clearinghouse Procedures and Standards Handbook.[21]

[a]Unhealthy eating is reverse-scored; higher scores reflect less unhealthy eating.
[b]Male = 0, female = 1.
[c]Not significant and not computed for the full model.
[d]Compared with White students (reference group).
[e]Middle school = 0, high school = 1.
[f]Implementation sites = 1, comparison sites = 0. Comparison sites did not have SBHCs; implementation sites had SBHCs that had been in operation for less than 1 year at time 1.
[g]established sites = 1, comparison sites = 0. Comparison sites did not have SBHCs; established sites had SBHCs that had been in operation for at least 6 years at time 1.
[h]Nonuser = 0, user = 1. Participants reported lifetime use of the health center.
[i]Given the primary interest in user effects, the effect size was computed comparing female users and nonusers.
*P < .10; **P < .05.

physical discomfort at time 2. No significant differences emerged between students at schools with SBHCs and students at schools without SBHCs.

Among students with access to an SBHC in their school, there were no differences in physical discomfort at time 2 between SBHC users and nonusers. However, the gender by user status interaction was significant ($\gamma=-0.14$; $P<.05$). For females, health center users had lower physical discomfort at time 2 than did nonusers ($\gamma=-0.10$; $P<.05$). For health center nonusers, females had significantly higher physical discomfort at time 2 than did males ($\gamma=0.19$; $P<.05$). Finally, we tested whether there was a difference in the user effect depending on the type of SBHC. No significant interaction effect was detected.

Emotional Discomfort

Being female ($\gamma=0.14$; $P<.05$), being in high school ($\gamma=0.17$; $P<.05$), and having higher levels of emotional discomfort at time 1 ($\gamma=0.50$; $P<.05$) were associated with greater emotional discomfort at time 2. Among students with access to an SBHC in their school, tests comparing emotional discomfort levels between SBHC users and nonusers revealed no significant differences. Neither the gender by SBHC user status interaction nor the SBHC type by SBHC user status interaction were significant.

Physical Activity

Being male and having higher levels of physical activity at time 1 were significantly related to higher levels of physical activity at time 2 ($\gamma=-0.25$; $P<.05$ and $\gamma=0.57$; $P<.05$, respectively). No significant differences emerged between students at schools with SBHCs and students at schools without SBHCs. Among students with access to an SBHC in their school, health center users reported significantly more physical activity at time 2 than did nonusers ($\gamma=0.20$; $P<.05$). Neither the gender by user interaction nor the SBHC type by SBHC user interaction were significant, suggesting that the effect of being a health center user on physical activity did not differ by gender or SBHC type.

Nutrition

Being White (compared with being African American; $\gamma=-0.23$; $P<.05$) and eating healthier at time 1 ($\gamma=0.42$; $P<.05$) were significantly related to higher levels of healthy eating at time 2. No significant differences emerged between students at schools with SBHCs and students at schools without SBHCs. Among students with access to an SBHC in their school, health center users reported eating significantly more healthy food at time 2 than did nonusers ($\gamma=0.17$; $P<.05$). We found no significant interaction effects for gender by SBHC user status or SBHC type by SBHC user status for healthy eating at time 2.

Being African American ($\gamma = -0.29$; $P < .05$) and reporting more unhealthy eating at time 1 ($\gamma = 0.35$; $P < .05$) were significantly related to higher levels of unhealthy eating at time 2. No significant differences emerged between students at schools with SBHCs and students at schools without SBHCs. Among students with access to an SBHC in their school, there were no significant differences in unhealthy eating between SBHC users and nonusers. Similarly, there was no significant interaction between SBHC use and gender or SBHC use and SBHC type.

DISCUSSION

We studied the impact of SBHCs on the health outcomes of middle and high school students. Using multilevel modeling, we analyzed both the school-level effect of SBHC type (comparison, implementation, established) and the individual-level effect of user status (user vs nonuser) on health outcomes.

School-Based Health Center Type

Despite the involvement of SBHCs in schoolwide activities such as health education campaigns, we found no school-level effects of SBHC type on student health outcomes. There were no significant differences in health outcomes among students who attended schools with no SBHCs, newly implemented SBHCs, or established SBHCs.

User Status

Although the mere presence or absence of SBHCs did not have schoolwide effects on student health, health outcomes did differ at schools with SBHCs, depending on whether students used the SBHC. Consistent with the work of Wade et al.[5]—but inconsistent with the work of Kisker, Brown, and Hill[11]—SBHC use was associated with an improved subjective sense of overall health. This inconsistency in results may be attributable to differences in study design. Whereas our study and the study conducted by Wade et al. differentiated between users and nonusers in schools with SBHCs, the Kisker, Brown, and Hill study did not; thus, the absence of benefits for nonusers may have masked the health benefits for users.

Because SBHC use is associated with greater satisfaction with health, one would expect that SBHC use would also be associated with fewer symptoms of physical discomfort. Although SBHC users in general did not experience significantly fewer physical symptoms compared with nonusers, female SBHC users experienced significantly fewer symptoms of physical discomfort at time 2 than did female nonusers. Given the greater satisfaction with health reported by SBHC users at time 2, one might also expect that SBHC users would be more likely to engage in the kinds of health behaviors that contribute to better health. As expected, health center users reported engaging in more physical activity and eating more healthy food at time 2 than did nonusers. These user effects were not dependent on how long the SBHC had been in operation, as shown by the nonsignificant findings for all of the SBHC type by SBHC use interactions.

The association of SBHC use with increased physical activity and increased consumption of healthy foods is noteworthy, given recent concerns about the epidemic of obesity among youths in the United States.[22-24] Our results indicate that SBHC use is associated with a behavior that counteracts a primary contributing factor to obesity among children and adolescents: physical inactivity.[25-28] The fact that SBHC use appears to be a component of a healthy lifestyle that includes more physical activity and greater consumption of healthy foods suggests that SBHCs might play a significant role in reducing obesity among children and adolescents. These findings highlight the importance of efforts to promote parental awareness of SBHCs and student use of SBHCs as ways to enhance these potential benefits.

Although our analyses found that SBHC use had statistically significant associations with a variety of positive self-reported health-related behaviors and health outcomes, it is worth noting that the effect sizes, which ranged from 0.20 to 0.22, were at the low end of the small-to-medium effect-size range (0.20–0.50), according to the conventions established by Cohen.[29]

Limitations

Because students were not randomly assigned to groups, selection bias resulting from unmeasured preexisting differences among students attending the 3 types of schools is a potential threat to the internal validity of this study. We attempted to address this limitation by reducing selection bias at the school level through careful matching of established and comparison sites. However, the overall impact of matching is limited by the inclusion of the implementation sites in the analyses, which were not matched to comparison sites. By controlling for time 1 outcomes and for race, gender, and SES, we sought to further reduce any preexisting differences across groups.

Conclusions

We examined the health-related impact of SBHCs and distinguished between the direct effects of SHBCs on students who used their services and indirect effects on all students in schools with SBHCs, including health center nonusers. Our findings support other studies' findings that SBHC use was associated with self-reported positive health outcomes for middle and high school students, including overall sense of health and health-promoting behaviors. Further research is needed to delineate the causal mechanisms mediating the relationship between the use of SBHCs and health outcomes. Such studies would employ more refined measures that quantify the frequency of SBHC use, the types of services used, and their relationship to both self-reported and documented health outcomes.

REFERENCES

1. Allison MA, Crane LA, Beaty BL, Davidson AJ, Melinkovich P, Kempe A. School-based health centers: improving access and quality care for low-income adolescents. *Pediatrics.* 2007;120(4):e887–e894.

2. Health Foundation of Greater Cincinnati. *Evaluation of Health Outcomes of Students Using School-Based Health Centers.* Cincinnati, OH: Health Foundation of Greater Cincinnati; 2005.

3. Kisker EE, Brown RS. Do school-based health centers improve adolescents' access to health care, health status, and risk-taking behavior? *J Adolesc Health.* 1996;18(5):335–343.

4. Crespo RD, Shaler GA. Assessment of school-based health centers in a rural state: the West Virginia experience. *J Adolesc Health.* 2000;26(3):187–193.

5. Wade TJ, Mansour M, Line K, Huentelman T, Keller K. Improvements in health-related quality of life among school-based health center users in elementary and middle school. *Ambul Pediatr.* 2008;8(4):241–249.

6. Wade TJ, Mansour M, Guo J, Huentelman T, Line K, Keller KN. Access and utilization patterns of school-based health centers at urban and rural elementary and middle schools. *Public Health Rep.* 2008;123(6):739–749.

7. Mavis B, Pearson R, Stewart G, Keefe C. A work sampling study of provider activities in school-based health centers. *J Sch Health.* 2009;79(6):262–268.

8. Guo JJ, Jang R, Keller K, McCracken A, Pan W, Cluxton R. Impact of school-based health centers on children with asthma. *J Adolesc Health.* 2005;37(4):266–274.

9. Webber MP, Carpiniello KE, Oruwariye T, Lo Y, Burton WB, Appel DK. Burden of asthma in inner-city elementary school children. *Arch Pediatr Adolesc Med.* 2003;157(2):125–129.

10. Webber MP, Hoxie A, Odlum M, Oruwariye T, Lo Y, Appel D. Impact of asthma intervention in two elementary school-based health centers in the Bronx, New York City. *Pediatr Pulmonol.* 2005;40(6):487–493.

11. Kisker EE, Brown RS, Hill J. *Healthy Caring: Outcomes of the Robert Wood Johnson Foundation's School-Based Adolescent Health Care Program.* Princeton, NJ: Mathematica Policy Research; 1994.

12. Starfield B, Riley AW, Green BF, et al. *Manual for the Child Health and Illness Profile: Adolescent Edition*. Baltimore, MD: Johns Hopkins University School of Hygiene and Public Health; 2000.

13. Starfield B, Bergner M, Ensminger ME, et al. Adolescent health status measurement: development of the Child Health and Illness Profile. *Pediatrics*. 1993;91(2):430–435.

14. Starfield B, Riley AW, Green BF, et al. The adolescent Child Health and Illness Profile: a population-based measure of health. *Med Care*. 1995;33(5):553–566.

15. Williams DR, Jackson PB. Social sources of racial disparities in health. *Health Aff (Millwood)*. 2005;24(2):325–334.

16. Lasser KE, Himmelstein DU, Woolhandler S. Access to care, health status, and health disparities in the United States and Canada: results of a cross-national population-based survey. *Am J Public Health*. 2006;96(7):1300–1307.

17. Murray CJL, Kukarni SC, Michaud C, et al. Eight Americas: investigating mortality disparities across races, counties, and race-counties in the United States. *PLoS Med*. 2006;3(9):e260.

18. Satcher D, Higginbotham EJ. The public health approach to eliminating disparities in health. *Am J Public Health*. 2008;98(3):400–403.

19. Ensminger ME, Forrest CB, Riley AW, et al. The validity of measures of socioeconomic status of adolescents. *J Adolesc Res*. 2000;15(3):392–419.

20. *Hierarchical Linear and Nonlinear Modeling* [computer program]. Version 6.03. Lincolnwood, IL: Scientific Software International; 2005.

21. Institute of Education Sciences, US Department of Education. *What Works Clearinghouse Procedures and Standards Handbook*. Washington, DC: Institute of Education Sciences, US Dept of Education; 2008.

22. Hedley AA, Ogden CL, Johnson CL. Prevalence of overweight and obesity among US children, adolescents, and adults, 1999–2002. *JAMA*. 2004;291(23):2847–2850.

23. Ogden CL, Flegal KM, Carroll MD. Prevalence and trends in overweight among US children and adolescents, 1999–2000. *JAMA*. 2002;288(14):1728–1732.

24. Ogden CL, Carroll MD, Curtin LR. Prevalence of overweight and obesity in the United States, 1999–2004. *JAMA*. 2006;295(13):1549–1555.

25. Gordon-Larsen P, Adair LS, Popkin BM. Ethnic differences in physical activity and inactivity patterns and overweight status. *Obes Res*. 2002;10(3):141–149.

26. Gortmaker SL, Must A, Sobol AM, Peterson K, Colditz GA, Dietz WH. Television viewing as a cause of increasing obesity among children in the United States, 1986–1990. *Arch Pediatr Adolesc Med*. 1996;150(4):356–362.

27. Jeffery RW, French SA. Epidemic obesity in the United States: are fast foods and television viewing contributing? *Am J Public Health*. 1998;88(2):277–280.

28. Tremblay MS, Willms JD. Is the Canadian childhood obesity epidemic related to physical inactivity? *Int J Obes Relat Metab Disord*. 2003;27(9):1100–1105.

29. Cohen J. A power primer. *Psychol Bull*. 1992;112(1):155–159.

About the Authors

Miles A. McNall, PhD – is the Associate Director of the Community Evaluation and Research Collaborative at Michigan State University. Miles has conducted evaluations of a variety of health and human service programs, including HIV case management for young men, integrated services for individuals with HIV and comorbid mental health and substance abuse disorders, school-based health centers, centralized billing services for school-based health centers, and home-based services for children with severe emotional disturbances. Miles holds a PhD in Sociology from the University of Minnesota.

Lauren F. Lichty, PhD – is a Visiting Assistant Professor in the Psychology Department at Michigan State University. She received her Doctorate in Ecological-Community Psychology from Michigan State University with a specialization in Quantitative Methods and Evaluation Science. Her research interests include innovative, participatory, and mixed-method research, youth empowerment, and promoting adolescent health and well-being through individual- and setting-level interventions.

Brian Mavis, PhD – received his PhD in Community Psychology from Michigan State University in 1988. He is associate professor and director of the Office of Medical Education Research and Development (OMERAD) in the College of Human Medicine at Michigan State University. Since that time, he has worked primarily on issues of assessment and evaluation in professional education settings. He has been involved in the evaluation for a variety of organizations such as the March of Dimes Foundation, School-Community Health Alliance of Michigan, National Board of Veterinary Medical Examiners, Henry Ford Health System, and the Statewide Autism Education Center. Additionally, he has been an evaluator for federally funded university programs, including Health Resources and Services Administration–funded minority recruitment and retention programs and National Institute of General Medical Sciences–sponsored educational programs.

Training School Health Nurses to Recognize and Refer Student Behavioral and Mental Problems in a Post-Disaster Setting

Marsha Broussard, Sarah Kohler Chrestman, and Colleen Kudla Arceneaux

INTRODUCTION

The mental health needs of children were significant post-Hurricane Katrina in the New Orleans Metropolitan area, including Jefferson, Orleans, Plaquemines, and St. Bernard Parishes (Metro Area). In 2006, Louisiana State University Health Sciences Center (LSUHSC), Department of Child Psychiatry, screened 2,192 students, grades 4 to 12, from Orleans and St. Bernard Parish public schools. Of the students screened, over 50% met the threshold for a possible mental health referral.[1] In July 2009, the US Government Accountability Office reported persistent barriers for accessing mental health services among Metro Area children. These barriers included poor access to mental health services due to a shortage of mental health providers; family priorities that prevented care seeking, such as the need to address extensive home damages, rebuilding challenges, financial problems, employment changes, and lack of transportation; and stigmatization around using mental health services.[2]

School health nurses (SHNs) were some of the first health care professionals to witness the disaster's effects on primary and secondary students' behavioral and mental health status. They were often the first line of defense in helping students cope with the pressures from displacement.[3] School Health Connection (SHC), a program of the Louisiana Public Health Institute (LPHI), convened a meeting of mental health providers working in Metro Area schools to develop solutions to assist overtaxed staff with burnout, and subsequently developed a training program for SHNs.

LPHI is a private nonprofit organization that addresses public health issues in Louisiana, convening public and private organizations and resources to bring forth solutions. The SHC program, launched in 2006 with W. K. Kellogg Foundation funds, was developed by LPHI to improve access to health services for students attending public schools in the Metro area. The SHN training program referenced in this article was conducted by SHC staff at LPHI, and was funded by the Robert Wood Johnson Foundation.

DEVELOPMENT OF THE SCHOOL HEALTH NURSE DISASTER RESPONSE TRAINING PROGRAM

In March 2007, a needs assessment was conducted at the Louisiana School Nurses Organization annual meeting to assess SHNs' knowledge and skills with addressing behavioral and mental needs of students experiencing post-disaster mental trauma. From a statewide audience of SHNs, 127 of approximately 234 attendees (54%) participated in a needs-assessment survey issued at their annual luncheon. The results indicated that they were observing three symptomatic student behaviors that they believed were associated with students' post-traumatic distress, including verbal confrontation, poor school performance, and physical altercations. SHNs also identified their own work-related stressors, including uncertainty regarding identifying varied student behaviors immediately post-hurricane, professional limitations regarding delivery of mental and behavioral health care, and unclear referral processes/lack of relationships to area mental and behavioral health providers.

In response to the survey results, SHC designed a comprehensive, five-component program to address the primary needs identified. The first two components were addressed through a training program designed to enhance SHNs' skills to recognize, treat, and provide appropriate referrals for students who were experiencing post-disaster depression, anxiety, and traumatic stress. The second goal of the training program was to improve SHNs skills to educate and inform teachers and parents regarding recognizing and referring children with post-disaster anxieties and behavioral difficulties. Teachers and parents could make referrals to the school nurse or to other professionals such as community mental health and medical providers. This component of the program was subjected to an internal evaluation, the results of which will be discussed later in this chapter.

A third component was the development of a tool kit that included information regarding age-specific warning signs in children post-disaster, age-specific guidelines for talking to traumatized children, a sample behavioral health referral process for schools, a sample behavioral health referral form, a regional resource guide, and instructions to assist SHNs in educating other school staff and parents on student mental health issues. These tools were developed by the LSUHSC nursing school faculty and reviewed by the group of community mental health providers before finalization. These tools are available on the SHC website (http://www. schoolhealthconnection.org).

A fourth program component was to provide SHNs access to professional mental health consultation using telemedicine to assist with SHNs with difficult cases. This component could not be developed due to an inability to find a mental health provider and lack of telemedicine access among SHNs. As a substitute, the SHC program developed a mental health resource manual that identified community-based mental health agencies and referral opportunities. SHNs were encouraged to utilize a listserv that was established for Metro Area school mental health providers to share information and support each other's informational and referral needs. These components were not evaluated.

A fifth component was initially designed as a daylong resiliency workshop to support SHNs in addressing burnout caused by the intense needs of students as well as attending to their personal and family concerns in the aftermath of the disaster. This workshop was designed and conducted by a special team from the Center for Mind and Body Medicine.[a] It incorporated self-help, meditation, and relaxation techniques and included demonstrations and practice sessions of these techniques. The workshop also emphasized increased self-awareness, how to conduct self-care, how to understand the mind–body connection, and how emotions affect physical being. Because of the costs associated with the daylong event and the unpredictability in participation, the trainings that were developed by LSUHSC School of Nursing eliminated this separate resiliency component and incorporated resiliency techniques in the main training program for SHNs.

The SHN disaster response training program was designed to assist SHNs with recognizing the signs and symptoms of post-traumatic stress disorder (PTSD) and associated behavioral health problems and to provide recommendations for early interventions and effective referral. This intervention was initially developed in 2008 by a team that included a registered mental health nurse contracted from LSUHSC and a clinical social worker from the LPHI staff. Due to staff turnover at LPHI and the resignation of the original team leader from the LSUHSC Department of Psychiatry, SHC contracted with the LSUHSC School of Nursing to deliver the program. The program content incorporated cognitive behavioral support techniques for diagnosing and providing early treatment for SHNs who had limited mental health training. SHNs were recruited for the training by LPHI staff who worked closely with school district personnel. Nurses from charter schools that were not connected to school districts were recruited through direct outreach to those schools.

---

[a] The Center for Mind and Body Medicine, founded by Dr. James Gordon, provides teaching and techniques to empower people to deal with stress and trauma after a natural disaster. More information is available at http://www.cmbm.org.

EVALUATION OF PROGRAM COMPONENTS

An internal evaluation of the SHN Disaster Response Trainings and other program components was conducted by staff from LPHI's evaluation division to assess the program successes and to document lessons learned from the project. Each training session included pre- and post-test surveys that assessed SHNs' knowledge and confidence with using training content. Knowledge was tested regarding developmental outcomes, trauma symptoms, and psychological first aid. SHNs also rated their level of confidence in conducting specific disaster response behavioral health skills on a scale from 1 ("Very Confident") to 4 ("Not at All Confident"). The post-test survey included SHNs' satisfaction with the training.

If the SHNs agreed, a follow-up survey was conducted five months after the initial training via email or telephone. Fifty-four (75%) of the 72 participating SHNs agreed to participate in the follow-up survey. The survey included a question to assess whether participating SHNs had received additional training on similar mental health topics since attending the "Disaster Response Training for School Health Nurses." All results from the three surveys were aggregated and analyzed for significant changes in knowledge and confidence by using the χ^2 test in SPSS version 15.0 (SPSS Inc, Predictive Analytics Software Statistics, Chicago, IL). Due to questionnaire modifications after the initial training, responses from Orleans parish SHNs pertaining to trauma symptoms and warning signs of suicide were separated from the other parish's responses. Otherwise all parish responses were aggregated.

EVALUATION FINDINGS

Demographics

A total of 72 SHNs, representing approximately 119 public schools in the Metro area and impacting at least 59,000 students, participated in the trainings. Because multiple school systems were operating in a post-disaster setting, the total number of SHNs for each parish was not available.

Pre-Test Findings

The pre-test was completed by 72 SHNs. In the knowledge component, correct responses were provided by 80% of the SHNs (Table 4.1). The overall mean of self-reported confidence levels was 2.23 (Table 4.2). The lowest levels of self-reported confidence were in providing resources to help parents work with traumatized children, assisting teachers working with traumatized children, and identifying the "red flags" for children of all age groups.

TABLE 4.1—SCHOOL HEALTH NURSES' (SHNs') KNOWLEDGE COMPONENT FINDINGS FROM THE PRE-TEST, POST-TEST, AND FOLLOW-UP SURVEYS

Question	Pre-Test (% Correct Responses)	Post-Test (% Correct Responses)	Change in % Correct Responses	P Value[b]	Follow-up (% Correct Responses)
Developmental Outcomes	97.2	100.0	+2.8	0.496	96.6
Trauma Symptom					81.0
Orleans Parish[a]	29.2	38.1	+8.9	0.526	
Other Parishes	38.1	86.7	+48.6	**0.02**	
Referring	94.2	89.9	−4.3	0.346	86.2
Warning of Suicide					100.0
Orleans Parish[a]	95.8	90.9	−4.9	0.6	
Other Parishes	97.9	95.6	−2.3	0.613	
Psychological First Aid	82.9	94.2	+11.3	**0.036**	89.7

[a]The questionnaire was modified slightly after the Orleans training. Because of these modifications, Orleans Parish SHNs had to be extrapolated from the other parishes.

[b]Bolded P values are statistically significant.

Post-Test Findings

Post-tests were completed by 70 SHNs and the percentage of correct responses increased in the areas of developmental outcomes, trauma symptoms, and psychological first aid (Table 4.1). Although the results are presented in aggregate format for Plaquemines and St. Bernard Parishes, the increase in correct responses for identifying PTSD symptoms was significant for all four parishes, $P = .036$; the increases in correct responses for psychological first aid were significant in three parishes (Table 4.1). A noticeable increase in confidence of SHNs was observed from pre-test to post-test in every area (see Table 4.2; P values range from <.001 to .001). Almost half of respondents reported that this was the first training they had ever received on children's reactions to trauma. The training satisfaction was very high.

Follow-Up Findings

Among participants, 54 (75%) SHNs agreed to a six-month follow-up assessment, of whom 30 participated. The percentage of correct responses was higher at follow-up than on the pre-test for three of five knowledge topics (Table 4.1). SHNs' confidence levels also remained strong several months after training, with the average confidence level at 1.80. Statistical significance was found in six of nine areas

TABLE 4.2—SCHOOL HEALTH NURSES' SELF-REPORTED CONFIDENCE LEVELS

Question	Pre-Test Mean	Post-Test Mean	P Value[a]	Follow-up
Help children cope with traumatic/stressful events	2.17	**1.80**	**<.001**	1.86
Distinguish between normal and abnormal reactions to stress in children	2.13	**1.72**	**<.001**	1.76
Identify the "red flags" for children of all age groups	2.28	**1.67**	**<.001**	1.90
Recognize the indicators of trauma in children	2.27	**1.70**	**<.001**	1.76
Provide resources to help parents work with their children who might be traumatized	2.39	1.69	**<.001**	1.86
Assist teachers in working with traumatized children	2.38	1.82	**<.001**	1.86
Recognize the warning signs of suicide ideation	2.15	1.62	**<.001**	1.76
Know when to refer a child for behavioral health consultation, evaluation, or services	2.03	1.57	**<.001**	1.55
Know where to effectively or efficiently refer a child for behavioral health consultation, evaluation, or services	2.23	1.64	**<.001**	1.75
Average	2.22	1.69		1.78

Note. Higher values indicate lower confidence levels.

[a]Bolded P values are statistically significant.

at follow-up (see Table 4.2). Over half of the participating SHNs (55.2%) reported using the "Disaster Response Training for School Health Nurses" training materials at follow-up. When asked if they had received any additional training on similar topics from other agencies, 17.2% of SHNs reported receiving additional training.

DISCUSSION

In Katrina's aftermath, mental health service needs in schools were exacerbated. Arming SHNs with enhanced capability to recognize and provide early treatment and referral for mental/behavior health issues was a strategy identified for reaching SHNs who were providing services to students. There was a significant increase in knowledge from pre- to post-test (including the three areas where confidence levels were the lowest during pre-training [see Table 4.2]), and the follow-up survey showed that "Disaster Response Training" knowledge was mostly retained—the percentage of correct responses remained higher at follow up than at pre-test for three of five knowledge topics. The follow-up survey also showed that confidence levels remained strong with an average confidence level of 1.78, which was still better than the average 2.22 from the pre-test. Through effective coordination with five school districts, over 20,000 students were potentially impacted by this training.[4]

CONCLUSIONS AND RECOMMENDATIONS

The evaluation process was not based upon an experimental design but did provide useful information to inform the program staff and program partners regarding next steps in improving future mental programs targeting SHNs and schools. Since 2006, SHC has hosted a consortium of Metro Area school mental health providers that have met bi-monthly to address students' mental health needs and prepare for future disasters. They reviewed the results of the SHN Disaster Response Training in addition to other programs and interventions that were provided post-Katrina in order to address the mental health issues of Metro Area students.

They generally observed that training SHNs was a good strategy for sustainability and for potentially impacting a large number of students, and recommended that there would be additional benefit to training more school personnel. They also recommended that future programs should focus on preventive mental health strategies through emphasizing holistic approaches to mental health that impact the entire school community and that are aimed at creating a positive school climate. The goal of such an approach would be to create a supportive environment and a sense of security for students prior to disasters, particularly those from distressed communities who are disproportionately impacted.[5] This approach would involve training the entire school staff to promote positive and supportive interactions between students, staff, and parents, which can be transformational, be preventive, and result in the creation of mental health protective factors.[5]

REFERENCES

1. Osofsky HJ, Osofsky JD, Harris WW. Katrina's children: social policy considerations for children in disasters. *Soc Policy Rep.* 2007;21(1):3–18.

2. US Government Accountability Office. *Hurricane Katrina, Barriers to Mental Health Services for Children Persist in Greater New Orleans, Although Federal Grants Are Helping*

to *Address Them: Report to Congressional Requesters.* Washington, DC: US Government Accountability Office; 2009. GAO-09-563.

3. Broussard L, Myers R, Meaux J. The impact of hurricanes Katrina and Rita on Louisiana school nurses. *J Sch Nurs.* 2008;24(2):78–82.

4. Louisiana Department of Education. Multi-Stats—Feb 1, 2008—By Site—Total Reported. Available at: http://www.doe.state.la.us/offices/infomanagement/student_enrollment_data.html. Accessed September 16, 2009.

5. Cahill WJ, Holdsworth R, Rowling L, Carson, S. Mindmatters, a whole school approach to promoting mental health and wellbeing. *Aust N Z J Psychiatry.* 2000;34(4):594–601.

About the Authors

Marsha Broussard, DrPh, MPH–is a public health leader who serves as the Program Director and Principal Investigator for the School Health Connection program and the Orleans Teen Pregnancy Prevention Program at the Louisiana Public Health Institute (LPHI). LPHI, an independent nonprofit public health organization, strives to improve health and quality of life in Louisiana. Under Dr. Broussard's leadership, LPHI has become a key stakeholder in school health services, including school-based health centers, health and wellness programs, and risk reduction programs, all targeting adolescents. Success has required coalition building across state and local governmental agencies, universities, foundations, and local partners.

Sarah Kohler Chrestman, MPH–serves as an Evaluation Coordinator for LPHI. She has spent the last four years evaluating SHC, a local effort to rebuild and create school-based health centers. Through SHC she has evaluated the Disaster Response Mental Health Training, where she assessed knowledge and confidence gained among school nurses, and the school-based health center electronic medical records (EMR) project, where she monitored progress and outcome indicators in the implementation of an EMR in the school-based health center network. She currently works with Louisiana Positive Charge evaluating efforts to link people living with HIV/AIDS to medical care.

Colleen Kudla Arceneaux, MPH–is a Program Manager for School Health Connection (SHC) at the LPHI. In this position, she coordinated the implementation and evaluation of the school nurse training program. Currently, Ms. Arceneaux is managing School Health Connection's school wellness initiative. This initiative, guided by the coordinated school health framework, is taking place in public schools throughout New Orleans to improve the health and well-being of the students, their families, and faculty. She also serves on the boards of two local nonprofits whose missions are to increase physical activity and improve health outcomes of students.

School-Based Female-Specific Substance Use Prevention: Lessons From a Massachusetts Demonstration Project

Leslie A. Mandel and John W. Kulig

INTRODUCTION

Patterns of adolescent substance use and abuse, as well as risk and protective factors, outcomes, and approaches to prevention can vary by gender.[1-4] Yet, gender is not typically considered in substance use health promotion. One reason may be that substance use among adolescents has been declining.[5] Emerging evidence, however, suggests that not only have improvements slowed,[6] but substance use among female adolescents, in particular, is increasing.[7-10] New data reveal that females are using substances at rates that equal or exceed male use (Table 5.1).[7-11] In response, some researchers recommend tailoring prevention programming to girls.[12,13]

Female adolescents use substances for different reasons than males and have greater vulnerability than males to the physical health impacts of substances.[13] For example, among girls daily marijuana use is associated with depression, but not among boys.[14] Girls, unlike boys, use stimulants and cigarettes to control weight[13,15] and deal with depression, anxiety, and stress.[16] Low self-esteem is correlated with cigarette use in female but not male adolescents.[17] Girls are more likely than boys to use substances to cope with life transitions.[13] Peer and family influences impact girls' substance use more than they do for boys.[12,18] Differences in gender role identity and expectations influence adolescents' receptivity to pro-drinking messages.[2] Finally, substance abuse among girls is often accompanied by increased risk of sexual and physical assault,[19] unintended pregnancy, HIV, and other sexually transmitted infections.[20]

The experiences of female adolescents cannot be understood or addressed by using theoretical constructs of adult women or strategies developed for males.[21] Given multiple personal, social, and environmental factors related to female

TABLE 5.1 — PREVALENCE OF ALCOHOL, TOBACCO, AND OTHER DRUG USE AMONG YOUTHS AGE 12–17 YEARS, BY GENDER: 2002–2006

YEAR	Current Alcohol Use[a]		Cigarette Smoking in Last Month[a]		Cigarette Smoking Initiation[a]		Marijuana Initiation[a]		Misuse of Prescription Drugs[a]		Inhalant Use in Past Year[b]	
	Girls 12–17	Boys 12–17	Girls 12–17	Boys 12–17	Girls 12–17	Boys 12–17	Girls 12–17	Boys 12–17	Girls 12–17	Boys 12–17	Girls 12–17	Boys 12–17
2002			13.6%	12.3%	7.4%	6.1%	6.7%	6.3%				
2003			12.5%	11.9%	7.5%	5.8%	6.2%	5.2%				
2004	18.0%	17.2%	12.5%	11.3%	7.8%	5.8%	6.3%	5.3%	10.1%	7.6%		
2005	17.2%	15.9%	10.7%	10.8%	7.1%	6.3%					13.5%	11.3%
2006	17.0%	16.3%	10.7%	10.0%	6.9%	5.7%						

Sources: [a]*Data compiled from the national findings for the 2004, 2005, and 2006 National Survey on Drug Use and Health.*[8–10]

[b]*Data from the 2005 Youth Risk Behavior Surveillance.*[11]

adolescent substance use and abuse, effective prevention efforts must be gender-specific and involve students, families, schools, and communities.[22,23]

Located within schools, school-based health centers (SBHCs) have ongoing access to youth, families, and school personnel; deliver comprehensive health services[24]; and have exceptional potential for prevention, early intervention, and health promotion.[25] Students with a history of current or past substance use are more willing to consult an SBHC than any other type of health care facility.[26] SBHC users have also been identified as having high prevalence of substance abuse issues.[27-29] SBHCs improve access to[30,31] and utilization of[32] mental health and substance abuse services for extremely high-risk adolescents. Further, female students are more likely to use SBHC services than males.[26,33,34] Thus, SBHCs may be uniquely suited to addressing female adolescent substance use prevention.

Notwithstanding compelling data on the appropriateness of SBHC services for addressing substance use, there is a dearth of published research on specific SBHC substance use prevention efforts or gender-based approaches to school-based health care. This chapter describes findings from a longitudinal demonstration project that aimed to prevent, reduce, or delay substance use among multicultural female adolescents aged 14–18 years who attended a Boston, Massachusetts, public secondary school from 1994–1999. The project was designed to augment the services of an existing SBHC. While this cutting edge initiative occurred a decade ago, recent national trends in female adolescent substance use in conjunction with recent health care reform give this model new currency.

METHODS

The Young Women's Health Initiative (YWHI) was developed in response to one school's concerns over increased violence and drug use among female students. Girls were becoming perpetrators, as well as victims of violence, and were involved in the sale, use, and abuse of substances. Table 5.2 offers a summary of the demographics of the female student population in the school. Families of students in the school ranked higher on objective measures of poverty than did students of any other school in Boston. In addition, communities in which students attending the intervention school reside reported the highest percentage of risk factors for adverse health outcomes in the city and the state.[35]

School administrators, in collaboration with a neighboring academic medical center operating an SBHC within the school, devised a longitudinal intervention that included a continuum of primary and secondary prevention services delivered on site by a multidisciplinary clinical team.

TABLE 5.2—YOUNG WOMEN'S HEALTH INITIATIVE TARGET POPULATION

Target:	450 girls enrolled in the study school
Race	14% White 52% Black 27% Latino 3% Asian 1% American Indian 3% Other
Age	14% — 11–14 years old 82% — 15–18 years old 4% — 19–20 years old
Grades	13% — 9th graders 28% — 10th graders 30% — 11th graders 28% — 12th graders 1% — graduates

Risk and protective factors were aimed at five domains known to affect substance use significantly among adolescent females. These domains include: (1) individual factors, (2) peer influence, (3) intimate partners, (4) families, and (5) the school.[22] The intervention was comprised of 10 components. Each component, offered individually or in small groups, provided services aimed at multiple domains of impact, not necessarily just one (Table 5.3).

Comparisons were made between the study school students receiving any YWHI individual services (treatment), study school students receiving no YWHI services or only classroom-based group services (control group 1), and students at another high school that had no access to SBHC services (control group 2). There were two hypotheses for the study: (1) at baseline, females seeking individual treatment will demonstrate higher substance use levels than those in comparison groups, and (2) at follow-up, females receiving individual clinical services will demonstrate greater positive substance use change from baseline than those in the comparison groups.

Data were gathered on the dosage and types of services provided to all females (Table 5.4). Results and discussion of these findings are presented more fully elsewhere.[36] Also, at four points over 30 months, a cohort of ninth graders at the study school and the comparison school completed the National Youth Survey,[37] a 113-item instrument measuring: **risk factors** (personal factors, family environment, neighborhood environment, social influences), **resiliency factors**

TABLE 5.3—YOUNG WOMEN'S HEALTH INITIATIVE—LOGIC MODEL

Program Inputs	Activities	Intermediate Outcomes	Ultimate Outcomes
1. School administrative support and resources 2. Academic medical center support and resources 3. Existing school-based health center (SBHC) with basic primary care services and staff 4. State and private funding for basic SBHC services, as well as third-party billing 5. Federal funding for gender-specific demonstration project 6. Evaluation team	• Mental health counseling • Dating violence education and counseling • Reproductive health education • Tobacco health education and cessation • Parenting life-skills education • Case management for pregnant and parenting students • Peer leadership and peer education • Vocational case management • Mediation counseling • Media literacy • Teachers, administrators, parent, and service provider training in early identification of students in need of assistance with substance use risk factors or actual substance use	**Reduce Associated Risk Factors:** • Depression • Suicidal behavior • Violent relationships • Early initiation of sexual activity • Unprotected sexual activity • Unintended pregnancy • Repeat pregnancy • Interpersonal violence • Peer group norms valuing violence, drug and alcohol use, and unsafe sexual activities **Enhance Associated Protective Factors:** • Academic performance and high school completion • Sexual abstinence • Effective use of contraception • Life-skills and career planning • Self-esteem • Social coping • Effective parenting • Health knowledge and disease prevention • Refusal skills • Parental awareness and involvement in teens' academic, health, and life planning • Positive assertiveness • Responsive school climate	**Prevention, Reduction, Delay in:** • Alcohol, tobacco, and other drug use (as measured by lifetime use, 30-day use, and age at initiation) • Alcohol use • Heavy alcohol use • Street drug use • Cigarette smoking • Heavy cigarette smoking

TABLE 5.4 — EXPOSURE TO HEALTH CENTER SERVICES, BY YEAR

Program Year	Number of Girls at Treatment School (Midyear Estimate)	Percentage and Number of Girls Exposed to Services	
		Individual Services	Group Services
1994–1995	440	35% (n=153)	48% (n=212)
1995–1996	460	38% (n=176)	63% (n=290)
1996–1997	513	31% (n=163)	44% (n=226)
1997–1998	553	24% (n=133)	46% (n=254)
1998–1999	434	38% (n=168)	47% (n=202)

(school and family bonding, self-concept, self-control, self-efficacy, positive outlook, confidence, cooperation), and **substance attitudes and use** (tobacco, alcohol, marijuana, inhalants, other drugs). Survey cohorts mirrored the racial and ethnic demographics of the target population of all girls in the study school. The survey was available in Spanish for students as needed. School absenteeism presented challenges in reaching all students. However, efforts were made to locate and administer surveys at other times to those not present during regular collection periods. At least one follow-up survey was completed by over 90% of those who took the baseline survey (Table 5.5).

TABLE 5.5 — SURVEY COMPLETION, BY TREATMENT AND CONTROL GROUPS

Survey Status of 9th Grade Girls in the Study	BASELINE (September 1996; Month 0)	EXIT (May 1997; 6–12 mo)	FOLLOW-UP 1 (January 1998; 15–19 mo)	FOLLOW-UP 2 (December 1998; 25–31 mo)
Treatment	n=45	n=41	n=34	n=32
Control 1: Classroom group services only	n=63	n=51	n=38	n=40
Control 2: Comparison school, no services[a]	n=104	n=93	n=67	n=57

[a]Although the treatment school population was at highest risk for adverse health outcomes among all area high schools, the comparison school population that was chosen had the most similarities to the treatment school.

Using the Statistical Package for Social Sciences, Version 9.0 (1998), survey sections were treated as scales, with descriptive and frequency statistics providing summary data. For descriptive purposes, each group's mean scores were plotted at every time point. Analysis of variance was used to compare the group means at each time point, and when the overall test was significant at the $P \leq 0.05$ level, subsequent pairwise comparisons between the group means were done.

RESULTS

Girls seeking individual services demonstrated higher baseline substance use than those in the control groups. After at least two years follow-up, study students showed marijuana-use reduction when compared with the comparison group (Figures 5.1 and 5.2).

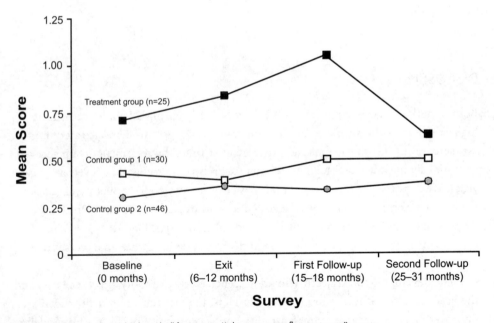

Note. Results shown are from girls who took all four surveys. High mean scores reflect greater marijuana use.

Figure 5.1 — Marijuana use scale, by group.

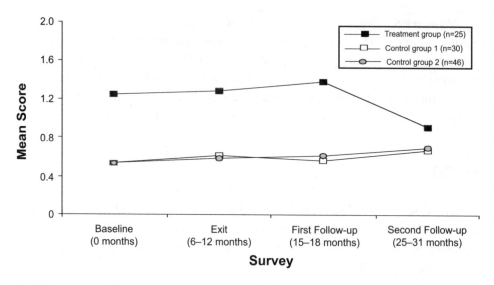

Note. Higher mean scores reflect greater use.

Figure 5.2—Daily use scale for alcohol, tobacco, and other drugs, by group.

DISCUSSION

Both hypotheses were supported. YWHI successfully enrolled female students at highest risk for substance use. While both comparison groups demonstrated modest increases in substance abuse as expected over time, the treatment group showed an initial significant increase in marijuana use, returning to baseline levels after two years. We hypothesize that through the YWHI intervention, complex psychosocial issues, such as sexual abuse, were revealed and addressed over time. Identifying these issues may have temporarily increased substance use. Had the study concluded before two years, it would have appeared to demonstrate an adverse treatment outcome.

The developmental trajectory in adolescence is toward more substance use, and the best predictor of future use is past use. Thus, the fact that treatment students improved over time suggests the feasibility and acceptability of the YWHI model. An ongoing, comprehensive substance use prevention program addressing risk and protective factors is more likely to produce sustainable outcomes than are categorical school-based educational efforts, but such a program may require two or more years to show positive effects.

Although this study offered an in-depth look at female adolescent substance use prevention in an SBHC setting, the findings are based on only one SBHC. Thus, it may be over-reaching to say that the findings will have implications for all SBHCs. Nevertheless, there are elements of the study that suggest that a similar model could be implemented in other SBHCs. The following are some critical lessons and future recommendations from the YWHI experience for other SBHCs looking to develop a gender-specific program and enhance their service delivery potential:

1. The support and partnership of school administration and faculty are essential for a successful longitudinal school-based prevention effort.

2. Most existing SBHCs have the infrastructure, resources, and access to female students to facilitate the development of a gender-specific, multidimensional substance use prevention program.

3. The recent passage of health care reform policy has resulted in a resurgence of national interest in SBHCs coupled with newly available federal funding for SBHCs. This interest may offer a unique window of opportunity to consider enhancing SBHC services to address the growing substance use by female adolescents.

4. Future studies should determine the dose–response relationship to the various interventions employed and extend longitudinal follow-up. Demonstration of positive program effects on school attendance and academic achievement would further educators' support for broad implementation of the model.

REFERENCES

1. MacDonald M, Wright NE. Cigarette smoking and the disenfranchisement of adolescent girls: a discourse of resistance? *Health Care Women Int.* 2002;23(3):281–305.

2. Thomas BS. The effectiveness of selected risk factors in mediating gender differences in drinking and its problems. *J Adolesc Health.* 1995;17(2):91–98.

3. Robbins C. Sex differences in psychosocial consequences of alcohol and drug abuse. *J Health Soc Behav.* 1989;30(1):117–130.

4. Robbins C, Martin S. Gender, styles of deviance, and drinking problems. *J Health Soc Behav.* 1993;34(4):302–321.

5. Centers for Disease Control and Prevention. Trends in the prevalence of selected risk behaviors for all students National YRBS: 1991—2007. Available at: http://www.brhpc.org/files/yrbs07_us_summary_trend_all.pdf. Accessed October 13, 2009.

6. Johnston LD, O'Malley PM, Bachman JG, Schulenberg JE. *Monitoring the Future: National Results on Adolescent Drug Use: Overview of Key Findings,* 2005. Bethesda, MD: National Institute on Drug Abuse, Department of Health and Human Resources; 2006. NIH Publication No. 06-5882.

7. Johnston LD, O'Malley PM, Bachman JG, Schulenberg JE. *Monitoring the Future: National Results on Adolescent Drug Use: Overview of Key Findings,* 2006. Bethesda, MD: National Institute on Drug Abuse, Department of Health and Human Resources; 2007. NIH Publication No. 07-6202.

8. Substance Abuse and Mental Health Services Administration. *Results From the 2006 National Survey on Drug Use and Health: National Findings.* Rockville, MD: Office of Applied Studies, Substance Abuse and Mental Health Services Administration, Department of Health and Human Services; 2007. NSDUH Series H-32, DHHS Publication No. SMA 07-4293.

9. Substance Abuse and Mental Health Services Administration. *Results From the 2005 National Survey on Drug Use and Health: National Findings.* Rockville, MD: Office of Applied Studies, Substance Abuse and Mental Health Services Administration, Department of Health and Human Services; 2007. NSDUH Series H-30, DHHS Publication No. SMA 06-4194.

10. Substance Abuse and Mental Health Services Administration. *Results From the 2004 National Survey on Drug Use and Health: National Findings.* Rockville, MD: Office of Applied Studies, Substance Abuse and Mental Health Services Administration, Department of Health and Human Services; 2007. NSDUH Series H-28, DHHS Publication No. SMA 05-4062.

11. Department of Health and Human Services, Office of Minority Health and Health Disparities. Youth Risk Behavior Surveillance System. Highlights in Minority Health and Health Disparities: September, 2006. Available at: http://www.cdc.gov/omhd/highlights/2006/HSept06YRBSS.htm. Accessed March 14, 2010.

12. Schinke SP, Fang L, Cole KCA. Substance use among early adolescent girls: risk and protective factors. *J Adolesc Health.* 2008;43(2):191–194.

13. Poole N, Dell CA. *Girls, Women and Substance Use.* Ottawa, Ontario: Canadian Centre on Substance Abuse; 2005. Available at: http://www.ccsa.ca/2005%20CCSA%20Documents/ccsa-011142-2005.pdf. Accessed August 15, 2009.

14. Patton GC, Coffey C, Carlin JB, Degenhardt L, Lynskey M, Hall W. Cannabis use and mental health in young people: cohort study. *BMJ.* 2002;325(7374):1195–1198.

15. Johnston LD, Bachman JG, O'Malley PM. *Monitoring the Future: A Continuing Study of American Youth (12th-Grade Survey), 1997.* Ann Arbor: Institute for Social Research, University of Michigan; 1997.

16. Schoen C, Davis K, Scott Collins K, et al. *The Commonwealth Fund Survey of the Health of Adolescent Girls.* New York, NY: The Commonwealth Fund; 1997.

17. Amos A. Women and smoking. *Br Med Bull.* 1996;52(1):74–89.

18. Griffin KW, Botvin GJ, Doyle MM, Diaz T, Epstein JA. A six-year follow-up study of determinants of heavy cigarette smoking among high-school seniors. *J Behav Med.* 1999;22(3):271–284.

19. Silverman JG, Raj A, Mucci LA, Hathaway JE. Dating violence against adolescent girls and associated substance use, unhealthy weight control, sexual risk behavior, pregnancy, and suicidality. *JAMA.* 2001;286(5):572–579.

20. Philips L. *The Girls Report: What We Know and Need to Know About Growing Up Female.* New York, NY: The National Council for Research on Women; 1998.

21. Cousins LH, Mabrey T. Re-gendering social work practice and education: the case for African-American girls. *J Hum Behav Soc Environ.* 1998;1(23):91–104.

22. Kumpfer KL, Turner CW. The social ecology model of adolescent substance abuse: implications for prevention. *Int J Addict.* 1990–1991;25(4A):435–463.

23. O'Donnell L, Stueve A, San Doval A, et al. Violence prevention and young adolescents' participation in community youth service. *J Adolesc Health.* 1999;24(1):28–37.

24. National Assembly on School-Based Health Care. National census school year 2004–05. Available at: http://ww2.nasbhc.org/RoadMap/Public/EQ_2005census.pdf. Accessed August 1, 2011.

25. Weist MD, Schlitt J. Alliances and school-based health care. *J Sch Health.* 1998;68(10):401–403.

26. Santelli J, Kouzis A, Newcomer S. School-based health centers and adolescent use of primary care and hospital care. *J Adolesc Health.* 1996;19(4):267–275.

27. Knight JR, Harris SK, Sherritt L, et. al. Prevalence of positive substance abuse screen results among adolescent primary care patients. *Arch Pediatr Adolesc Med.* 2007;161(11):1035–1041.

28. Mason MJ, Wood TA. Clinical mental health training within a multidisciplinary school-based health clinic. *J Health Soc Policy.* 2000;11(3):45– 65.

29. Jepson L, Juszczak L, Fisher M. Mental health care in a high school-based health service. *Adolescence.* 1998;33(129):1–15.

30. Anglin TM, Naylor KE, Kaplan DW. Comprehensive school-based health care: high school students' use of medical, mental health, and substance abuse services. *Pediatrics.* 1996;97(3):318–330.

31. Kaplan DW, Calonge BN, Guernsey BP, Hanrahan MB. Managed care and school-based health centers: use of health services. *Arch Pediatr Adolesc Med.* 1998;152(1):25–33.

32. Juszczak L, Melinkovich P, Kaplan D. Use of health and mental health services by adolescents across multiple delivery sites. *J Adolesc Health*. 2003;32(6 Suppl):108–118.

33. Pastore DR, Murray PJ, Juszczak L, Society of Adolescent Medicine. School-based health center: position paper of the Society for Adolescent Medicine. *J Adolesc Health*. 2001;29(6):448–450.

34. Massachusetts Department of Public Health. Massachusetts School-Based Health Centers—Fact Sheets 1996–2006, "State-Funded SBHC Reports & Links." Available at: http://www.ma4sbhc.org/whatis.html. Accessed August 11, 2011.

35. Boston Public Health Commission. *The Health of Boston 1998*. Boston, MA: Office of Research, Health Assessments and Data Systems; 1998.

36. Stone D, Ruthazer R, Mandel L, Kulig J. *The Young Women's Health Initiative at Boston High School, Final Report submitted to Center for Substance Abuse Prevention*. Boston, MA: Center for Substance Abuse and Prevention; 2000.

37. Center for Substance Abuse Prevention. *National Youth Survey: Baseline Questionnaire (12–18 Version)*. Washington, DC: US Department of Health and Human Services; 1999. OMB No: 0930-0178.

About the Authors

Leslie A. Mandel, PhD, MA, MSM–is currently an independent program evaluator specializing in advocacy and policy change. She is also an instructor in the community health program at Pine Manor College. Dr. Mandel's dissertation explored organizational issues of partnerships between school-based health centers (SBHCs), health care systems, and public schools in Massachusetts. She is actively involved in national-level associations dedicated to evaluation and quality of SBHC programs. She was one of the founders of the Massachusetts Association for School-Based Health Centers. Finally, she was part of the management team at The Student Health Center at Boston High School.

John W. Kulig, MD, MPH–is currently Director of Adolescent Medicine at Tufts Medical Center's Floating Hospital for Children and Professor of Pediatrics, Public Health, and Community Medicine at Tufts University School of Medicine in Boston. Dr. Kulig developed the Adolescent Medicine program at Tufts Medical Center and started one of Boston's first school-based clinics. The Student Health Center at Boston High School received grant support from the W. K. Kellogg Foundation, the Center for Substance Abuse Prevention, and the Bureau of Primary Health Care. He currently sees patients and precepts trainees in the Adolescent Clinic and an outpatient treatment program for opioid-dependent youth.

School-Based and Linked Health Centers Immunization Project: A State-Funded Effort to Improve Adolescent Immunization Rates

Jennifer Salerno

The Michigan Department of Community Health (MDCH), Child and Adolescent Health Center (CAHC) Program is committed to providing preventive services and improving the health status of Michigan's highest-risk children and adolescents. The CAHC Program consists of 57 school-based and linked health centers (SBLHCs) located throughout upper and lower Michigan.[1] SBLHCs eliminate many common barriers to health care for children and adolescents by delivering comprehensive preventive and primary care in or very near schools. Staffed by nurse practitioners, physician assistants, and physicians, SBLHCs are safe, confidential health care centers ideally situated to improve access and quality of health care provided to underserved adolescent populations.[2] By residing inside or very near schools, these health care centers are able to reach adolescents who lack access to traditional sources of preventive medical care or who receive fragmented care.[3] Additionally, surveys indicate that SBLHCs are well received by the medical community. A 2001 survey of US physicians concluded that most physicians supported adolescent immunization efforts and school-based immunization programs.[4]

Adolescents are the lowest users of preventive health care and often do not have an identified medical home.[5] Because of these factors and many others, it has been a challenge to communicate and facilitate new vaccine recommendations effectively. In 2006, immunization rates in the United States were nearly 80% for young children, but rates for adolescents were significantly lower. When new vaccine recommendations for adolescents are added and immunization requirements change, trends in overall immunization compliance rates for adolescents drop. In addition to these trends, children and adolescents who live at or below the federal poverty level are even less likely to be immunized than are their peers.[6]

When adolescents present for care through avenues such as emergency departments, urgent care centers, and sexually transmitted infection clinics, the adolescent's actual immunization status is difficult to verify and often neglected as part of their health visit.[7] Effective delivery of recommended vaccines and innovative outreach programs are important in the prevention and control of vaccine-preventable diseases and in the reduction of health disparities. In response to this need, the MDCH implemented an immunization project designed to improve child and adolescent immunization rates and to develop recommendations for SBLHCs across Michigan.

As of 2002, Michigan school districts are required to assess immunization status and report immunization-deficient students who were entering kindergarten, entering sixth grade, and new entrants to a school district. All other students are exempt from this reporting requirement, and parents do not receive notification from their schools that their children may be deficient in their immunizations. This is especially problematic when new immunization recommendations are established for adolescents beyond the sixth grade. There are no school-required statewide processes in place to identify and notify adolescents or their parents of these changes. If the adolescent is not seeking regular or routine medical care through their primary care provider, they remain unaware of current immunization status and new recommendations.

PROJECT GOALS

The goal of the immunization project was to improve the immunization rates of the SBLHC populations by increasing awareness, developing partnerships, identifying deficiencies, and providing the necessary immunizations, thus reducing or eliminating the morbidity and mortality that may result from vaccine-preventable diseases. In addition, the immunization project was to achieve an immunization compliance percentile that was higher than reported national averages and approaching *Healthy People 2010* goals. Vaccine delivery was maximized through providing universal access to adolescents attending the schools in which the SBLHCs were located in or linked to without disparities among subgroups in the population. The foundation of this project was the Centers for Disease Control and Prevention's (CDC's) National Vaccine Advisory Committee's (NVAC's) recommendations for immunization practice.[8]

METHODS

Twelve newly opened SBLHCs serving elementary, middle, high school, and alternative school students in communities across Michigan were designated as the project sites. The project timeline was September 2006 through June 2007. The goals of the immunization project and the CDC list of revised standards for child and adolescent immunization practices[8] were reviewed with the 12 project sites. These CDC revised standards focus on making vaccines easily accessible, effectively communicating vaccination information, implementing strategies to improve vaccination rates, and developing community partnerships to reach target patient populations. The project sites were charged with improving child and adolescent immunization rates in the students enrolled in and attending the schools in which the SBLHCs are physically located in or linked to.

Immunization records were reviewed and activities to improve immunization rates were planned and implemented. The Michigan Care Improvement Registry (MCIR) school and provider view was used to review entire student population records when available. MCIR was created in 1998 to collect reliable immunization information and benefits Michigan's youth serving agencies and citizens by obtaining and consolidating immunization information in an online format, which allows providers to access up-to-date patient immunization histories.[9] School districts across Michigan were just beginning to use this statewide immunization tracking system to monitor and report their students' immunization statuses at the time of this project. If MCIR was not being used, the current tracking system used by each school district was reviewed. SBLHC staff and/or school personnel reviewed these immunization records. School population numbers and the number of immunization-deficient students were reported to MDCH in September or October 2006 and again in June 2007. Activities to increase immunization rates were planned and implemented by each site during this time period (Table 6.1). Challenges and recommendations were reported to and discussed with MDCH staff throughout the project implementation.

RESULTS WITH DISCUSSION

Identified Barriers and Solutions
ACCURATE IMMUNIZATION RECORDS
Barriers: During this process we learned that many school districts did not include all students in their immunization databases or rosters. Only those students required to be reported for school entry (as previously described) were included in many of the school immunization databases. In addition, many schools did not have

TABLE 6.1 — ACTIVITIES PERFORMED BY SCHOOL-BASED AND LINKED HEALTH CENTERS (SBLHCS) AND/OR SCHOOL PERSONNEL TO INCREASE ADOLESCENT IMMUNIZATION RATES

Established a positive working relationship between the health center staff and school staff responsible for immunization review (nurses, secretaries, and counselors).
Reviewed Michigan Care Improvement Registry and school records for immunization-deficient students and updated records as information was received or immunizations given.
Created an accurate database of immunization records and lists of immunization-deficient students if these were not already in existence.
Sent letters, consents, and vaccine information sheets to parents of students with incomplete immunizations. Information also given directly to students to take home.
Used a recall system to remind parents of students who were incomplete.
Called parents and/or met individually with students to follow up on letters and verify immunization status.
Outreached to fifth grade students to assess for sixth grade immunization requirements.
Made announcements at school open houses.
Attended assemblies to educate and encourage students to get immunizations.
Included articles in school newsletters on new Centers for Disease Control and Prevention vaccine recommendations for adolescents.
Provided immunization information at school events that parents attended including parent/teacher conferences.
Posters, brochures, and fliers in Child and Adolescent Health Center (CAHC) Programs on adolescent immunizations.
Continual review of list of incomplete students and attempts to obtain records or consent to give necessary immunizations.
Notated immunization status on every CAHC visit. Audited this as part of a chart review to ensure notation of immunization status on every visit. Gave feedback to providers and other staff responsible for checking immunization status.
Had the problem list on the front of the chart with a blank for "Immunizations Current Until_____" that was reviewed at every visit.
Asked parents to send immunization records when scheduling CAHC appointments.
Immunization Days planned and implemented.
Staff recognition/incentives for identifying and immunizing deficient adolescents.
Encouraged return of vaccine records and update of immunization status by giving a coupon to students for a free treat when immunization status was up to date.
Entered adolescents into a drawing for a pizza party if they had their vaccines up to date.

updated immunization records beyond kindergarten entry for students that had never left the district. Other schools had no records at all for nonreportable students.

Solutions: MCIR, provider view, was used to access student immunization records for those who were missing information or identified as deficient. MCIR was limited because not all health care provider offices were entering immunizations into the MCIR web-based system at the time of this project. School and MCIR records were compared to create an accurate immunization database. Once this database was created and immunization-deficient students identified, letters to parents requesting updated vaccine records due to deficiencies were sent home via students and US mail. Consent forms for the SBLHCs to administer recommended immunizations were also sent with information about the deficiencies using the CDC Vaccine Information Sheets.

ACCESS TO SCHOOL IMMUNIZATION RECORDS

Barriers: It was challenging to access school immunization records if the student had not provided a signed parental consent form allowing the SBLHCs access to school immunization records.

Solutions: This was overcome by language in SBLHC contracts with school districts, on school emergency cards, and on SBLHC registration forms allowing access to school immunization records. In addition, school district personnel reviewed immunization records and sent deficiency letters/packets to parents of immunization-deficient students. SBLHC staff assisted school personnel by putting the information packets together including vaccine information sheets and SBLHC consent forms for immunization administration.

NONELIGIBLE VACCINE FOR CHILDREN STUDENTS

Barriers: SBLHCs have difficulty obtaining reimbursement from private insurance companies for medical services provided in the centers including vaccine administration. The high cost of vaccines makes it difficult for SBLHCs to purchase and provide vaccines for students who are insured and do not qualify for the federal vaccines for children (VFC).

Solutions: Various funding sources including private donations, small grants, and state funding were used for purchasing vaccines to give to students who did not qualify for the VFC program, reducing costs to the SBLHCs.

Recommendations for Improving Child and Adolescent Immunization Rates

During the implementation and evaluation phases of the immunization project, SBLHC staff were surveyed as to what made the project activities—identifying immunization-deficient students, notifying and effectively communicating vaccination information to staff and parents, making vaccines easily accessible through the SBLHCs, and implementing strategies to improve vaccination rates—easier and/or more difficult. School environment and project commitment from SBLHC staff impacted the difficulty of the project activities. Survey information was compiled into eight recommendations for improving immunization rates:

1. Partner with the school principal, secretaries, school nurse, or other designated staff. Enlist their efforts to obtain current immunization records, identify immunization-deficient students, send information packets home, and make phone calls to parents.
2. Provide education and training to SBLHC staff on current recommendations for adolescent immunizations. Include adolescent immunization status as a quality improvement indicator.
3. Develop effective communication strategies to enable parents and adolescents to become knowledgeable about vaccines and preventable diseases as well as ways to access the SBLHC for vaccinations. Use these strategies to promote other preventive health services offered through the SBLHC.
4. Require parents to bring current immunization records to fall orientation/registration days for all students.
5. Have individual student immunization information (found in MCIR or school records) at fall orientations to identify students with incomplete records or deficiencies. This will allow school or SBLHC staff to inform parents of the deficiencies, obtain copies of records, and get consent for immunization to be given in the SBLHC on that day or in the near future.
6. Hold new semester schedules, grades, or sports participation until current immunization record is received and/or immunizations are up to date.
7. Add language in SBLHC consent forms to include parental consent for immunization administration.
8. Collaborate with local health departments to sponsor immunization clinics at the schools.

National adolescent immunization data were reported in 1997 and again in 2006. In 1997, National Health Interview Survey baseline estimates for adolescent immunization rates were 48% for hepatitis B; 89% for measles, mumps, and rubella (MMR); 93% for tetanus-diphtheria (Td); and 45% for varicella (for adolescents without history of disease and 1 dose of vaccine) based on a phone survey of parents. Provider-reported vaccination records were used to obtain 2006 estimates for adolescent immunization rates, which were 81.3% for hepatitis B; 86.9% for MMR; 60.1% for Td or tetanus, diphtheria, and pertussis (Tdap); and 89.6% for varicella (for adolescents with history of disease or 1 dose of vaccine). National goals for vaccination coverage for adolescents aged 13–15 years were included in *Healthy People 2010* with targets for 90% coverage specified for existing routine recommendations.[10]

The SBLHC sites involved in this project were asked to report students with up to date immunizations (compliance rates) at two points in time, September 2006 and June 2007. Students were considered compliant if they had received three doses of hepatitis B vaccine, two doses of MMR, one booster of Td or Tdap at age 11–12 years or within the last 5 years, and varicella disease or one to two doses of vaccine (based on age) as identified by *Healthy People 2010*. Overall immunization rates, not rates specific for each vaccine type, were collected for this project. At the end of the project, 76% of the project sites achieved near or above 70% immunization compliance rates for youth attending the schools in which the SBLHCs were located or linked, and 30% of these project sites achieved 90% or higher immunization compliance rates (Figure 6.1).

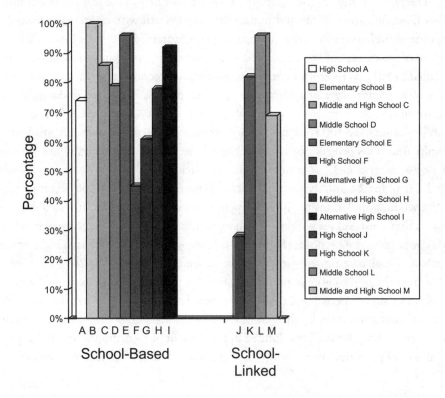

Note. Complete vaccines were three doses hepatitis B; two doses measles, mumps, and rubella; one booster of tetanus-diphtheria or tetanus, diphtheria, and pertussis at age 11 to 12 years or within the last five years; and varicella disease or one dose of vaccine.

Figure 6.1—Percentage of school population with complete vaccines in June 2007.

There were many variables related to achieving high rates of immunization compliance within school populations. In schools with large numbers of students, it was more difficult to impact overall immunization compliance rates, but these SBLHCs were able to make an impact on larger numbers of youth individually. Elementary school sites in this project began with much higher compliance rates than did high school sites and had smaller student populations, allowing them to show greater overall school population compliance rates at the end of this project. SBLHCs that were unable to target entire school populations and SBLHCs that began the immunization project late in the school year were limited in their ability to impact the school population immunization compliance rates. One high school's school-linked health center's opening was delayed until the spring of 2007, limiting the time available to implement the immunization project's activities and therefore only minimally impacting adolescent immunization rates.

The positive impact of this project is better reflected in the improvement in school immunization status and in the number of youth with improved immunization compliance rates when compared with September 2006 to June 2007. Increased awareness of recommended vaccines by parents/guardians and students resulted in SBLHC receipt of current immunization records, and vaccine administration by primary care providers or by SBLHC providers resulted in documented improved student immunization compliance rates. Forty-six percent of the project sites impacted over 100 students; 23% of these sites impacted over 200 students (Figure 6.2). This project positively impacted the immunization compliance status of 1,494 students in 12 communities across Michigan.

Nine of the 12 SBLHCs, with 10 schools participating, were able to target their entire school populations for improvement in immunization rates. It was demonstrated that these SBLHCs increased immunization compliance rates by as much as 70% at participating schools (Figure 6.3). These schools averaged an 83.9% immunization compliance rate postintervention, nearing *Healthy People 2010* goals of 90%, as compared to 60.3% preintervention, an increase of approximately 23.6%.

Project sites experiencing multiple barriers had lower overall impact on adolescent immunization rates by the end of the project. Inaccurate immunization records on entire student populations, limited access to school records, and limited support from school personnel were found to be the most difficult barriers to overcome.

CONCLUSIONS

Total school population immunization compliance rates increased by raising awareness and improving staff and parent knowledge of vaccines and preventable

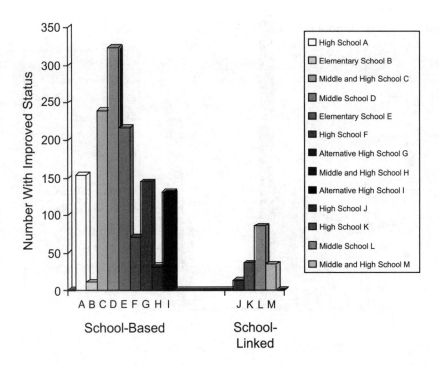

Figure 6.2 — Number of children and adolescents with improved immunization status in June 2007.

diseases through effective communication strategies, identifying immunization deficiencies, and providing immunizations in school through SBLHCs. The identified barriers, recommendations for improving immunization rates, and activities performed in this project have national implications for making a positive impact on immunization rates in schools, SBLHCs, and state-sponsored health plans. Quality indicators of adolescent immunization rates are likely tied to operational funding and financial incentives for all of these entities.

SBLHCs are key players in reducing vaccine-preventable morbidity and mortality among at-risk children and adolescents. Bringing the vaccines to the children and adolescents while they are in school is imperative to a successful immunization initiative. Any vaccination effort requires extensive support and collaboration from stakeholders, including school administrators and staff, state and local public health officials, parents, and health care providers. Model vaccination programs owe their success to multiagency collaborations and integration of vaccinations into existing school processes and SBLHC health care services. This can only be possible through true ownership and commitment from the entire team.

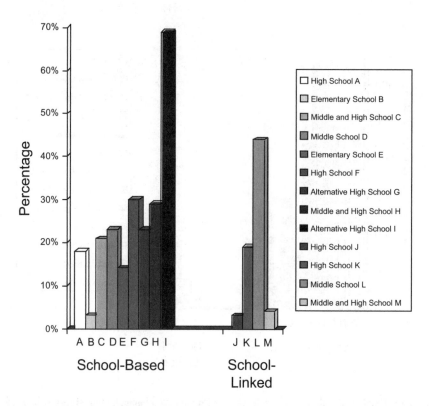

Figure 6.3—Improvement in percentage of the school population with complete vaccines in June 2007.

The *Healthy People 2010*[10] national goal is to ensure that 90% of our adolescents aged 13–15 years are fully immunized. Our results support the evidence that when the CDC's Standards for Immunization Practice are implemented fully and processes are in place to identify and overcome barriers, such high coverage rates can be achieved through SBLHCs.

REFERENCES

1. Michigan Department of Community Health. Child and Adolescent Health Center Program website. Available at: http://www.michigan.gov/mdch/0,1607,7-132-2942_4911_4912_44686-95368—,00.html. Accessed April 15, 2011.
2. Allison MA, Crane LA, Beaty BL, Davidson AJ, Melinkovich P, Kempe A. School-based health centers: improving access and quality of care for low-income adolescents. *Pediatrics.* 2007;120(4):e887–e894.

3. Schaffer SJ, Fontanesi J, Rickert D, et al. How effectively can health care settings beyond the traditional medical home provide vaccines to adolescents? *Pediatrics.* 2008;121(Suppl 1):S35–S45.

4. Schaffer SJ, Humiston SG, Shone LP, Averhoff FM, Szilagyi PG. Adolescent immunization practices: a national survey of US physicians. *Arch Pediatr Adolesc Med.* 2001;155(5):566–571.

5. Centers for Disease Control and Prevention. Adolescent immunization. 2007. Available at: http://www.cdc.gov/ncird/progbriefs/downloads/adolescent.pdf. Accessed April 15, 2011.

6. Reinberg S. US teens fall short on vaccine coverage. *Washington Post.* August 30, 2007. Available at: http://www.washingtonpost.com/wp-dyn/content/article/2007/08/30/AR2007083001329.html. Accessed April 15, 2011.

7. Centers for Disease Control and Prevention. Adolescent immunization. *Immunization Program Operations Manual.* Atlanta, GA: CDC; 2007. Available at: http://www.cdc.gov/vaccines/vac-gen/policies/ipom/downloads/chp-06-adolescent-iz.pdf. Accessed June 15, 2011.

8. National Vaccine Advisory Committee. Standards for child and adolescent immunization practices. *Pediatrics.* 2003;112(4):958–963.

9. Michigan Care Information Registry. About MCIR website. Available at: http://www.mcir.org/aboutmcircontent.html. Accessed June 15, 2011.

10. Centers for Disease Control and Prevention. Data 2010: The Healthy People 2010 Database website. Available at: http://wonder.cdc.gov/data2010/obj.htm. Accessed April 15, 2011.

About the Author

Jennifer Salerno, MS, CPNP – is a Nurse Practitioner/Director of the University of Michigan (UM), Regional Alliance for Healthy Schools (RAHS) School-Based Health Center program. Jennifer is also an adjunct faculty member at the UM School of Nursing and a consultant to the Michigan Department of Community Health, Child and Adolescent Health Center program. Jennifer's passion is to provide, promote, and mentor quality adolescent health care. She has expertise in adolescent risk assessment and risk behavior counseling using motivational interviewing strategies, and has developed the Rapid Assessment for Adolescent Preventive Services (RAAPS) risk screening tool used by hundreds of health professionals worldwide.

The Role of School-Based Health Centers in Addressing Behavioral Health in Post-Disaster New Orleans

Marsha Broussard, Lisanne Brown, Paul Hutchinson,
and Sarah Kohler Chrestman

INTRODUCTION

School-based health centers (SBHCs) aim to increase access to quality primary care and behavioral health services for the most vulnerable community members who may otherwise not have access to care. In New Orleans, Hurricane Katrina left an already vulnerable population without basic resources. The August 2005 storm devastated most private and governmental assets, including educational and health care facilities, housing, and other basic infrastructure.

School Health Connection (SHC), a program of the Louisiana Public Health Institute (LPHI), was established in 2006. The SHC program aimed to improve access to primary care and behavioral health services among students in the New Orleans Metropolitan Area (which includes four parishes/counties including Orleans Parish) by establishing a robust system of SBHCs. The SHC program sought to replace those SBHCs lost due to the storm and expand SBHCs in three additional parishes which were also affected. As a result of the SHC program and the generous contributions of the W. K. Kellogg Foundation, the Robert Wood Johnson Foundation, and many local education and health partners, 12 new SBHCs were opened between 2007 and 2011 to serve students throughout the Metro area. The opening of one additional SBHC in the City of New Orleans is anticipated in the fall of 2012.

New Orleans students, many living in poverty, faced difficult odds accessing health services in the pre-Katrina environment, and these circumstances were exacerbated post-Katrina. The new SBHC services targeted public high schools primarily due to their larger enrollments, the high proportion of at-risk students, and SBHC costs and scalability factors. This new system of care has amassed considerable expertise in adolescent health and in addressing youth's behavioral risk factors, which have serious health and social consequences. To measure the impact of these services provided by SBHCs, SHC conducted a survey of students in schools with SBHCs and those in schools that were planning to establish one.

ADOLESCENT BEHAVIORAL RISK FACTORS

Adolescence is a developmental period that is characterized by social, behavioral, cognitive, and emotional transitions. Between the ages of 12 and 18 years, youth make a multitude of decisions that impact both physical and emotional health and often have life-altering consequences. During this period of adolescence, high-risk behaviors result in major health and emotional risks. These behaviors include unhealthy dietary behaviors and physical inactivity; behaviors that contribute to unintentional injuries and violence; tobacco, alcohol, and other drug use; and sexual behaviors that contribute to unintended pregnancy and sexually transmitted diseases (STDs), including HIV infection.[1]

Violence is a fact of life for a considerable proportion of high school students in New Orleans. Youth and adult observations from a 2009 qualitative study revealed that youth violence was a significant issue in Orleans Parish that was further exacerbated when Katrina devastated facilities and programs that historically engaged youth, leaving few recreational and social outlets. Residents further stated that recovery efforts in many neighborhoods were slow, resulting in families living in neighborhoods with significant blight; and many residents remaining displaced and homeless, with household members living in close quarters. Some youth were still living with friends while displaced parents lived in other cities.[2]

Violence and teen dating, in particular intimate partner violence, was another social problem. According to the 2007 Orleans Parish Youth Risk Behavioral Survey (YRBS), which was completed by 2,034 public school students, 22% of students reported that they had been hit, slapped, or physically hurt on purpose by their boyfriend or girlfriend,[3] compared to 14% for Black, non-Hispanic, youth reported in the national 2007 YRBS.

Sexual activity places youth at risk for HIV infection and other STDs, as well as pregnancy. In the 2007 Orleans Parish YRBS, 56.4% of high school students reported ever having had sexual intercourse,[3] compared to 48% of high school students nationally. Further, 21.4% of Orleans high school students reported having had sex with four or more sex partners during their life, compared to 15% nationally.[4]

Cigarette smoking and substance use are two leading causes of preventable morbidity and mortality, including cancer, accidental death and dismemberment,

anti-social behaviors, and others. Despite anti-smoking and substance abuse education, 54% of high school students have tried cigarette smoking, 16% before the
age of 13; and 16% of 8th graders, 33% of 10th graders, and 44% of 12th graders
reported alcohol use.[5] Earlier onset of substance use is associated with greater
use in adulthood.[6,7] Although lower than national data, the Orleans Parish YRBS
reported that 47.4% of youth had tried smoking.

SCHOOL-BASED HEALTH CENTERS AS A SOLUTION

Students' use of SBHC services for screening and treatment of sexually transmitted
infections (STIs) among females,[8] medical care, mental health, and substance abuse
services[9] were shown to be higher in comparison to traditional sources for medical
care, community mental health, and substance abuse services. SBHCs are especially
effective in the treatment of school-age youth and are generally associated with
a high level of patient satisfaction.[10] Pastore et al. indicated that the majority of
students who used the SBHC were satisfied with the services received and were
using the SBHC as their regular source of care.[11] Studies have shown that despite
the stressors associated with youth living in poverty and distressed communities,
supportive school environments and school mental health programs can provide
needed support.[12] Use of SBHC services has been identified as potentially effective
strategies to reduce dropout rates associated with teen pregnancy, mental illness,
and emotional disturbances.[13]

STUDY PURPOSE

The purpose of this study was to measure the impact of the new Metro Area capacity of SBHC services on access to quality health care, including behavioral health,
and reduction of high-risk behaviors that lead to poor school performance.

METHODS

In spring 2009, a cross-sectional analysis study sampling 2,011 students was conducted in six public high schools in Orleans parish to collect information on their
health, health-care seeking behaviors, and other aspects of their lives that might
have an impact on their mental and physical well-being. A quasi-experimental
research design was utilized involving three intervention schools with SBHCs and

three comparison schools slated to have an SBHC eventually (hereafter "waiting list schools"). The overall goal of the research was to assess the effectiveness of SBHCs in increasing access to and utilization of essential health services (e.g., annual physicals, routine curative care, reproductive health counseling, behavioral health counseling and treatment), as well as to promote healthy lifestyles and good decision-making in a complex and often difficult urban environment.

A quantitative survey instrument was developed for this study based on the YRBS. Key components of the questionnaire included demographics (age, gender, race), substance abuse, sexual behaviors, body weight and exercise, mental health and treatment, STDs, other health issues (e.g., diabetes, hypertension, family planning, dental care, routine screening), use of SBHC health services, and satisfaction with such services.

Schools were selected for participation through their association with the SHC program and divided into two groups based upon whether they had an operational SBHC. In the 2009–2010 school year, when the data were collected, only three of the six participating schools had opened their SBHC, and three were on the waiting list. Therefore, for practical reasons, assignment of schools was not random and was largely determined by the administrative feasibility and timing for developing an SBHC. The student profiles of six participating schools were similar according to gender, race, family income, and free and reduced lunch enrollment (Table 7.1).

The survey administration method closely followed YRBS protocol previously administered in many of the participating schools. A survey coordinator was identified within each school, and he or she was responsible for training the necessary school staff to administer the survey, collect the surveys, and track the completed

TABLE 7.1 — PROFILES OF PARTICIPATING ORLEANS PARISH SCHOOLS

School	Total Enrollment	Response Rate, %	SBHC Status	No. Students Enrolled in SBHC	Total Patient Visits
School 1	324	79.9	Yes	365	2121
School 2	541	73.9	Yes	688	2583
School 3	730	47.5	Yes	289	1246
School 4	866	79.9	No	0	0
School 5	376	41.0	No	0	0
School 6	591	18.3	No	0	0
TOTAL	2562	76.2	—	1342	5950

Note. SBHC=school-based health center.

surveys. One week prior to the survey administration, passive parental consents were sent home with the students. If parents requested that their child not participate, the student was provided with an alternative activity by the school. Questionnaires were administered during a class period designated by the school on a specified day or over a few specified days, depending on the class schedule. A student consent form was administered with the survey to ensure that participation was voluntary. The questionnaire took about 30 to 45 minutes to complete and utilized a scantron answer sheet separate from the questionnaire form. The completed surveys were collected by SHC evaluation staff and identified by school and class before the data scanning and cleaning process. All schools received a stipend of $1,000, with $100 designated for the study coordinator. Any additional incentives for other staff assisting in the survey were at the school's discretion. All schools conducted the survey in April and May 2009. For the six surveyed schools, the response rate among all enrolled students—not just those present on the survey day—was 76.2%.

RESULTS

Description of Participants

As can be seen in Table 7.2, approximately 60% of the students in the public high schools surveyed were female, and approximately 90% were African American. Approximately 20% reported that the principal source of household income was welfare, social security, or unemployment benefits. Nearly two thirds—62%—reported receiving free lunches at school, and 12% reported being chronically hungry due to food shortages at home.

TABLE 7.2—KEY DEMOGRAPHIC CHARACTERISTICS OF SIX ORLEANS PARISH PUBLIC SCHOOLS, BY SBHC STATUS

	SBHC (n=980), %	Non-SBHC (n=944), %	Total (N=1,924), %	P Value
Female	61.3	58.2	59.5	.1
African American	87.0	94.3	90.0	<.001
Principal source of income is welfare, social security, or unemployment benefits	17.8	20.3	19.0	.162
Free Lunch	61.8	63.0	62.3	.742
Hunger in last 30 days	10.9	12.2	11.6	.378

Awareness, Enrollment, and Use of SBHCs

Table 7.3 presents overall awareness of SBHCs in all surveyed schools and enrollment among students in schools with an SBHC. Students in schools with an SBHC were significantly more likely to say that they have an SBHC (85.3%) compared with students in non-SBHC schools (26.2%). Students in non-SBHC schools were also much more likely to be unsure (28.4%) compared with SBHC schools (9.2%). There were no significant differences for awareness of SBHCs by age or sex of students (data not shown).

TABLE 7.3 — AWARENESS OF, ENROLLMENT IN, AND USE OF SCHOOL-BASED HEALTH CENTERS (SBHCs)

Variable	SBHC (n=980), %	Non-SBHC (n=944), %	Total (n=1,924), %	P Value
Does your school have a SHBC for its students to access?	85.3	26.2	56.3	<.001
Enrollment at SHBC	68.7	NA	NA	
During the past 12 months, used the SBHC for any reason at least once	71.9	NA	NA	
During the past 12 months, used the SBHC for behavioral health at least once	39.4	NA	NA	
Percentage who said they would use SBHC if they needed medical care	24.9	3.9	14.4	<.001
During the past 12 months percentage of respondents who said they were treated at an emergency room or hospital at least once	30.0	35.1	32.6	.019
Have you ever talked with a behavioral health (mental health) counselor, psychologist, or psychiatrist? (% yes)	29.8	23.0	26.4	.001
Percentage of respondents who said that source of professional counseling among those seeking care was a school clinic or nurse	39.3	23.4	32.3	<.001
In past 12 months have you talked with a behavioral health (mental health) counselor, psychologist, or psychiatrist? (% yes)	16.5	11.6	14.1	.002

Among students at SBHC schools, 68.7% reported that they were "enrolled" at their SBHC, and 71.9% percent of enrolled students reported having used the SBHC in the last year. Females were more likely to be enrolled than were males (74.5% and 60.6%, respectively; $P=.01$), and clinic use was not associated with age (data not shown).

Use of Health Services

Just over one fifth of students—22.3%—reported needing medical care in the last 12 months and not receiving it. The percentage was slightly lower among schools with an SBHC (20.8% versus 24.2%), but this was not statistically significant ($P=.14$). This outcome was also not associated with age or sex (data not shown). The top three reasons, besides "other," cited for not receiving medical care was because the wait was too long or the hours were inconvenient, it cost too much money, or they had no way of getting there.

Most students (55.4%) said that they would go to a doctor's office if they needed medical care, whereas 19.5% of students said that they would seek out the emergency room (ER). In schools having an SBHC, students, regardless of age or sex, were more likely to say that they would seek care at the school clinic (24.9% versus 3.9%) and less likely to seek care at a doctor's office or ER.

Almost one third of students (32.6%) reported visiting the ER in the past 12 months (Table 7.3), and 8.2% of students did so three times or more. Female students were more likely to have used the ER than were male students ($P=.01$). Students from schools with an SBHC were less likely to visit an ER than were students from schools without an SBHC (30.0% and 35.1%, respectively; $P=.019$). One in nine students (11.3%) reported having stayed overnight in the hospital in the past 12 months. Older students were more likely to have stayed in the hospital ($P=.01$), but this was not associated with sex or having a school clinic.

Use of School-Based Health Center Behavioral Health Care Services

Students reported a high prevalence of anxiety and depression-like symptoms. Just over 28% of students—including nearly 21% of males and a third of females—reported chronic feelings of sadness and inability to undertake normal tasks, and just over 10% reported that they had seriously considered suicide in the last year (Table 7.4). SBHCs played an important role in increasing access to and use of behavioral health services. For example, in schools with an SBHC, students with suicidal ideation were 8 percentage points more likely to have seen a behavioral health counselor in the last year than were similar students in schools without an SBHC. Further, SBHC students were more likely to have ever met with a behavioral health counselor (29.8% versus 23.0%; $P=.001$), and to have talked with a behavioral health counselor in the last 12 months (16.5% versus 11.6%; P=.002). SBHC students versus non-SBHC students were nearly 16 percentage points more likely to have been treated for a behavioral health issue by a school clinic or nurse (39.3% versus 23.4%; P<.001). The variable—whether or not a student had been treated for a behavioral health issue by a school clinic or nurse—is binary. When we are comparing outcomes for students in SBHC schools relative to students in non-SBHC schools, we are looking at the difference in mean (average) outcomes for the two groups—SBHC students versus non-SBHC students—and controlling for potential confounders.

Risk Conditions and Behaviors

Regarding high-risk behaviors (Table 7.4), SBHC students relative to non-SBHC students were less likely to have drunk alcohol (60.1% versus 70.5%; P<.001), less likely to have smoked marijuana (28.0% versus 38.3%; P<.001), less likely to have had sex (53.5% versus 60.5%; P=.002) and more likely to have been tested for an STD (28.5% versus 24.0%; P=.072). However, sexually active students in SBHC schools were less likely to use contraception (31.4% versus 35.9%; P=.041).

Violence and Threats of Violence

Regarding students and the potential for violence, 20% of male students (and 15% of students overall) had carried a weapon in the last month. Students in schools with an SBHC were less likely to carry a weapon in the past 30 days (12.6%) versus students with no access to an SBHC (16.7%). Over 10% of males and females had skipped at least one day of school in the past month because they felt unsafe at school or on the way to or from school. Over 10% of males reported having been threatened with a weapon on school property in the preceding 12 months. Of these, nearly a third reported that they had carried a weapon on school property in the last month, compared with only 4% of males who had not been threatened (data not shown). These latter results did not, however, differ if a student had a school with an SBHC or not. However, 30.5% of students in schools with SBHCs had been in a fight compared to 37.6% of students in schools without SBHCs (P=.001).

While nearly a third of students reported being so sad or hopeless for at least a two-week period in the last year that they stopped doing some usual activities, students who had been the victims of threats had nearly double the likelihood of such episodes of depression. They were nearly three times more likely to have seriously considered suicide in the last 12 months. Girls who reported having been physically forced to have sex were nearly three times as likely to consider suicide.

TABLE 7.4 — RISK BEHAVIORS AMONG STUDENTS, BY SCHOOL-BASED HEALTH CENTER (SBHC) STATUS

Reported Behavior or Risk Factor	SBHC (n=980), %	Non-SBHC (n=944), %	Total (n=1,924), %	P Value
Overweight or obese	33.9	33.1	33.5	.695
Told that he/she has diabetes	4.3	2.7	3.5	.047
Exercised to lose weight	53.9	52.3	53.1	.462
Sexually active	53.5	60.5	56.9	.002
Tested for sexually transmitted disease	28.5	24.0	26.2	.072
Currently using contraception	31.4	35.9	33.6	.041
Used drugs or alcohol during last sexual intercourse	12.0	10.8	11.4	.5
Used a condom during last sexual intercourse	72.3	73.3	72.8	.721
Ever been pregnant/Ever gotten someone pregnant	17.5	15.4	16.4	.617
Depression (last 12 months)	29.3	26.9	28.1	.817
Suicide ideation (last 12 months)	11.4	11.7	11.6	.177
Smoked in last 30 days	9.1	6.6	7.8	.042
Ever drank alcohol	60.1	70.5	65.2	<.001
Ever smoked marijuana	28.0	38.3	33.1	<.001
Carried a weapon (last 30 days)	12.6	16.7	14.6	.009
Carried a weapon on school property (last 30 days)	25.4	24.4	24.8	.864
Didn't go to school in last 30 days because of fear for safety	10.1	10.2	10.2	.937
In a fight (last 12 months)	30.5	37.6	34.0	.001
Physically abused by boyfriend/girlfriend (last 12 months)	7.9	6.8	7.3	.164

Multivariate Analysis

Separate multivariate logistic regressions were computed for each of the risk behavior variables (e.g., ever had sex, ever talked with a behavioral health counselor) using the full sample of students. Each risk behavior regression included a dummy variable for whether or not a respondent was in a school with an SBHC and a set of control variables. Control variables included the age of the respondent, gender (in the full sample regression), race (African American relative to all others), grade point average, and reporting of hunger in the last month (as a proxy for household socioeconomic status). Separate regressions were run for males, females, and the full sample.

TABLE 7.5—ADJUSTED ODDS RATIOS (ORs) FOR RISK BEHAVIORS FOR SBHC VERSUS NON-SBHC STUDENTS

	Male		Female		All	
	OR	P	OR	P	OR	P
Exercises more 4 or more days per week	0.7423	.059	1.3888**	.009	1.0920	.368
Ever had sex	0.5587**	.001	0.9344	.603	0.7821*	.018
Currently using contraception	0.8592	.366	0.8458	.221	0.8529	.131
Tested for STD	1.1925	.351	1.3569*	.033	1.2967*	.022
Ever drink alcohol	0.6102**	.002	0.6946**	.007	0.6569***	<.001
Ever smoke	0.7339	.464	1.8245	.123	1.1839	.552
Ever use pot	0.7194	.235	0.6964	.07	0.7146*	.037
Ever talked to a behavioral health counselor	1.7287**	.003	1.3597*	.028	1.4883***	<.001
If yes, source of counseling was school-based	2.1730***	<.001	2.5629***	<.001	2.1931***	<.001
Talked with behavioral health counselor in last 12 months	1.6299	.051	1.6394**	.004	1.6463***	<.001
Ever treated for a behavioral health issue	1.2738	.39	0.9671	.869	1.0795	.64
If yes, behavioral health treatment was at school	1.5058	.158	2.1775	.051	1.5059	.158
Treated in the ER at least once in last 12 months	0.7652	.128	0.8769	.312	0.8371	.087
Carried a weapon in last month	0.5311**	.002	0.8124	.314	0.6627**	.004
Was in a fight in last 12 months	0.7384	.06	0.8676	.294	0.8145*	.047

Note. SBHC=school-based health center. Logistic regressions were run with each outcome controlling for age of respondent, gender (in the full sample regression), race (African American relative to all others), grade point average, and reporting of hunger in the last month.

*P<0.05; **P<0.01; ***P<0.001.

Table 7.5 summarizes these results, presenting the adjusted odds ratio and P values for the association between SBHC participation and each successive risk behavior. Results are presented separately for males, females, and the combined sample. To test for differential effects by gender, fully interacted models—with a female dummy variable interacted with all of the models' covariates including the presence of an SBHC—were also estimated, but for ease of exposition, the results are not presented here.

The multivariate results largely corroborate the bivariate results described previously. Students in SBHC schools were less likely to have ever had sex (odds ratio [OR]=0.782; P=.018), drunk alcohol (OR=0.657; P<.001) or smoked pot (OR=0.715; P=.037), carried a weapon in the last month (OR=0.663; P=.004), and got in a fight in the last 12 months (OR=0.815; P=.047). They were more likely to have ever talked with a behavioral health counselor (OR=1.488; P<.001) and to have used a school-based source of behavioral health counseling (OR=2.193; P<.001). Females in SBHC schools were also more likely to have talked with a behavioral health counselor in the last year (OR=1.639; P=.004) and to have exercised (OR=1.388; P=.009). In the fully interacted models (not presented) in which the female dummy variable interacted with all of the models' covariates, there were no statistically significant differences in outcomes for females in SBHCs relative to males in SBHCs with the exceptions of: (1) exercising 4 or more days per week (OR=1.8410; P=.002) and (2) ever having sex (OR=1.6566; P=.019).

DISCUSSION

Although SBHCs were recently established in surveyed schools, general awareness among students of their presence was high. We noted that some students in schools without SBHCs (26.2%) responded positively to the question of having one; however, this may have been due to confusion because the comparison schools were in the process of developing an SBHC. Students also responded favorably to the new SBHCs in terms of enrollment and utilization of the services (Table 7.3).

Our study indicated that SBHC students made much greater use of behavioral health services than did students without SBHCs, which was positively associated with reductions in risk behaviors, some at statistically significant levels (Table 7.4). The need for mental and emotional support was exacerbated post-Katrina, and there was a lack of community providers. An important question for future analysis would be to examine if these behavioral health utilization patterns continue in a less stressful environment.

Adolescents are most likely to discontinue their education due to mental and behavioral health issues, which can lead to school suspension and dropout.[13] These study results showed a positive association between access to SBHCs and less fighting and less likelihood of carrying a weapon. These results also suggest that SBHCs may have a critical role to play in supporting students' efforts to complete secondary education by assisting them with behavioral and mental health issues that otherwise could result in suspensions and dropout. Further analyses to compare dropout and suspension rates in the study schools would be useful to support this inference.

Study Limitations

The SHC Student Survey had a number of limitations, which should be kept in mind when reviewing these study results. First, this was a cross-sectional survey, and thus only represented the situation at the six New Orleans high schools at one point in time. Although these study results were positive, they would also be strengthened if they are followed up with longitudinal analyses. Second, the responses of the students were self-reported, which depended on their ability to recall events. Third, we believe that many of the students in the schools without an SBHC may have stated that their school had an SBHC due to information in the school about a future SBHC. Alternatively, some students may have misidentified their school nurse office as a SBHC.

Conclusions

Orleans Parish SBHCs are located in public schools that serve largely African Americans, many of whom are economically and socially disadvantaged. The study results, indicating that this population's increased use of behavioral health services provided in SBHCs was positively associated with reductions in some risky behaviors, were promising. Further studies are needed to understand if SBHC services directly contribute to decreased substance use, delayed initiation of sexual activity, and provide protection for students from STIs. Further studies are also needed to determine if students' access to SBHC services can offset the exposure to community violence and threats and reduce fighting and use of weapons.

REFERENCES

1. Eaton DK, Kann L, Kinchen S, et al. Youth Risk Behavior Surveillance—United States, 2007. *MMWR Surveill Summ.* 2008;57(4):1–131. Available at: http//www.cdc.gov/healthyyouth/yrbs/pdf/yrbss07_mmwr.pdf. Accessed November 2009.

2. CommonHealth *Action.* New Orleans: community perspectives on the root causes of violence. Paper presented at: Violence Prevention Meeting; May 7, 2009; New Orleans, LA.

3. Louisiana Public Health Institute. Youth Risk Behavior Surveillance System (YRBSS) for Orleans Parish, 2007. Available at: http://lphi.org/home2/section/generic-362. Accessed January 30, 2011.

4. Centers for Disease Control and Prevention. Sexual Risk Behavior: HIV, STD, and Teen Pregnancy Prevention website. Available at: http://www.cdc.gov/healthyyouth/sexual behaviors/index.htm. Accessed September 30, 2009.

5. Eaton DK, Kann L, Kinchen S, et al. Youth Risk Behavior Surveillance—United States, 2005. *MMWR Surveill Summ*. 2006;55(5):1–108.

6. Escobedo LG, Marcus SE, Holtzman D, Giovino GA. Sports participation, age at smoking initiation, and the risk of smoking among US high school students. *JAMA*. 1993;269(11):1391–1395.

7. Breslau N, Peterson EL. Smoking cessation in young adults: age at initiation of cigarette smoking and other suspected influences. *Am J Public Health*. 1996;86(2):214–220.

8. Ethier KA, Dittus PJ, DeRosa CJ, Chung EQ, Martinez E, Kerndt PR. School-based health center access, reproductive health care, and contraceptive use among sexually experienced high school students. *J Adolesc Health*. 2011;48(6):562–565.

9. Anglin TM, Naylor KE, Kaplan DW. Comprehensive school-based health care: high school students' use of medical, mental health, and substance abuse services. *Pediatrics*. 1996;97(3):318–330.

10. Wade TJ, Mansour ME, Line K, Huentelman T, Keller KN. Improvements in health-related quality of life among school-based health center users in elementary and middle school. *Ambul Pediatr*. 2008;8(4):241–249.

11. Pastore DR, Juszczak L, Fisher M, Friedman, SB. School-based health center utilization. *Arch Pediatr Adolesc Med*. 1998;152(8):763–767.

12. Atkins MS, Frazier SL, Birman D, et al. School-based mental health services for children living in high poverty urban communities. *Adm Policy Ment Health*. 2006;33(2):146–159.

13. Freudenberg N, Ruglis J. Reframing school dropout as a public health issue. *Prev Chronic Dis*. 2007;4(4):1–11.

About the Authors

Marsha Broussard, DrPh, MPH–is a public health leader who serves as the Program Director and Principal Investigator for the School Health Connection program and the Orleans Teen Pregnancy Prevention Program at the Louisiana Public Health Institute (LPHI). LPHI, an independent nonprofit public health organization, strives to improve health and quality of life in Louisiana. Under Dr. Broussard's leadership, LPHI has become a key stakeholder in school health services, including school-based health centers, health and wellness programs, and risk reduction programs, all targeting adolescents. Success has required coalition building across state and local governmental agencies, universities, foundations, and local partners.

Lisanne Brown, PhD, MPH–received both degrees in Epidemiology from Tulane School of Public Health and Tropical Medicine. She is currently Director of the Division of Evaluation and Research at LPHI, with a staff of 10 evaluation specialists. As Division Director, Dr. Brown directs the evaluation of all LPHI programs including the School Health Connection Project, Louisiana Campaign for Tobacco-Free Living, and The Primary Care and Stabilization Grant. Dr. Brown has conducted a number of studies examining the effect of changes in health care delivery systems on population level outcomes.

Paul Hutchinson, PhD–is a health economist whose areas of expertise include econometric methods for program and impact evaluation, economic evaluations (e.g., cost-effectiveness analyses, cost-utility analyses), and health equity. He has led the design and implementation of large-scale population and health surveys in numerous countries, most recently South Africa, Jordan, and Bangladesh. He has nearly 20 years of experience working with Ministries of Health, universities, USAID, and UN Agencies (World Bank, UNICEF) in sub-Saharan Africa, Latin America, South Asia, and the Middle East.

Sarah Kohler Chrestman, MPH–serves as an Evaluation Coordinator for LPHI. She has spent the last four years evaluating School Health Connection (SHC), a local effort to rebuild and create school-based health centers. Through SHC she has evaluated the Disaster Response Mental Health Training, where she assessed knowledge and confidence gained among school nurses, and the school-based health center electronic medical records (EMR) project, where she monitored progress and outcome indicators in the implementation of an EMR in the school-based health center network. She currently works with Louisiana Positive Charge evaluating efforts to link people living with HIV/AIDS to medical care.

Weight Management and School-Based Health Care

Bethany W. van Helden

INTRODUCTION

According to *F as in Fat: How Obesity Policies Are Failing in America 2009*, a report released by the Trust for America's Health and the Robert Wood Johnson Foundation, 30.6% of Michigan's children are overweight or obese.[1] The children and adolescents visiting three school-based health centers (SBHCs) studied here are evidence of this growing public health emergency. Students registered at the health centers are coming in with headaches and injuries and are walking away with a referral to the Nutrition and Physical Activity Program. In 2008, over 200 students were referred to the staff registered dietitian for individual weight management counseling. The program utilizes motivational interviewing, a patient-centered approach to enhance intrinsic motivation to change health behavior.[2] Weight loss is not the focus; rather, developing healthy habits to maintain weight with an increase in height and resulting in a reduction in the individual's body mass index (BMI) is the program's goal.[3]

OBJECTIVE

The main objective of this study is to show that a multicomponent health promotion intervention for adolescents can be successful in influencing body composition and dietary and physical activity behavior.

METHODS

Setting

This study took place at three SBHCs (two middle schools and one alternative high school) in Ann Arbor and Ypsilanti, Michigan. Participants were recruited from students attending each of these schools.

Participants

A total of 90 overweight adolescents, 39 male and 51 female, 11 to 20 years of age, and with a BMI above the 85th percentile on BMI-for-age on the Centers for Disease Control and Prevention (CDC) growth charts, participated in individual counseling. A total of 133 students participated in the Walking Club, and 47 students participated in the Fitness Club.

Intervention

The ongoing program began in 2006, and the results described in this chapter are from data collected September 2007 through June 2008 at three SBHCs. Parent consent was obtained to provide health care services to all participants. Students participated in nutrition and physical activity counseling on a voluntary basis after being referred by a nurse practitioner and invited to participate by a registered dietitian. Students referred to the registered dietitian have a BMI at or above the 85th percentile on CDC BMI-for-age specific growth charts. This intervention uses the Transtheoretical Model of Behavior Change, which assesses an individual's readiness to act on a new healthier behavior and provides strategies, or processes of change, to guide the individual through the stages of change to action and maintenance.[4] If a student chooses to join the program, he or she participates in four weekly, 30-minute counseling sessions during the school day. The first session includes the identification of a health behavior goal by the student with help from the registered dietitian and the completion of a generic health behavior survey. The four counseling sessions also focus on expert committee recommendations endorsed by the CDC, Health Resources and Services Administration (HRSA), and the American Medical Association (AMA).[3]

1. Eat at least 5 servings of fruits and vegetables a day
2. Eat less junk food and no more than one sugary drink a day
3. Be physically active for 60 minutes a day
4. No more than 2 hours of "screen time" a day

The fourth and last session includes a post-assessment of BMI, stage of change regarding their chosen health behavior goal as well as the goals just listed, and nutrition and activity habits previously identified using the generic survey.

The Walking Club and Fitness Club are also facilitated by a registered dietitian and offered after school to all students registered at the SBHC, regardless of BMI percentile. The Walking Club consists of 8 weekly 60-minute sessions in the fall and spring months. Students walk in surrounding neighborhoods for 30 minutes, play active games for 20 minutes, and get a healthy snack before going home. The Fitness Club consists of 8 weekly 60-minute sessions in the winter months. Students identify health behavior goals to focus on for the 8 weeks. Each session consists of 30 minutes of nutrition and physical activity education and 30 minutes of active games, races, and exercise instruction.

Main Outcome Measures

The three main outcome measures for this study were BMI calculation, stage of change, and change in goals identified by the dietary and physical activity behavior survey.

RESULTS

Counseling Results

In the two middle schools, 20% of registered students are overweight (n=133), and 26% of registered students are obese (n=169). Out of a total of 63 students, post-intervention measurements showed that 70% moved positively in their stage of change (n=44), 40% decreased their BMI (n=25), and 25% maintained their BMI (n=16).

In the high school, 15% of students were identified as overweight (n=19), and 24% of students were identified as obese (n=30). Out of a total of 27 students, post-intervention measurements showed that 63% moved positively in their stage of change (n=17), 63% decreased their BMI (n=17), and 22% maintained their BMI (n=6).

Walking Club Results

In the two middle schools, a total of 12 sessions were offered throughout the school year, and 102 students participated. Of the 63 students who completed the post-intervention assessment, 39% increased the number of times they are physically active each week (n=25), 81% were meeting the goal of engaging in physical activity at least three times a week (n=51), 70% were in the "action" or "maintenance" stage of change (n=44), 32% decreased their average daily "screen time" (n=20), and 49% were meeting the goal of no more than two hours of daily "screen time" (n=31).

In the high school, a total of six sessions were offered throughout the school year, and 31 students participated in the intervention. Of the 15 students who completed the post-intervention assessment, 80% were meeting the goal of engaging in physical activity at least three times a week (n=12), 73% were in the "action" or "maintenance" stage of change (n=11), and 73% were meeting the goal of no more than two hours of "screen time" a day (n=11).

Fitness Club Results

In the two middle schools, a total of 15 sessions were offered throughout the school year, and 32 students participated. Of the 20 students who completed the post-intervention assessment, 70% were eating more fruits and vegetables (n=14), 90% were meeting the goal for no more than one sugary drink per day (n=18), 60% increased the number of times they were physically active each week (n=12), 90% were meeting the goal of engaging in physical activity at least three times a week (n=18), 75% were in the "action" or "maintenance" stage of change (n=15), 65% were meeting the goal of no more than two hours of daily "screen time" (n=13), 30% decreased their BMI (n=6), and 50% maintained their BMI (n=10).

In the high school, a total of nine sessions were offered throughout the school year, and 13 students participated. All students completed the post-intervention assessment, and the results showed that 57% of students were eating more fruits and vegetables (n=7), 100% were meeting the goal for no more than one sugary drink a day (n=13), 86% increased the number of times they were physically active each week (n=11), 63% were meeting the goal of engaging in physical activity at least three times a week (n=8), 63% of students were meeting the goal of no more than two hours of daily "screen time" (n=8), 38% of students decreased their BMI (n=5), and 22% of students maintained their BMI (n=3).

Success Story

One student participant describes the program in his own words.

Two years ago, I was 385 pounds, and I never thought about my weight, [or] the risks or dangers of obesity. Today, I am self confident and outgoing. So far, I have lost 137 pounds. I have more choices now. I have broken the cycle of obesity, but I did not do it alone.

Two years ago, I signed up for the Fitness Club on a dare with a friend. The Nutrition and Physical Activity Program was at my school-based health center. I remember being weighed before the group began and told that I weighed more than the scale could actually measure. The scale could only go up to 350 pounds. I was shocked, surprised, and scared.

The program consisted of weekly group meetings and two exercise classes every week. Having the class in the school made a big difference; I found that I was more energetic and willing to do the work. . . . The group meetings provided peer support. We could discuss nutrition, try new foods, and explore our personal strengths. I also started meeting individually with the dietitian for nutrition counseling. The counseling helped to teach me about the principle of "small changes." . . . I made my first change by switching from soda to water, without changing everything in my diet. Later, I started bringing my own lunches to school; this was my own way of practicing portion control.

I am still practicing these main exercise and nutrition principles today. I continue to make small changes towards a healthier lifestyle. When I make choices, I think about what will take me in a positive direction, instead of a negative one. Thanks to the health center I realized the amazing potential that was in me this entire time.[5]

This student was later invited in July 2008 by a US senator to testify before the Children and Families Subcommittee of the Senate Health, Education, Labor, and Pensions (HELP) Committee, in the second part of a public hearing on "Childhood Obesity: The Declining Health of America's Next Generation."

DISCUSSION

The SBHC's weight management program results showed that students participating in the program had success making positive changes in their health behavior. The success of the program is founded in the multicomponent approach that includes identification of overweight and obese students by a health care provider, individual counseling with a registered dietitian, and increased access to physical activity. Positive results related to individual counseling are tied to education, patient-centered goal setting, and weekly reinforcement. Success is evident by the combined result of weight loss and weight maintenance, which shows that 70% of participating students were no longer gaining weight following program participation. Another clear indicator of program success is the high percentage of walking and fitness club participants increasing physical activity sessions per week and decreasing consumption of sweetened beverages following program completion. It is evident that the SBHC's weight management program improved health behavior and reduced BMIs in adolescent students attending three schools in Michigan.

REFERENCES

1. Trust for America's Health. *F as in Fat: How Obesity Policies Are Failing in America 2009*. 2009. Available at: http://healthyamericans.org/reports/obesity2009/Obesity2009 Report.pdf. Accessed on August 27, 2011.

2. Resnicow K, Davis R, Rollnick S. Motivational interviewing for pediatric obesity: conceptual issues and evidence review. *J Am Diet Assoc*. 2006;106(12):2024–2033.

3. Barlow SE, and the Expert Committee. expert committee recommendations regarding the prevention, assessment, and treatment of child and adolescent overweight and obesity: summary report. *Pediatrics*. 2007;120(Suppl 4):S164–S192.

4. Prochaska JO, DiClemente CC. *The Transtheoretical Approach: Crossing Traditional Boundaries of Therapy*. Homewood, IL: Dow Jones-Irwin; 1984.

5. Miller J. Student participant testimony. Children and Families Subcommittee of the Senate Health, Education, Labor, and Pensions (HELP) Committee. July 23, 2008.

About the Author

Bethany W. van Helden, MS, RD–is a Public Health Nutritionist and Registered Dietitian. She obtained her Bachelor's degree from Michigan State University and Master's in Public Health Nutrition from Case Western Reserve University. She has worked in school-based health care with the University of Michigan's Regional Alliance for Healthy Schools in Ann Arbor, Michigan, and Ypsilanti, Michigan, since 2006.

SECTION II

Propelling the School-Based Health Care Movement: The W.K. Kellogg Foundation School-Based Health Care Policy Program

OVERVIEW

This section of the volume focuses on the W. K. Kellogg Foundation School-Based Health Care Policy Program (SBHCPP) and the lessons useful to the school-based health care movement. In the early 2000s, the W. K. Kellogg Foundation (WKKF) invested strategically in policy analyses, interim grants, and a prototype policy project to test the hypothesis that an investment in strengthening the network of school-based health centers (SBHCs) might be best served through a broad-based, multilevel, national policy advocacy initiative. At the time of the creation of the SBHCPP in 2004, state associations were tenuously funded (if at all) and were staffed by dedicated part-time or volunteering clinicians. They had loyal support from their clientele, but because they were not well known or understood by political decision-makers or even the educators who served in the same locations, they seemed to have no political base of support. Fundamentally, the WKKF believed that a substantive investment held the potential of bolstering the network of SBHCs' financial stability and, given the population they were most apt to serve, could also improve access to health prevention and promoting interventions, thereby reducing health disparities well documented in the nation's children and youth. As a result, the SBHCPP was born.[1]

It became clear early in the SBHCPP that, given the organizational characteristics of grantees, a support network of consultants was critical to facilitating the learning and development needed to actualize the vision of the SBHCPP. Figure Sec II.1 provides one way to visualize the core cognate support offered grantees that are expounded on in this section's chapters.

The eight chapters of this section advance some of the strategic underpinnings of the SBHCPP. We begin with Zimmerman's assessment of the comprehensive

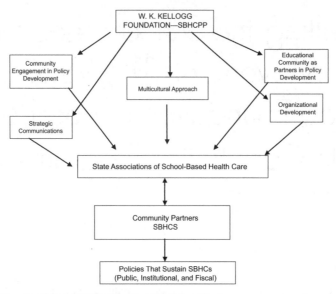

Note. SBHC=School-Based Health Center; SBHCPP=School-Based Health Care Policy Program.

Figure Sec II.1 — W. K. Kellogg Foundation core SBCHPP disciplines.

successes and lessons learned over the six-year tenure of the SBHCPP in Chapter 9. She discusses the design and the impact on SBHC policy through a programmatic lens. Policy advances include those at local, state, and federal levels. Articulation of lessons learned are particularly relevant to SBHC advocates, practitioners, and philanthropy. She ends with opportunities and challenges to policy implementation.

Lehmann and Zuckerman, in Chapter 10, delve specifically into federal policy advances fueled by the SBHCPP grantees, which included the National Assembly on School-Based Health Care (NASBHC). They share with readers the benefits and challenges of seeking to engage federal policy decision-makers in strategizing on behalf of SBHCs. The noted success of securing unprecedented national visibility and validation of SBHCs in statute has also been accompanied by disappointing delays and compromises. Some of the greatest lessons here are the need to be ever vigilant of the political tides, the validity of building bipartisan support, and, above all, the critical importance of relationship building that precede any political "ask."

Educational and health policy synergy prior to SBHCPP was a foreign concept to grantees. The authors of Chapter 11 detail the rationale for purposefully seeking educational community support in SBHC policy. Although SBHCs and schools are both committed to enhancing the lives of children, these institutions speak different languages and are accountable to very different types of public and private bodies.

This chapter provides an overview of the role of federal, state, and local governmental agencies in the development and implementation of public educational policy and funding in an effort to provide SBHCs the foundation for building a bridge between the health and educational lexicons.

As noted in Figure Sec II.1, a multicultural approach to all dimensions of the SBHCPP was an expectation. The W. K. Kellogg school-based health care initiative adopted a multicultural/racial equity (MC/RE) lens. The lens was key to nurturing a movement that emphasizes culturally appropriate practices, including engagement, organizing, and equity-focused advocacy. In Chapter 12, Batts, Capitman, and Weinstock describe the processes for applying the MC/RE lens to policy analysis, advocacy, and system change. As a specific example of how to operationalize a multicultural approach to policy advocacy, Campisteguy, in Chapter 13, provides a glimpse of program-related work in one Native American Community.

In Chapter 14, Campisteguy and Saverino explain the six-part strategic approach that helped grantees craft effective communication. Fundamental to planning around communication is the notion that by creating ones' own message one introduces the idea or point of view that correctly reveals the vision and goals of an institution. Restated, the premise was that if SBHCs did not create their own strategic messages, other organizations would create them in a less favorable light.

In support of the general tenets of strategic communications, the WKKF funded a national poll, which provided data and served as the basis for grantee policy advocacy communications. Chapter 15, "Messages Matter," provides the findings of the national poll and discusses how results can promote supportive legislation for SBHCs and inform the larger health community of the efficacy of empirical studies that test messages designed to advance policies.

Social movements have varying definitions. Common across them are the notions that these movements are change-oriented, they seek to introduce new ideas into the political and social discourse, and they tend to bubble up from grassroots identification of need. They also demonstrate a concerted effort to meet that need and reverse injustice or reduce a disparity. Rovner, in Chapter 16, provides a vivid example of how "all politics are local" and how the school-based health care movement has actually been fueled particularly by states embracing the model, which has then spilled over to federal recognition of SBHCs.

REFERENCE

1. Zimmerman JB, Campisteguy ME, Parks LS, Richardson JW. *The School-Based Health Care Policy Program: Capstone Evaluation Outcomes, Impact, and Lessons Learned 2004–2010*. Battlecreek, MI: W. K. Kellogg Foundation; 2011.

Lessons Learned From the School-Based Health Care Policy Program: Fueling the Movement for School-Based Health Care

Janet B. Zimmerman

VISION OF THE SCHOOL-BASED HEALTH CARE POLICY PROGRAM

"SBHCs will be financially stable, available and accessible to all children and families and supported as a consumer-centered model of quality care in communities throughout the United States"
— *W. K. Kellogg Foundation*

More than seven million children in the United States have no health insurance,[1,2(Table HC1),3] and many more have limited access to health care because of other systemic and structural barriers to care.[4–6] Uninsured children are more likely to have no usual source of care,[2(Table HC2),7] to receive late or no care for health problems, and to report unmet health needs than are children whose families have health insurance.[8] Low-income children and children of color face particular inequities.[9–11] Not only is quality health care more difficult for them to obtain than it is for other children, but they also are disproportionately exposed to the environmental risks that cause poor health in the first place.[12]

There are solutions to these problems. School-based health centers (SBHCs) provide one. SBHCs reflect the convergence of public health, primary care, and mental health care in a setting that students can easily access—schools. SBHCs have grown from a handful of projects in the early seventies to over 1,900 centers serving two million students per year in 48 states and territories.[13,14] SBHCs serve some of the most vulnerable populations of children and youth in the country, including significant numbers of uninsured and underinsured youth with limited access to health care. This model of health care delivery has won the endorsement of numerous professional organizations and is supported by the majority of the public (W. K. Kellogg Foundation, unpublished data, 2007).[15] SBHCs have proven their ability to provide access to preventive, primary, mental health, and oral health care, providing a cost-effective way of reducing unmet needs among some of the nation's most historically underserved children.[16-20]

Despite their track record of success, SBHCs have faced a challenging time maintaining the revenue base needed to sustain and expand their services. This difficulty reflects several factors: the historical absence of federal and state policies designed to build and broaden access to SBHCs, inadequate reimbursement from public and private insurance, insurance policies that fail to cover needed services, and the absence of an organized national, state, and community voice that demands policy change.

PROGRAM DESIGN

In 2004, the W. K. Kellogg Foundation implemented a multistate, multilevel initiative to advance policies that would sustain school-based health care in communities throughout the United States. A core strategy for achieving the program's vision, consistent with a guiding philosophy of the Foundation, was to engage communities, including youth, in advocacy for policies that favor school-based health care. To help build the school-based health care associations' capacities for community engagement and policy advocacy, the Foundation engaged a team of expert consultants to provide training and technical assistance services in several core strategies:

- Applying a multicultural lens throughout organizational development and policy advocacy.
- Building organizational infrastructure and capacities to support policy advocacy.
- Engaging communities, including youth, in organizational development and policy advocacy.
- Building skills in strategic communication for policy advocacy.
- Building bridges between health and educational communities to support policy advocacy.
- Strengthening skills in resource development to sustain the SBHC associations' work.
- Strengthening collaborative work between the national policy arena and state, local, tribal partnerships.
- Using evaluation research to inform policy advocacy and strengthen policy outcomes and impact.

The Foundation awarded over $26 million to national, state, and local entities to participate in this six-year initiative. Nine geographically and politically diverse state school-based health care associations and the National Assembly on School-Based Health Care (the "National Assembly"), the sole national organization representing SBHCs, received funding. State-level grantees included associations at different levels of organizational development: some had stronger infrastructures than others, and some had made at least initial steps into policy advocacy and showed significant potential for growth. Participating states included California, Louisiana, Maine, Maryland, Massachusetts, Michigan, New Mexico, New York, and Oregon. The state grants included funding for 40 community partners, including the Navajo, Laguna Pueblo, and Acoma Pueblo sovereign nations in New Mexico. Each community partner, in turn, developed partnerships with youth and other local groups to engage in community-based advocacy campaigns.

Data used to inform this chapter are drawn from multiple sources, including the school-based health care associations' progress and evaluation reports from 2004 through 2010.

IMPACT OF THE SCHOOL-BASED HEALTH CARE POLICY PROGRAM ON POLICY

The School-Based Health Care Policy Program (SBHCPP) played a key and often leadership role in contributing to several major policy outcomes at the federal, state, and local levels.

1. SBHCs **are now recognized in federal law as a potential provider of health care.** In a precedent-setting accomplishment, the Children's Health Insurance Program Reauthorization Act (CHIPRA), signed into law by President Obama shortly after his inauguration, defines and recognizes SBHCs as a potential provider of services, establishing, for the first time, a legal basis for being reimbursed for their services. Among other things, CHIPRA specifically identifies tribal entities and governments as potential providers of SBHCs. This achievement paves the way for SBHCs to be more adequately and consistently reimbursed for the services they provide.

2. **The Patient Protection and Affordable Care Act, signed into law in March 2010, includes authorizing legislation for SBHCs.** The Act includes two important provisions for SBHCs: language authorizing a federal SBHC grant program, and an emergency appropriation that would provide $200 million for SBHCs over four years. This law paves the way for federal

legislation to appropriate designated funds for SBHCs, a vitally important policy change needed to sustain and expand SBHCs nationwide.

3. **State funding for SBHCs increased in every participating state in the SBHCPP.** Funding for SBHCs in one state grew from $2.5 million in 2004 to $7.0 million in 2010, for example; in another, the budget for SBHCs grew by almost $4.5 million between the 2005 and 2009 legislative sessions, despite the dire economic outlook in most states. Through leveraging state dollars to obtain a federal Medicaid match on federal funds, another state's funding for SBHCs more than tripled, increasing from $3.7 million in 2004 to $14.2 million by 2010. In addition, a state that historically did not have a school-based health care state office now has a grants program for SBHCs that sets the foundation for continued advocacy to establish a state school-based health care office and to secure appropriations to fund SBHCs.

4. **Local policy, including policies in schools and SBHCs, grew more responsive to the demands and needs of local communities.** Community advocates, which included youth, made significant strides in establishing consumer-centered policies in schools, school districts, and SBHCs. Youth made inroads in protecting their rights to privacy and confidential services and in establishing healthier nutritional choices in their schools, for example. As is typical of nationwide trends, SBHCs in the SBHCPP are providing participating states access to expanded behavioral/psychosocial health care, care aimed at encouraging healthy behaviors, risk/disease prevention, reproductive health care, oral health care, health education, and other community-wide services such as screening for tuberculosis and H1N1 vaccinations.

As will be described later, the SBHCPP also made major strides in building capacity for policy advocacy among the national and state school-based health care associations and their community and strategic partners.

LESSONS LEARNED

The six years of experience in the SBHCPP offer a range of lessons for philanthropy in supporting major policy initiatives for school-based health care associations in their ongoing work to advance SBHCs nationwide, including the following.

Philanthropy serves as an essential catalyst for policy and systems change. The SBHCPP underscored the critical role that philanthropy plays in building broad-based community-driven policy initiatives through taking calculated investment risks that few institutions, including government, are usually willing to take. These risks include

- Providing significant amounts of funding and support to build nascent and largely untested organizations as a primary structure for mobilizing systemic change.
- Investing heavily in an emergent model of health care that adopts policies that are sometimes controversial.
- Having the confidence that historically marginalized populations will step forward and serve as a powerful force for social change, if given the opportunity and means to do so.

When national, state, and community-based partnerships are equipped for policy advocacy, they can serve as potent agents of change. The policy outcomes described in this chapter highlight the depth of the transformation of school-based health care associations from small, primarily volunteer membership-driven organizations into organizations capable of mobilizing policy change on a large scale. When the SBHCPP began, most of the participating state associations operated as informal organizations, many without staff, and many with governing boards consisting of a few nurse clinicians. The National Assembly and the state associations' work focused primarily on serving their members and responding to policy threats to funding rather than on building proactive policy campaigns to advance sustainable SBHCs. In general, SBHCs remained low on the radar screen; while they were important to the students and community members they served, they were often of limited relevance or interest to others.

This low profile changed significantly in the course of the program. Most associations expanded and diversified their staffs and governing boards to represent more specifically the multicultural populations they exist to serve, as well to broaden their base of expertise in advocacy. Most of the associations established legal independence from fiduciaries to enable greater autonomy over the development and implementation of their organizational priorities and policy. Most adopted more participatory, inclusive, and democratic practices to empower their stakeholders, including youth, to help guide organizational decisions and practices. The school-based health care associations and their stakeholders also became increasingly proficient in utilizing the core strategies for policy advocacy. Driven by their mission to improve the lives of vulnerable children—and fueled by the resources, technical assistance, opportunities, and expectations of philanthropy— these associations and their partners helped build and strengthen the foundation of support needed to achieve the kinds of federal, state, and local policy outcomes observed in the course of the SBHCPP.

Achieving the level and pace of change in the SBHCPP depends on visionary, entrepreneurial leadership. The SBHCPP associations helped set the stage for building nationwide capacity for policy advocacy. The impact of a few SBHC associations in particular helped to achieve federal and state policy change in a very short amount of time. Organizations that made a particularly striking impact on federal and state policy had leaders who stood out in several ways. Their leaders showed unusual skill at analyzing the political landscape for opportunities for policy change and then following up with persistence on those that seemed most promising. They created an organizational climate of openness, inclusion, and self-reflection, joined by a readiness to adjust their strategic approach midcourse, as needed. They regularly looked beyond the associations' borders for opportunities to develop relationships and to collaborate with other leaders, whether among the power base in Congress, their staff members, other organizations, or youth and other communities.

Achieving transformative change in a major policy initiative also depends upon vision-driven leadership from philanthropy. It goes without saying that directing a multisite, multilevel initiative intrinsically requires greater oversight and leadership than does managing a traditional grants-based program. The SBHCPP underscored the role that philanthropy can play in influencing the depth and pace of the work. Among other things, this work included helping grantees identify opportunities for policy change; maintaining a consistent commitment to the program's vision and to the core strategies for achieving it, and expecting others to do the same; and maintaining high expectations for well-developed and well-implemented plans for policy advocacy and, when these expectations were not met, intervening to support their correction.

Community partners and youth serve as powerful forces for change when given the opportunity and support. A key component of the SBHCPP was to build the capacities of communities, including youth, to become leaders for policy change in support of SBHCs. While seasoned policy consultants and advocates played a crucial role in the SBHCPP and in achieving program outcomes, the power of the communities' voice was felt as well; communities played a vital role in increasing the visibility of and support for SBHCs in local, state, and federal policy circles. The SBHCPP community partners, who often were staff members from the SBHCs or the organizations that sponsored them, played a pivotal role in connecting the national and state associations to youth, parents, local community groups, and local policy officials. They also played a major role in equipping local community advisory boards and youth advisory boards to become influential and self-directing forces in policy advocacy. Youth played a particularly active role, and often a leadership role, in the SBHCPP. They provided testimony at state and federal legislative hearings, hosted site visits to local SBHCs, led letter writing and signature campaigns, and helped design and participate in advocacy days and other legislative rallies. They served as spokespersons for their communities and for SBHCs in media interviews on behalf of their local SBHCs, served a variety of formal and informal advisory capacities, and mobilized other youth to join in the advocacy campaign and become policy leaders.

Findings from project-level evaluations, as well as from the SBHCPP's "Youth Voice Project," a multistate series of videotaped interviews and conversations designed and implemented by youth, provided a compelling portrait of the youth experience in the SBHCPP and how deeply their work in this program came to matter to the program and to the youth themselves. Youth described the program's impact on their sense of connection with school, their motivation to do well academically, and building their sense of confidence and efficacy in influencing policy decisions. As one community partner commented, "Youth have taken what we've given them and run with it. It's a movement being driven by the youth." Community-driven policy change in the SBHCPP would not have occurred at the level and pace it did without the support, leadership, and expectations of philanthropy.

Philanthropy can play a significant role in leveraging relationships between historically isolated communities—including building bridges between the health and education communities. Even though health status and educational outcomes are inextricably interrelated, members of the health and education community rarely joined forces in advocacy to support and sustain SBHCs in the past. This lack of collaborative advocacy began to change in the course of the SBHCPP. The program made it a priority and expectation that school-based health care associations and their partners would develop a bridge between these two communities and work together in policy advocacy on behalf of school-based health care. The Foundation also engaged a specialist in educational policy to work with the associations in the process of strengthening relationships and "building bridges" with members of the education community. Without philanthropy's expectations for change, it is unlikely these relationships would have taken shape at the pace they did.

The impact of broad-based policy initiatives is enhanced by "Project Grant Rule" established by the United States Internal Revenue Service (IRS). The SBHCPP is a complex initiative designed to achieve multilevel policy and systems change. As such, it is subject to the rules as well as the opportunities that govern policy advocacy by the IRS. The IRS prohibits private foundations from using their resources to support lobbying (influencing legislation). They also include special circumstances that allow private foundations to make general support grants to nonprofit organizations whose work may include lobbying if those grants are not earmarked in whole or in part for lobbying (under various provisions in what are known as "Project Grant Rules").[21] The Project Grant Rules provide important opportunities for philanthropy to support an array of organizations whose skills in policy advocacy are essential for broad-based social change movements.

IMPLEMENTATION LESSONS

Alongside the program's progress and achievements were several challenges that offer useful lessons for other large-scale policy initiatives.

Analyzing the factors and dynamics that explain variations in the rates of progress among grantees in large-scale policy initiatives is important in facilitating productivity and reducing barriers to success. Although the SBHCPP intentionally selected school-based health care associations at different levels of organizational readiness for policy advocacy, two of the original nine associations did not progress at a level the Foundation deemed sufficient to warrant funding for the duration of the program. As a result, they were funded for only a portion of the six-years— one for four years, and the other for five. Beyond that, two of the remaining seven school-based health care associations ended the program with significant limitations in their organizational infrastructures and capacities for policy advocacy. These difficulties could reflect mismatched training and technical assistance with the needs of the organizations, organizational or leadership issues, the interaction of these or other factors with broader environmental conditions, or inevitabilities in large-scale, complex policy work. Understanding the reasons some organizations struggle in policy advocacy and others excel is important in preventing and managing problems early, as well as in attracting organizations and leadership that can serve to model and inspire innovative strategies for others.

Finding the "right" level, intensity, and venues for cross-site networking and communication requires joint planning between grantees and funders. Large-scale policy initiatives, which assume a more expansive role for philanthropy in guiding and overseeing grantees' work than exists with traditional grants, bear the inherent advantages of creating opportunities for policy change and cross-site learning that exceed what usually is possible through single projects. The SBHCPP organized several forums to foster programwide training and cross-site learning. However, grantees often called for more frequent opportunities for sharing and networking, as well as for increased opportunities for interacting with and learning about collective program progress from the Foundation. Establishing mechanisms for regular collaborative planning would assist in determining the most productive and cost-effective strategies for building the network of communication among members within large-scale initiatives.

Achieving long-term engagement from community partners requires reducing the challenges they face in fulfilling their expected roles. The state associations' community partners often struggled to find the capacity and resources needed to support their role in policy advocacy in the SBHCPP. Community partners were often viewed as the backbone of the SBHCPP and the force that enabled the community-driven campaign for SBHCs to occur in the first place. Yet, these partners often found it difficult to comfortably sustain their other full-time jobs—which were often to serve as clinical or administrative staff in busy SBHCs—while also playing a leadership role in supporting and sometimes directly participating in policy advocacy. Strategies for balancing expectations and supporting these local partnerships are important in building on this core component of a broad-based advocacy campaign.

Ensuring seamless advocacy requires preparation for staff turnover and leadership changes. The complex work of policy advocacy often made it difficult to sustain continuity and momentum when staff, particularly executive directors, left the organizations and new directors arrived. Staff turnover presented challenges for many of the associations given the significant learning curves required to maintain timely and well-conceived strategies for policy advocacy. To reduce the disruption of staffing changes, several of the associations developed secession plans—plans designed to reduce the organizations' reliance on their directors and program staff.

The associations and their partners faced similar challenges in maintaining continuity of impact and strength of relationships with the departure and influx of new legislative officials, governors, and executive appointments because of term limits, electoral changes in state and national executive leadership, and shifts in majority parties. Often, just as strong relationships were taking off, new officials or aides/staffers would arrive, requiring building relationships all over again. This ability to accommodate leadership change proved of essential importance in sustaining an effective, coherent strategy for policy advocacy.

Skills in strategic communication are essential in advancing a broad-based movement for school-based health care. As was abundantly evident in the early years of the program, SBHCs were not on the radar screen of most policymakers or decision-makers at any level, whether local, state, federal, tribal, or institutional. The school-based health care associations and their partners made significant strides in building their capacities for strategic communication, including developing effective messages, strategically identifying messengers and channels for communication, and researching and tailoring these strategies to particular audiences.

Additional evaluation research on the value and impact of school-based health care is needed to increase the power and reach of strategic communication. One of the challenges SBHC advocates faced in building well-defended communication campaigns was the relative absence of a well-developed base of data on which to support the case behind the messages. Though growing, the limited pool of evaluation research on SBHCs places a premium on making the most of opportunities for evaluation in ongoing work for school-based health care. Discussions between grantees and funders would help sort through how best to utilize evaluation to meet project-level management needs while helping to fill systemwide gaps in the data needed for effective policy advocacy.

Increasing the visibility of SBHCs and strengthening support for policies that favor them remain a major need. Although advocates of school-based health care made progress in penetrating the political dialogue about SBHCs, SBHCs remain unknown to many. Developing a comprehensive, multilevel, and sustained national campaign for school-based health care aimed at building public and policymaker support remains a critical need, and is one that affords substantial opportunity to fuel school-based health care policy advocacy in the next phase of growth and expansion.

Accelerating tribal policies that support the expansion and sustainability of SBHCs for Native Americans requires advocacy that is informed by and responsive to complex tribal structures, organizations, policies, and culture. Advancing tribal policies that favor SBHCs proved complicated for several reasons: the insufficient strength of relationships, knowledge, resources, and expertise needed to work within a system that was unfamiliar to most mainstream stakeholders of school-based health care; a frequent lack of understanding of and confusion surrounding tribal policies that govern Native American organizations and sovereign entities; the complexity of jurisdictional bureaucracies and boundaries of mainstream and tribal health and education systems; the continuing repercussions of historical tensions created by oppressive US policies toward Native Americans; and underfunding of tribal programs and the Indian Health System. Assuring sustainable SBHCs for all children requires designating adequate resources, including time, to overcome these barriers.

MOVING FORWARD: BUILDING ON THE MOMENTUM OF THE SCHOOL-BASED HEALTH CARE POLICY PROGRAM

Accelerating progress toward expanding sustainable school-based health care is likely to be supported by several things: encouraging "transformative" rather than transactional advocacy; encouraging multiculturalism throughout policy advocacy; casting school-based health care in a public health frame; and utilizing lessons learned from past social movements to guide continued advocacy.

Engaging in "transformative" rather than transactional advocacy. Many of the associations had a tendency, especially in the SBHCPP's early years, to engage in "transactional" advocacy—advocacy comprised of activities or events that, while often productive, did not tend to build off of one another to support and advance an integrated strategic plan. A model of "transformative advocacy," as conceived in the SBHCPP, was developed to emphasize the potential for more synergistic and holistic policy advocacy—policy advocacy that builds off of and weaves together the accomplishments and lessons learned from each strategic activity or event into the next opportunity for growth, lasting change, and success. In this approach policy outcomes or accomplishments are viewed as inputs for continued development, not as endpoints unto themselves.

Transformative advocacy was encouraged when associations utilized the guiding vision as the center of the work and primary criterion for decision-making. When policy advocacy was not grounded in the overarching vision, the work tended to take a stop-and-start and disconnected quality, responding to short-term needs that may or may not have ultimately helped to increase the likelihood of longer-term improvements or SBHC sustainability.

Transformative advocacy also was encouraged when members of the SBHCPP consultant team adopted a more integrated, collaborative, multidisciplinary, and applied approach to training and technical assistance itself. The consultants modified their approach to provide support to the school-based health care associations by working increasingly as a unit, identifying opportunities for developing integrated approaches for policy advocacy. This shift in approach, though emerging, showed promise for fostering strategic planning for policy advocacy in integrative and ultimately more productive ways.

Expanding and accelerating favorable policy outcomes through engaging multicultural stakeholders in all aspects of policy advocacy. Participants in the SBHCPP made significant strides in strengthening and supporting multiculturalism in policy advocacy for SBHCs. Extending and deepening this work may be encouraged in a range of ways: by recognizing and appreciating how multiculturalism affects the interpretation and operationalization of policy advocacy; by identifying the form of outreach and engagement strategies that are most meaningful, credible, and attractive to youth and/or adults from multicultural populations; by specifying the kinds of communication strategies and methods of implementation that are most meaningful and persuasive in different cultural contexts; and by understanding the range of implications of multiculturalism for designing and implementing evaluation research, for example.[22]

Reframing school-based health care in a public health model. SBHCs are often likened to "a doctor's office in schools" for the diagnostic and treatment services they provide to individual students in need. SBHCs can also be framed in a broader light that focuses on their potential role in preventing problems and promoting health for populations of children. Because SBHCs are located in schools—

institutions that are responsible for advancing the educational achievement of all students—SBHCs are in a unique position to advance the health, well-being, and readiness to learn of all students as well. By applying a public health frame to SBHCs' role in schools, SBHCs can be understood not only for the role they play as a clinical provider of diagnostic and treatment services to individual students (the parallel of remedial educational services for individual children who have difficulties with learning) but also for the role they can play in preventing ill health and promoting quality health for all children (the parallel of teaching all students to learn and prosper academically). The public health model encourages SBHCs to develop interventions aimed at preventing problems and improving all students' health and well-being, whether that means working to prevent environmental and social threats related to youth's exposure to violence, hunger, or school dropout; developing overall school wellness plans; or providing health care to victims of natural disasters or trauma, for example. It is this more expansive role as an agent for securing the health of all children for which the school-based health care policy campaign may wish to reposition itself in the future.

Utilizing a social movement frame to propel the work forward. The social movement's literature offers a body of empirical and theoretical work on the factors that create broad-based movements for change. One thing these approaches share in common is what activist Grace Lee Boggs calls "the construction of power from below."[23] How thoroughly school-based health care associations have built a base of support, leadership, and infrastructure to "construct power from below" may be subject to question. Whether they have the population base and reasons to build a groundswell call for change, however, is not.

The disparities in health and inequities in access to health care based on racial, ethnic, and socioeconomic status are evident in communities in every state throughout the country. As the entities organized to represent SBHCs and the children and families they serve, school-based health care associations are in a uniquely powerful position to mobilize a groundswell of support on behalf of expanding SBHCs nationwide. The evidence of SBHCs' abilities to reduce health disparities and improve health equity is growing, as is a readiness of communities to join in the advocacy campaign in a collective call for change. Virtually all of the characteristics of social movements[24] have implications for broadening the reach of policy advocacy for SBHCs. The continuing need is to make the connections between what is known about building a social movement and what these points suggest for building a broad-based campaign for children. An "SBHC movement" can continue to build a sense of social will and societal responsibility for eliminating unfair and unjust health inequities through advancing a simple solution: providing health care at a place where all populations of children can access it, in schools.

CONCLUSIONS

It is, perhaps, easy to overlook how short the duration of the SBHCPP is in light of the distance traveled and the magnitude of its accomplishments. Whatever the challenges and roadblocks that may have prevented further action, the SBHCPP has left a mark on federal, state, and local policy that few might have imagined possible just six years ago, particularly in a climate of significant economic retrenchment and major pendulum swings in the political arena. SBHCs have gone from a model that few policymakers understood or cared much about to one that is winning support, even from the country's most conservative members of the policy community, not only at the local level but in state and federal policy circles as well. In addition, school-based health care associations and their partners are building their capacities, relationships, and networks necessary to develop a sustained campaign for effective policy change.

The call by young people for policies that support SBHCs has also been heard in their communities, in their schools and districts, in state legislatures, governors' offices, and by members of Congress. Youth have helped to obtain funds in support of mental health and suicide prevention programs, swayed the views of politicians to support their local centers, and held Congressional committee members in close attention as they shared their stories about how their local SBHC helped them cope with difficult circumstances. The hope, of course, is that these voices will continue to be heard and magnified as the SBHC model of care takes root throughout the country, improving quality and equity of health for generations of children, youth, families, and communities for years to come.

> *"SBHCs are a remarkable part of our nation's health care safety net for the kids. . . . School health centers are going to be a part of our national policy. And for the first time, we're going to see to it that we're putting money into that."*
>
> —*Senator John Dingell,*
> *Chairman of the House Energy and*
> *Commerce Committee*[25]

REFERENCES

1. Lynch V, Phong S, Kenny G, Macri J, and the Urban Institute. Uninsured Children: Who are they and where do they live? New national and state estimates from the 2008 American Community Survey. 2010. Available at http://www.rwjf.org/files/research/67668.pdf. Accessed April 11, 2011.

2. Federal Interagency Forum on Child and Family Statistics. *America's Children: Key National Indicators of Well-Being, 2009*. Washington, DC: US Government Printing Office; 2009:21. Available at: http://www.childstats.gov/pdf/ac2009/ac_09.pdf. Accessed April 11, 2011.

3. Centers for Disease Control and Prevention. Health insurance coverage: early release of estimates from the national Health Interview Survey, January–September 2010. Page 10. Available at: http://www.cdc.gov/nchs/data/nhis/earlyrelease/insur201103.pdf. Accessed April 11, 2011.

4. US Department of Health and Human Services, Centers for Disease Control and Prevention, National Center for Health Statistics. Summary health statistics for US children: National Health Interview Survey, 2009. *Vital and Health Statistics*. 2009;10(247):101. Available at: http://citeseerx.ist.psu.edu/viewdoc/download;jsessionid=5B62082AB4FE2 C9354DFD16A589CE104?doi=10.1.1.172.6210&rep=rep1&type=pdf. Accessed April 11, 2011.

5. Center for Health Care Strategies, Inc. Reducing barriers to health care: practical strategies for local organizations. Covering kids & families access initiative toolkit. 2007. Available at: http://www.chcs.org/usr_doc/CKF-AI_Toolkit.pdf. Accessed April 11, 2011.

6. Medicaid and CHIP Payment and Access Commission. MACPAC March 2011 Report to the Congress on Medicaid and CHIP. Available at: http://docs.google.com/viewer?-a=v&pid=sites&srcid=bWFjcGFjLmdvdnxtYWNwYWN8Z3g6NTZmYjU1ZDcwMTQ zMDc0MA. Accessed April 11, 2011.

7. ChildStats.gov, Forum on Child and Family Statistics. America's Children in Brief: Key National Indicators of Well-Being, 2011. Available at: http://childstats.gov/americaschil dren/care2.asp. Accessed July 11, 2011.

8. Guendelman S, Pearl M. Children's ability to access and to use health care. *Health Affairs*. 2004;23(2):235–244. Available at: http://content.healthaffairs.org/ content/23/2/235.full. Accessed April 11, 2001.

9. Satcher D. Disparities in children's health: major challenges and opportunities. Institute of Medicine Roundtable on Health Disparities. 2008. Available at: http://www.iom. edu/~/media/Files/Activity%20Files/SelectPops/HealthDisparities/Satcher_Childrendis paritiesinhealthchallengesandopportunities124082.pdf. Accessed April 11, 2011.

10. National Institute for Health Care Management Foundation. Reducing health disparities among children: strategies and programs for health plans. 2007. Available at: http:// www.nihcm.org/pdf/HealthDisparitiesFinal.pdf . Accessed April 11, 2011.

11. Institute of Medicine of the National Academies. *Focusing on Children's Health: Community Approaches to Addressing Health Disparities. Workshop Summary*. Washington, DC: National Academies of Science; 2009. Available at: http://www.iom.edu/ Reports/2009/FocusChildrensHealth.aspx. Accessed April 11, 2011.

12. PBS. *Unnatural Causes . . . Is Inequality Making Us Sick?* 2009. Available at: http:// www.pbs.org/unnaturalcauses/hour_01.htm. Accessed April 11, 2011.

13. Strozer J, Juszczak L, Ammerman A. 2007–2008 National School-Based Health Care Census. Washington, DC: National Assembly on School-Based Health Care; 2010. Available at: http://ww2.nasbhc.org/NASBHCCensusReport07-08.pdf. Accessed April 11, 2011.

14. Tucker C. School settings a boon to student health: school-based health centers improving access for youth. *The Nation's Health*. April 2011:1, 20. Available at: http://the nationshealth.aphapublications.org/content/41/3/local/complete-issue.pdf. Accessed April 11, 2011.

15. Center for Health and Health Care in Schools. Parents speak out on health and health care in schools. Available at: http://www.healthinschools.org/Publications-and-Resources/Polls-and-Surveys/Public-Opinion-Polls/Parents-Speak-Out-on-Health-and-Health-Care-in-Schools.aspx. Accessed April 11, 2009.

16. General Accounting Office. Report to the Chairman, Committee on Government Operations, House of Representatives. *Health Care Reform: School-Based Health Centers Can Promote Access to Care*. 1994. GAO/HEHS-94-166. Available at: http://archive.gao.gov/t2pbat3/151636.pdf. Accessed April 11, 2011.

17. US Government Accountability Office. *School-Based Health Centers: Available Information on Federal Funding*. 2010. GAO-11-18R. Available at: http://www.gao.gov/products/GAO-11-18R. Accessed April 11, 2011.

18. *American Journal of Public Health*. Special issue on School-Based Health Care. 2010;100(9):1556–1805.

19. Allison MA, Crane LA, Davidson AJ, Melinkovich P, Kempe A. School-based health centers: improving access and quality of care for low-income adolescents. *Pediatrics*. 2007;120(4):e887–e894.

20. Guo JJ, Jang R, Keller KN, McCracken AL, Pan W, Cluxton RJ. Impact of school-based health centers on children with asthma. *J Adolesc Health*. 2005:37(4):266–274.

21. Center for Lobbying in the Public Interest. Funding nonprofit organizations that lobby. Available at: http://www.cof.org/files/Documents/Legal/IRS_Letter_on_Funding_Non profits_That_Lobby_Explained.pdf. Accessed April 11, 2011.

22. Chouinard JA, Cousins JB. A review and synthesis of current research on cross-cultural evaluation. *Am J Eval*. 2009;30(4):457–494.

23. Boggs GL. Seven great ideas for movement builders. *Yes! Magazine*. Posted May 24, 2005. Available at: http://www.yesmagazine.org/article.asp?ID=1260. Accessed April 11, 2011.

24. Grassroots Policy Project. Strategy for social change. 2007. Available at: http://www.grassrootspolicy.org/system/files/strategy_for_social_change.pdf. Accessed April 11, 2011.

25. Dingell J. Quoted from: National Assembly on School-Based Health Care. *School-Based Health Care Policy Program Capstone Report. 2006–2010*. Battle Creek, MI: W. K. Kellogg Foundation; 2010.

About the Author

Janet Zimmerman–served as an evaluation consultant in the School-Based Health Care Policy Program to the W. K. Kellogg Foundation and the primary evaluator for the multisite program-level evaluation. She currently serves as an evaluation consultant to the American Public Health Association's Center for School, Health, and Education. Prior to this work, Zimmerman served as a Senior Research Scientist and Program Director at the Michigan Public Health Institute, where she directed and participated in a range of state- and federally funded evaluation studies, and as an independent Research Evaluator, in which capacity she conducted evaluations at the national, multistate, state, and community levels.

Strategic Engagement With Policymakers

Brooke Lehmann and Megan Zuckerman

Strategically engaging policymakers is critical if one's goals are to influence federal and state legislation. Policymakers often have their own agenda and therefore in order to persuade them to consider your cause, you must accomplish several things. First, members of the US Congress must be educated about the topic or cause. The issue must be one of substance, importance, and value; additionally, empirical data must exist to support its efficacy—particularly since, as with most issues brought before Congress and/or a State legislative body—the "ask" is for access to public money. Secondly and perhaps most crucially, a commonality between the issue and the members of Congress must be established in order for them to be truly engaged in the cause. This commonality most often exists in the form of constituents; illustrating the issue's impact on the member's constituents or forging a personal link between the issue and the member, all of which are pivotal determinants of success. Lobbying one's legislature is a fluid process that takes dedication, determination, and in the end a bit of luck, but it can also be one of the most effective tools for creating positive change if executed properly.

In the case of school-based health centers (SBHCs), it took several years before members of Congress were willing to propose federal legislation in support of this health care model, and nearly seven more years before these clinics were finally included in a bill signed into law. Obtaining that goal was far from easy and required multiple strategies in order to move incrementally closer to this goal. However, as this chapter will illustrate, with perseverance, a well-crafted strategy and the ability to remain flexible, challenging political and economic hurdles can be overcome.

Framing the work of the National Assembly on School-Based Health Care (NASBHC) as a case study, this chapter outlines six steps for attempting to influence a legislative body and create policy changes. Over the course of seven years,[a] NASBHC and its state affiliates worked to achieve the first-ever authorization[b] for SBHCs, a health care safety-net provider for children and adolescents who had never been the beneficiaries of federal support. NASBHC labored to make SBHCs a federally authorized program to ensure a long-term sustainable relationship with the federal government, as opposed to pursuing a short-term appropriation of federal funds for a single fiscal year. This case will illustrate how one can move a legislative body from being opposed to an idea to embracing and codifying it through a thoughtful process of strategic engagement and a bit of good timing.

The following six steps helped to secure the SBHC federal legislation:
1. Educating Congressional staff and members,
2. Recruiting committed, well-placed champions,
3. Obtaining diverse and bipartisan support,
4. Avoiding or managing controversy,
5. Providing Congressional staff with timely information, and
6. Demonstrating a willingness to compromise while staying focused on the big picture objective.

It is important to note that in all of these endeavors, NASBHC worked hand-in-hand with its state affiliates,[c] another essential element in achieving success, since the state organizations are the links to constituents, and constituents are the link to the members of Congress.

EDUCATION OF CONGRESSIONAL STAFF AND MEMBERS

As with any legislative strategy, the first step is to gauge the knowledge and interest of key Congressional members and to educate those members and their staff accordingly. A simple initial step that can be taken to educate policymakers is

---

[a] NASBHC and several of its state affiliates were W. K. Kellogg Foundation School-Based Health Care Policy Program grantees during this period. The program had at its core an expectation to advance local, state, and federal policies supportive of SBHCs.
[b] An authorization bill is a proposed public law that permits the federal government to carry out various functions and programs. Authorization bills are generally contrasted with appropriations bills, which are laws that provide funding for discretionary programs that are already authorized; for the federal government to legally carry out an action, it must both be authorized and have money available to fund any required expenditures. For more information, see Davidson RH, Oleszek WJ, Lee FE. *Congress and Its Members, 11th ed.* Washington, DC: CQ Press; 2008.
[c] Referred throughout as both state assemblies and state associations.

to have the constituent reach out to their Congressional member by requesting a meeting in the district, requesting a meeting in that member's office, making a phone call, and/or sending an introductory email.

Once the relationship with a policymaker is established, consistent communication and the ongoing exchange of ideas strengthens the relationship along with the hope of turning the casual observer into a champion of the cause.

RECRUITMENT OF COMMITTED, WELL-PLACED CHAMPIONS

As with all legislative endeavors, selection of well-placed, committed Congressional champions is integral to successes. In order to secure such an individual, one must first recognize the Congressional committees that have jurisdiction over the particular issue and then identify members of the committees that may have an interest (or could be persuaded to take an interest) in the cause. One means of accomplishing this goal is to identify and capitalize on any personal or professional relationships between constituents or advocates and members of Congress. These relationships help move a Congressional member from being disinterested to being interested and, perhaps one day, acting as a champion.

During the authorization campaign conducted by NASBHC, the personal appeals by friends to key members of Congress—also known as a "grass tops" approach—were essential to gaining the support and strengthening the commitment of two well-placed members. "Grass tops" contacts should not be overused, but when appropriately targeted, the friend can often gain access to and influence a Congressional member at crucial junctures and at times of impasse. In addition, an SBHC site visit by the policymaker, particularly in the district or state, is a powerful tool; during the authorization process, one such visit successfully turned two members of Congress into champions.

OBTAINING DIVERSE AND BIPARTISAN SUPPORT

It is important to demonstrate a broad range of support for an issue and, when possible, gain buy-in that is bipartisan. Members of both the majority and minority party are of equal importance and it should not be forgotten that the United States House of Representatives and one third of the United States Senate are subject to elections every two years. Therefore, the majority and minority parties are often changing; in order to be successful at both obtaining and retaining support, it is imperative to forge connections with both sides of the aisle. In the case of SBHCs, the support of a "pro-life" member of Congress and Republican support helped to avert controversy surrounding reproductive health issues, making advancement of the authorization legislation much more likely.

AVOIDING OR MANAGING CONTROVERSY

While no one can truly predict the actions of Congress, successful advocates can often anticipate opinions, issues, and possible actions that opponent members might use to thwart momentum. It is important to try to prepare for possible attacks by developing talking points, factual one-pagers, example op-eds, and other communication tools that could be utilized. The more quickly a controversy can be resolved, the more likely it is that legislative efforts will move forward.

In the case of SBHCs, reproductive health has always been a sensitive subject with policymakers. Many strategies have been employed to help move legislators beyond their concerns regarding SBHCs and reproductive health care services, including educating Members about the types of reproductive health care services actually provided in SBHCs, as well as emphasizing SBHC strengths, such as the clinics' ability to address childhood obesity, expanding the capacity of the health care system to handle the greater patient load expected from increased health insurance coverage, and the benefits SBHCs provide to the education system.

PROVIDING STAFF WITH TIMELY INFORMATION

Policymakers and their staff spend their days gathering as much valuable information as possible in a concise manner in order to make informed decisions while adhering to tight schedules and constant deadlines. Requests for information from staff can occur precipitously and must be addressed in a manner that reflects this fast-paced environment. Advocates will be served well by having data available and staff or volunteers identified to address various requests from Congressional staff.

OPENNESS TO COMPROMISE WHILE STAYING FOCUSED ON THE OBJECTIVE

It is not uncommon for legislation to be rewritten in the middle of the night and for negotiations and deals to be struck early and late in the day. It is therefore important for advocates to venture into the legislative process with a very thoughtful and specific request, while also maintaining an appreciation for and acceptance of the fact that the ask may take many forms from its inception to conclusion. Compromise is the name of the game and while no one wants to lose the essence of their legislative request, it is often necessary to give up on some of the details as opposed to the risk of losing everything altogether.

The SBHC legislation that was obtained by NASBHC's efforts throughout the health care reform debate is riddled with compromises that were required for a host of political reasons. However, the ultimate goal—a federal program supporting SBHCs—remained very much in tact as the later narrative will illustrate.

INITIAL PURSUIT OF APPROPRIATIONS FOR A DEMONSTRATION PROJECT

The authorization strategy was an outgrowth of activities that took place between December 2004 and July 2005. During those months, both NASBHC and the state assemblies focused their federal activities on the pursuit of an appropriation for a demonstration project.[d] The idea of the demonstration project was offered by staffers in Senator A's (D)[e] office who thought that it would be a quick and perhaps easier way to get immediate funding for SBHCs as well as to build awareness among Congressional members regarding the centers' financial plight. It was an arduous undertaking both because of the field's lack of experience and the timing of the appropriation process, but both NASBHC and the field accepted the challenge with enthusiasm.[f] Unfortunately, the appropriation was not included in the spending bill that year, and so it was after this round of activity that NASBHC resolved to pursue an authorization.

NASBHC came to appreciate that an authorization, although very difficult to obtain, would be the best strategy to pursue for the field at large rather than launching another appropriations campaign. First, NASBHC had learned much more about the federal funding process over the course of the previous months and understood that an appropriation would be something that they and their field would need to pursue every year. The authorization, on the other hand, was

---

[d] A demonstration project is a mechanism for Congress to sample the success of a program by picking a program located in one or more states for the federal government to fund to test the program's effectiveness.

[e] For purposes of anonymity, all members' of Congress names have been identified by a letter with their political party designation after, identified with a (D) for Democrat and (R) for Republican.

[f] At one point during this campaign, NASBHC staff conducted over 100 congressional visits in a six-week period, which culminated in two legislative briefings outlining the appropriations request and offering more detailed information on SBHCs.

something that, if obtained, would have a longer federal life span (although it would also need to be appropriated).

Secondly, the authorization, unlike an appropriation, would create a much more significant relationship between the federal government and SBHCs—something for which the need was clear, as demonstrated during the summer of 2005 after Hurricane Katrina hit the Gulf Coast. Several members of the Louisiana delegation sought federal support for the Louisiana SBHCs that survived the storm and for those that were administering care to the surge of children and adults who had fled north. However, the Health Resources and Services Administration (HRSA) said that because SBHCs were not an authorized program, any emergency funds utilized for recovery efforts could not be directed their way. Hence, while the authorization would hopefully lead to increased funding for SBHCs through an established grant program, it would also forever alter the type of relationship that SBHCs had with the federal government and expand the opportunities for funding and resources for years to come.

In order to obtain an authorization, NASBHC needed to follow the basic "recipe" that all new programs and organizations must follow when seeking such a bill.[g] However, even before NASBHC began to undertake the actions required to obtain an authorization, they first needed to work with fellow nonprofit coalition partners.

THE LEGISLATIVE VEHICLE DICTATES FINDING COMMON GROUND WITH A NEEDED ALLY

To begin, the most likely legislative vehicle advancing through Congress during this time period was the community health center (CHC) reauthorization. In order to proceed and gain Congressional support for the insertion of SBHCs in the CHC reauthorization, NASBHC needed to mend the relationship that existed between itself and a national nonprofit intricately involved with CHCs. Historically, the CHC nonprofit had feared that their federal funding could be carved up in order to support the expansion of SBHCs—not an outcome that they welcomed. Why was this relationship so important to the advancement of NASBHC's strategy? Because CHCs had become the hallmark of the Bush Administration's efforts to support health care and vulnerable populations and,

---

[g] Generally, this "recipe" is as follows: seek strategic members of Congress who will support and introduce an authorizing bill, identify a legislative vehicle for the bill, create as much support throughout Congress for the bill as the legislative vehicle is debated, work with partners, networks, and/or fields to promote the issue/bill, "survive" the legislative process that the vehicle must go through (markup, votes), and then hope the vehicle passes.

as such, they had widespread bipartisan support and received millions of federal dollars. Additionally, while there was little concern that the CHC reauthorization would not pass, given the broad acceptance of the program, the CHC nonprofit hoped for an easy passage, and, at this time, SBHCs remained very controversial due to reproductive health concerns.[h]

A STATE SCHOOL-BASED HEALTH CARE ASSOCIATION PROVIDES A BRIDGE

NASBHC knew that they would need to gain the CHC nonprofit's support for their federal efforts—or at least an agreement by them not to obstruct those efforts—before they could move forward in any meaningful way. To that end, NASBHC worked with a mutual friend,[i] a state SBHC-related association, to obtain a meeting with the CHC nonprofit to discuss the details of NASBHC's strategy and receiving the CHC nonprofit's "consent." The meeting served as the beginning of a dialogue that ultimately produced a strong partnership between these two organizations, with the common goal of seeking a separate federal program for SBHCs. The ability of NASBHC now to go to the Congress and, when asked, indicate the CHC nonprofit's support for an SBHC authorization, moved the conversation regarding an SBHC authorization to the next level.

FINDING CHAMPIONS AND ALLIES FOR AUTHORIZATION LEGISLATION: SENATE

Simultaneously, NASBHC continued to seek champions for the proposed authorization bill with the hope of it being inserted in the CHC reauthorization. At the time, Congress was under Republican control. Despite the fact that NASBHCs strongest supporters were Democrats, these policymakers were well-positioned on committees of jurisdiction. For example, Senator B (D)[j] had been a long time supporter of SBHCs, so NASBHC staff naturally contacted staff in his office, in

---

[h] As used here, "reproductive health" refers to access to contraception, treatment of sexually transmitted diseases, and the extent to which students can receive such services without parental consent. "Reproductive health" also includes the issue of abortion, since some policymakers fear that abortions may be provided or promoted by SBHCs.

[i] *Friend* denotes an organization that shared a working relationship with both the CHC nonprofit and NASBHC.

[j] Senator B was the Ranking Member of the Subcommittee on Children and Families, second only to the Chairman of the full Health, Education, Labor and Pensions (HELP) Committee.

partnership with the relevant state SBHC association, to see how willing he would be to sponsor a bill.

As for Republicans, NASBHC's strategy for securing a Republican sponsor of the bill focused on Senator C (R), given his interest in mental health and the strength of his state's SBHC association. Initially, his office proved to be more difficult to obtain support from than had been anticipated. In the end, however, the state assembly launched a very successful grassroots movement, and the senator committed to the sponsorship.

FINDING CHAMPIONS AND ALLIES FOR AUTHORIZATION LEGISLATION: HOUSE OF REPRESENTATIVES

On the House side, the options for sponsors were more limited. NASBHC and its field were still making great efforts to educate House members and staff by making constituent and site visits, for example, in hopes of reducing and/or eliminating some of the old stigmas regarding SBHCs, particularly reproductive health care controversies.[k]

NASBHC's original Republican target in the House was Representative D (R), for several reasons; he had signed onto the appropriations request made in 2005, he was a member of the Energy and Commerce Committee, and, given Senator C's[l] support in the Senate, NASBHC and the relevant state assembly assumed they could persuade him. To accomplish this, NASBHC and the Assembly held constituent meetings in Washington, DC (state constituents flew in), launched a grassroots campaign similar to that used to secure Senator C's support, and even asked Senator C's office to engage in outreach efforts. All of these activities were taking place during the midterm elections and, ultimately, Representative D was unwilling to commit during the election period. As NASBHC would learn, the elections would alter the balance of power.

A SCHOOL-BASED HEALTH CENTER VISIT SWAYS A CONGRESSIONAL OPPONENT'S SUPPORT

Meanwhile, a southern SBHC assembly had taken advantage of a trip to Washington, DC, to convene staff from the office of each member of the state's

---

[k] It should be noted that NASBHC was also pursuing opportunities to educate Senate staff about SBHCs.
[l] Both Representative D and Senator C were from the same state.

Congressional delegation and transport them on a bus to a local SBHC. Surprisingly, Representative E (R), who had not been supportive of SBHCs because she is particularly conservative on reproductive health care issues, decided to join the group. However, upon seeing the clinic and having the opportunity to ask questions of the clinic staff, the Congresswoman declared herself a supporter and offered to assist in the development of legislation to support SBHCs. While this was certainly a more positive outcome than NASBHC had anticipated, it was not entirely unprecedented. Frequently, once a Congressional member and/or staffer actually views a clinic and sees how it functions, his/her support often grows exponentially.

MIDTERM ELECTION CHANGES AND OPPORTUNITIES

The midterm elections concluded and significantly altered the course of events for the SBHC authorization. Both the House and Senate "flipped," which meant that now the Democrats were in majority and NASBHC's legislative sponsors would be strategically positioned to move the SBHC authorization forward.

The year 2007 began with a new Congress, a new majority, and NASBHC hosting a very successful legislative briefing (one for the House and one for the Senate) that focused on SBHCs as well as disaster preparedness and emergency relief. A key testimony of the briefing was a military family whose son had received mental health services from the center during his father's third deployment to Iraq. Both the father and son spoke to a packed room in the House as well as the Senate and, in the end, their testimony elevated the conversation regarding SBHCs. The briefing illustrated that SBHCs not only serve children in schools but also have a more flexible and broader application that can serve many needs. In fact, subsequent to this briefing, SBHCs were mentioned in pieces of legislation outside of the CHC reauthorization, including a large disaster preparedness bill in the House.

INTRODUCTION OF THE HOUSE AND SENATE BILLS

On February 14, 2007, Senator C introduced the Senate bill, S. 600, titled the "School-Based Health Clinic Establishment Act." The bill was originally co-sponsored by six senators—three Democrats and three Republicans.

NASBHC took a "grass tops" approach to secure the support of Senator F (R) and worked with one of their board members, a former high ranking government official and former colleague of the senator's. Senator F's support of the bill was crucial as the Ranking Member on the subcommittee with jurisdiction over the bill—the Subcommittee on Children and Families of the Committee on Health, Education, Labor, and Pensions (HELP Committee)—which was chaired by Senator B. Through communications between Senator F and his "friend," NASBHC was able to secure Senator F's support and co-sponsorship of the bill in October 2007. By the end of that month, there were a total of 20 bill co-sponsors (in addition to Senator C).

In addition, a new sponsor—Representative G (D)—was identified in the House with the assistance of Representative H's[m] (D) staff. NASBHC then worked with staff from that office and Representative E's office to introduce the House companion to S. 600. That bill, H.R. 4230, was introduced on November 15, 2007, with 17 original co-sponsors. Eventually the bill would have a total of 29 co-sponsors (in addition to Representative G) although Representative E would remain the only Republican on the bill.

Although the majority now in Congressional control was one that was generally much more favorable to SBHCs, there were several other factors complicating NASBHCs efforts to move the authorization bill forward. To begin, NASBHC had to disentangle SBHCs from issues surrounding fraud and abuse in billings related to school-based health services for children with disabilities. In addition, an influential health care system was attempting to use the CHC reauthorization as a means of removing the community board requirement[n] from the next iteration of the bill. Since the community board is seen as the hallmark of the CHC program, this initiative was met with strong resistance and concern on the part of both the CHC nonprofit and other CHC supporters. NASBHC was placed in a rather awkward position after being approached by the health system: what they were seeking would actually benefit many SBHCs across the country, but supporting them could lead to the demise of NASBHC's relationship with the CHC nonprofit. In the end, NASBHC was able to stay silent on the issue.

Last, while the Senate was debating the CHC reauthorization and S.600, an SBHC in a northeastern middle school decided to offer reproductive health care services. This decision made national news, and SBHCs were thrust into a national dialogue that had not been foreseen.

In the end, between the negative media attention and the fact that the health system ended up with a Government Accountability Office (GAO) study[o] in the

---

[m] Representative H was another influential House member, the chairman of a committee of great relevance whose support was gained by the work of his state's SBHC assembly—as the chairman, he would not sponsor the bill directly so he pledged his support by asking his colleagues to sponsor and support the bill.

[n] Having a board that includes members of the community is a criterion for becoming a federally recognized CHC.

[o] A GAO study is one commissioned by Congress and conducted by the GAO.

CHC reauthorization, the Senate subcommittee asked that NASBHC also accept a GAO study instead of the authorization. Thus, when the CHC reauthorization passed in the Senate, it included a GAO study which, at its conclusion, would hopefully document the efficacy of the SBHC model and the need for additional support.

THE BEGINNING OF A NEW AUTHORIZATION STRATEGY

The CHC reauthorization became law in the Spring of 2008 without an SBHC authorization. NASBHC decided it was best to keep the SBHC authorization bill alive to await a new legislative vehicle; however, it would need to find a new House sponsor since Representative G would be retiring when that Congress ended. Internally, NASBHC identified several Congressional members, including Representative I (D) and Representative J (D). Representative I had been added to the list of Congressional members who were critical to NASBHC's success because of his position as the head of the Democratic pro-life caucus. In partnership with his state's assembly, NASBHC worked tirelessly with his staff to win his support and, after his assembly was able to get the Congressman to visit a center in his district, he declared himself a supporter, yet not a co-sponsor. Despite his unwillingness to sponsor the bill, Representative I did allow NASBHC to inform other members of Congress of his support, enabling NASBHC to obtain additional sponsors and supporters and providing supporters with a greater sense of security in avoiding a battle over reproductive health care.

Knowing now that Representative I would not lead the authorization bill, NASBHC worked with the relevant state assembly to win the support of Representative J, who had a long history of supporting school health services (she had been a school nurse) and was well positioned on the Energy and Commerce Committee. By the end of the year, Representative J had confirmed her willingness to sponsor the authorization and NASBHC began to look at the new Congress and the new opportunities it presented.

A NEW ADMINISTRATION EQUALS CHANGE

The November 2008 elections brought the new Obama Administration and an increase in the margin of majority for the Democrats in both the House and Senate. Not long after the elections, Congress continued its work on a stimulus package that was aimed at ameliorating some of the economic woes of the country at the time. As a still unauthorized program, NASBHC was unable to secure any dollars for SBHCs; nevertheless, in hopes of finding loopholes, NASBC reached out to various Congressional staff to ascertain the possibilities. As a consequence of this, NASBHC staff had a conversation with Senator B's staff, anticipating that they would discuss both the stimulus and the chance that the Senator might use his position on the banking committee to find some additional funding for SBHCs. However, Senator B's staffer called to share the news that Senator B had decided to prioritize the SBHC authorization in the new Congress and wanted to make sure that NASBHC would be there to support him. This decision by Senator B appeared to be prompted by both his impending retirement and his understanding that health care reform, something that was already being discussed, would provide a vehicle for him to help SBHCs.

The next steps therefore became reintroducing the bill in the Senate and the House and identifying a legislative vehicle. One of the first events to reshape NASBHCs authorization strategy in the new Congress was the replacement of Representative H as Chairman of the Energy and Commerce Committee. While this was upsetting to NASBHC—given all the years they had put into cultivating this relationship, his replacement, Representative K (D), was probably the longest supporter of SBHCs and, in fact, had put out the first ever SBHC legislation back in the 1980s. So, while it was a loss in some ways for SBHCs, it was also a gain. The Congressional agenda for the year took shape and health care reform was front and center.

CHAMPIONS PAVE THE ROAD TO HEALTH CARE REFORM

Health care reform would prove to be *the* event that would finally lead to the authorization of SBHCs; it provided not only an appropriate legislative vehicle but also a sizeable portion of the bill focused on the creation of new delivery system programs. Because Representatives H and K would chair health care reform in the House—a tremendous win for SBHCs—Senators L (D), B, and M (D) (Chair of the Finance Committee) would oversee this process in the Senate. With Senators L and B, NASBHC knew that they had supporters. However, at the time, no relationship existed with Senator M, and NASBHC did not have any SBHCs in his state, so efforts were made to find connections that would lead to conversations with his staff.

In the Senate, the authorization would be under the control of the HELP Committee. Discussions took place on a regular basis between NASBHC staff and Senator B's subcommittee staff, and it was decided that instead of reintroducing S. 600, they would just write the language of the bill into their section of the health care reform bill. This was performed so as not to bring too much attention to the provision and to avoid any undue controversy.

In the House, on the other hand, it was decided that the authorization bill should be reintroduced, with Representative J as the new lead sponsor and Representative E as the lead Republican. Notably, an original cosponsor of that bill was Representative N (R), a senior member of his state delegation known for his conservative views. While his support may not have been necessary, given that Democrats had a majority, SBHCs had become a bipartisan issue, and it was worthwhile that he would be a Republican member to count on in the future.[p]

COMPROMISES SECURED FOR SCHOOL-BASED HEALTH CENTERS

NASBHC's strategy during the Senate's consideration of the health care reform bill was (1) to survive and (2) to maintain the fundamental integrity of the SBHC provision. During the HELP Committee's mark-up of the relevant section of the health care reform bill, committee members filed 22 amendments to weaken the SBHC provision. NASBHC worked with Congressional staff and strategic partners, particularly those from the pro-choice community, to draft talking points that could be used by other members to reject those amendments which were unacceptable and to draft compromise amendments for those that were deemed politically necessary to accept.

Specifically, NASBHC staff worked with individuals from several nonprofits and think tanks to modify language offered by Senator O (R), which would ensure that clinics followed all local, state, and federal reporting laws related to the provisions of health care delivery. This amendment was significant for several reasons. Senator O had been courted by NASBHC and his state assembly for a very long time, since he was a member of the HELP Committee and came from a state with a strong SBHC network. With the exception of Senator F, Senator O was the only Republican member on the committee that NASBHC stood a reasonable chance of winning over. Thus, in order to maintain the developing relationship with his office, NASBHC and Congressional staff agreed that every attempt should be made to accept Senator O's amendment. However, the amendment was significant in that it was the first time that a member of Congress had resorted to such a sophisticated

---

[p] Another very significant Republican to join those supporting SBHCs was Representative P (R), although he did not become a cosponsor of the Representative J bill. Representative P had expressed opposition to the SBHC model during the CHC reauthorization hearing. However, Representative P's exposure to the model in his district turned him into a supporter. In fact, Representative P and two other House members from his state wrote a letter to their colleagues touting their local SBHCs at a time when other Republicans were questioning the value of SBHCs.

method of addressing the reproductive health care issue in SBHCs. Fortunately, through the diligence of NASBHC's partners, language was crafted that both appeased the SBHC field and Senator O. By the conclusion of the markup, the SBHC authorization provision remained in the bill. It was slightly altered from its original version, but not in ways that were unacceptable or that NASBHC and Congressional staff did not believe could be worked through in a House–Senate conference.

Meanwhile, the House continued to work on its version of the health care reform bill and NASBHC staff worked with the Energy and Commerce Committee staff to ensure that the authorization language was written in that bill as well. The Committee staff included a more robust SBHC provision in their bill, which included not only the language from Representative J's bill, but also money for technical assistance and wording that made reimbursing SBHCs by public health insurance programs mandatory.[q]

As of late July 2009, the SBHC provision had made it through markup in the House and was now in the base bill.[r] It was assumed at this point that the differences between the two provisions—House and Senate—would be worked through in conference committee, so the goal of NASBHC at this point was to ensure support on both sides for the exact language that was preferred as well as obtaining and maintaining the reimbursement provisions still at play in the Senate.

However, by the fall of 2009, the health care reform bill itself was in jeopardy and there were significant questions as to whether or not Congress could actually get the bill passed. Senator L passed away in August leaving Senator B in charge of the bill in the Senate, along with Senator M and leadership. By late fall, the controversies surrounding the bill were far beyond particulars as small as the SBHC provision and were focused on more major concerns around cost, abortion, and personal mandates. After the new year, it started to become clear that the only way the bill would pass into law would be if the House agreed to accept the Senate version—the version most supported by the Obama Administration and the more conservative of the two bills. In early March, the House agreed to the Senate bill and both chambers drafted and passed a smaller reconciliation bill. The debate had come to an end.

---

[q] These two provisions were supported in the Senate by various members but not included in the Senate bill for several reasons. First, the technical assistance provision was stripped when the HELP and Finance Committees merged their bills because there were concerns that the SBHC provision was too long. Second, the reimbursement provision had not been considered by the committee of jurisdiction, the Finance Committee.

[r] In contrast to the Senate, there was only one amendment concerning SBHCs during the House markup. That amendment was proposed by a southern Republican representative. It was eventually modified in cooperation with Representative H and accepted by the committee.

VICTORY FOR SCHOOL-BASED HEALTH CENTERS

On March 23, 2010, President Obama signed into law the Patient Protection and Affordable Care Act, and SBHCs finally had a federally authorized grant program. While the Senate authorizing language was not the preferred version (as mentioned earlier, the House provision included technical assistance money and the public insurance reimbursement provision), it was, and is, the first federal recognition of SBHCs as an important health care model for children and youth.

CONCLUSION

As illustrated in securing the SBHC authorization, strategically engaging policy-makers is an arduous, carefully devised yet unpredictable process. Through implementation of the six steps—educating Congressional staff and members, recruiting committed individuals, creating well-placed champions, obtaining diverse and bipartisan support, avoiding or managing controversy, providing staff with timely information, and demonstrating a willingness to compromise while staying focused on the big picture goal—the legislation that the advocate is seeking may be successful.

About the Authors

Brooke Lehmann–is a clinical social worker and public interest attorney who has spent two decades providing direct clinical and advocacy services to children and families. Ms. Lehmann is a principal with Childworks and a founder of two not-for-profits whose missions are to advance the health and educational needs of vulnerable populations of children. As a recognized child advocate, she has managed multimillion dollar advocacy campaigns, provided policy analyses, strategic guidance, and consultative services on pediatric health systems' design and development and education system reform. She is a graduate of University of Pennsylvania, Yale University, and American University.

Megan Zuckerman, JD–received her JD from Brooklyn Law School and her BA in Communication and Art History from Tulane University. After a number of legislative positions on and off Capitol Hill representing issues varying from First Amendment to mental health, Megan ultimately served as Health and Education Legislative Assistant for Senator Mary L. Landrieu (D-LA) and served the senator during the aftermath of Hurricanes Katrina and Rita. Megan is currently a legislative advocate at Childworks, PLLC, representing children's health and education issues. In addition, Megan is a certified mediator earning her practice hours at Volunteer Lawyers for the Arts NYC- MediateArt.

Health and Educational Policy Synergy

*Jeanita W. Richardson
and Terri D. Wright*

School-based health centers (SBHCs) create an effective framework for the health and well-being of all children, but the greatest potential impact of SBHCs is for children in poverty. The rationale to locate health care clinics in schools goes far beyond the issue of accessibility of health care, and SBHCs have the potential to address the multifaceted needs of children in poverty.

As a policy change initiative, the W. K. Kellogg Foundation's (WKKF's) School-Based Health Care Policy Program (SBHCPP) required grantees to develop core partnerships between the SBHC and education communities by virtue of the common challenges and missions of both the health and education disciplines. Collaboration yields great mutual benefits for organizational partners, including higher academic achievement, fiscal sustainability for SBHCs, and more importantly the creation of a holistic web of support for children and youth. This chapter describes why and how applying educational policy knowledge was key to enhancing alliances with schools that ultimately yielded benefits in both the health and educational arenas.

RESPONDING TO THE NEEDS OF CHILDREN IN POVERTY

The needs of children in poverty are far more complex than education and health disciplinary silos might imply. Children, because of their unique developmental processes and their inability to care for themselves, are most susceptible to the multiplied disadvantages associated with poverty.[1-3] Food insecurity, housing insecurity, low-performing schools, exposure to violence, and inaccessible health care are seemingly discrete conditions that amalgamate to shape the environment of children in poverty.

Economically challenged youth also are more likely to experience environmental exposures, which have negative implications for their health. For example, poor children are more than twice as likely as nonpoor children to live in a household with someone who smokes in the home (32% vs. 12%). Also, given the tendency for older homes to have lead-based paint, poor children are twice as likely as nonpoor children to have blood-lead levels of at least 2.5 micrograms per deciliter (30% vs. 15%), levels that are associated with adverse health outcomes.[4]

In addition to environmental exposures, children in poverty experience disparities in access to health care and health outcomes as compared to youth with greater financial status.[2,5,6] The uninsurance rate for poor children is twice that of nonpoor children (16% vs. 8%), and also these youth are less likely to have access to primary and preventive care. Within every age group, poor children are more likely to be overweight and obese than are nonpoor children. Poor children are also more likely than nonpoor children to have been diagnosed with asthma (18% vs. 13%). Finally, poor parents are more than twice as likely as nonpoor parents to report their child has "definite to severe" emotional, behavioral, or social problems (10% vs. 5%).[4]

The aforementioned income-sensitive health issues also trickle into schools. Poor children are more likely to have missed five or more days of school in the past year for health-related reasons (20% vs. 15%).[4] Many of the health outcomes just cited have direct consequences for cognitive and behavioral development, so it should come as no surprise that the longer children live in poverty, the lower their educational achievement and the slower their general maturation processes, not necessarily because of innate deficits, but because of susceptibility to preventable and chronic diseases, toxic exposure, and malnutrition.[3,7]

School systems serving substantial numbers of low-income and minority youth are documented as disproportionately underfunded.[8] To exasperate school funding challenges, the cognitive and behavioral health outcomes that youth in poverty experience require additional spending on educational interventions; unfortunately, high poverty schools are the very institutions commanding the fewest resources.[3]

Children faced with inadequate health care and toxic environmental exposures experience concomitant threats to childhood educational potential because of the schools they attend. Rather than schools being a haven from the challenges of economic depravation, they are instead magnifiers of the inadequacies of the very social systems designed to mitigate dimensions of low status.

Stressors to child health ("social determinants" in the public health lexicon) are also hindrances to learning readiness ("at-risk factors" in the educational lexicon).

Thus in a real sense, the children in greatest need of health support tend to be the same children at-risk of performing poorly in school.[2,9–12] Increasingly, researchers from both health and education disciplines are coming to the realization that health and academic prowess are inextricably linked. Consider a recent article in *Pediatrics* that argues disparities in health and education are perpetuated because of the lack of health and educational policies supporting one another.[2]

As per the Foundation for Child Development, good health, cognitive and literacy skills, and motivation are key predictors of academic achievement in the third grade. Third grade performance in turn is an important predictor of future educational success, including high school graduation. Furthermore, this report and others point out that childhood access to health services is crucial to facilitating transition to productive adulthood.[2,3,13]

Two poignant examples of health and educational reciprocity are the high school dropout rates and the prevalence of asthma. Only half of Native American, African American, and Hispanic/Latino American youth graduate from high school.[2,14–16] Youth do not complete high school for a number of reasons, two of which are health challenges and the need to contribute to family income. Dropping out of high school is associated with higher likelihood of joblessness, uninsurance, limited residential choices, earlier onset of chronic disease, and early adoption of risk behaviors, such as sexual activity.[2,17–19] Among women, failure to complete high school is linked to poor maternal health and maternal economic disadvantage. As these discussions illustrate, health challenges are often a causal factor of dropping out, and as a continuation of that cycle, dropping out is associated with poor health outcomes later in life. Cycles of familial disadvantage often yield similar challenges for the next generation of youth, particularly as it relates to limited access to preventive care.[2]

Asthma prevalence and its disproportionate diagnosis in economically challenged youth provides another example of the nexus between poverty, schools, and health.[10] Asthma is the most common chronic disease children experience and it affects over nine million youth under 18 years of age. Approximately three million hospital visits and 200,000 hospitalizations are associated with childhood asthma annually. Relative to schooling, asthmatic youth tend to be absent from school three times more than nonasthmatic children.[5,20,21] Medication prescribed to ease symptoms may interfere with the learning process because of side effects such as diminished ability to concentrate and feelings of agitation, depression, or anxiety.[21] Given the cognitive diminishing impact of ill health, children may demonstrate difficulty coping academically and behaviorally in traditional school settings. If children are not in school or do not feel well, their prospects of learning and performing optimally are diminished.

SCHOOL-BASED HEALTH CENTERS AS A SAFETY NET

In short, poverty and the limitations it breeds are the greatest predictors of health and educational risk. Despite the grim statistics, the spiral of health disparities negatively impacting learning and academic achievement and vice versa is a cycle that can be broken.[5] SBHCs are a critical safety-net provider for the children they serve because they are largely concentrated in schools serving high need populations.[12,22,23] More than 50 million students spend time in schools each day, many of whom suffer from disproportionate disadvantage.[5] School buildings are effective sites to deliver a comprehensive range of services that empower youth to become productive, healthy adults because they are a familiar and stable social context.

While neither SBHCs nor educators control educational risk or social determinants of health, public health professionals possess a critical skill set that enables them to promote preventative interventions, early detection, and management of health outcomes that positively accrue to both school-level personnel, students, and their families. SBHC interventions promote early diagnoses of preventable or treatable health problems, thereby theoretically improving the quality of academic interactions. For example, in one longitudinal study, students who used their SBHC to help manage chronic illnesses, such as asthma, improved their attendance rates, while students who used the mental health support services at their SBHC demonstrated increases in their grade point average. The spillover effect of chronic disease management was decreased use of emergency services.[23]

Childhood poverty stressors are undeniably relevant to SBHCs and schools as they attempt to maximize the potential of youth who encounter many obstacles as they strive to become productive healthy citizens. Furthermore, SBHCs make important contributions because they mitigate health disparities that are a function of income and, in partnership with schools, could have a profound effect on learning readiness.

SCHOOL-BASED HEALTH CARE AND SCHOOL COLLABORATION

The WKKF's School-Based Health Care Policy Program (SBHCPP) grantees were challenged to foster core partnerships between the SBHC and education communities by virtue of the common challenges and missions of both disciplines. As with any relationship, the key to enhancing collaborations with schools is the ability to articulate challenges common to SBHCs and schools that might be more effectively addressed if both groups worked together.

SBHCPP grantees were advised to frame the benefits of their services not solely as health service delivery but also as facilitating the ways in which SBHCs could aid schools in meeting their accountability objectives. In order to do that, grantees needed to understand educational financing and governance, as well as the mandates established in the No Child Left Behind (NCLB) Act (now referred to by its original name, the Elementary and Secondary Education Act [ESEA]) that dictate the priorities of educators.

It was the belief of the WKKF program director that a fundamental understanding of the role of federal, state, and local bodies in policy development and implementation would aid grantees in establishing mutually beneficial partnerships that would advance policies supportive of child and adolescent health and learning. However, it became evident that by and large the grantees and their partners lacked specific expertise in educational policy because of the "silo"-ing of public health and educational policy expertise. As a result, specific strategies promoted grantee understanding of and skill in engaging educators in policy advocacy. To begin, deconstruction of educational policy making was necessary.

EDUCATION POLICY 101

Schools as institutions are charged with more responsibility than they could possibly accomplish, particularly given the numbers of their unfunded and underfunded academic and health mandates. Rhetorically, educators acknowledge that health matters to their students even if they are unaware of the causal relationships between health and learning readiness. What they do not possess is the time to manage much more than the strict curricular and testing schedules associated with legislated accountability. Yet, their time is compromised by having to also manage the health-related issues presented in the classroom.

If efforts are to be efficient and effective, it is germane to know which decision-makers are relevant to any particular policy target and the scope of their authority. Early in the tenure of the program, monographs were commissioned that detailed the role of federal, state, and local governments and agencies in setting school priorities and funding (see Figure 11.1).

The information provided in Figure 11.1 was new to many grantees. For example, it was not common knowledge that public education is not governed at the federal level (as dictated by the Constitution), but rather by each state. There is no explicit reference to education in the Constitution. On average only six to ten percent of public school budgets tend to be supported with federal funds. Federal legislative

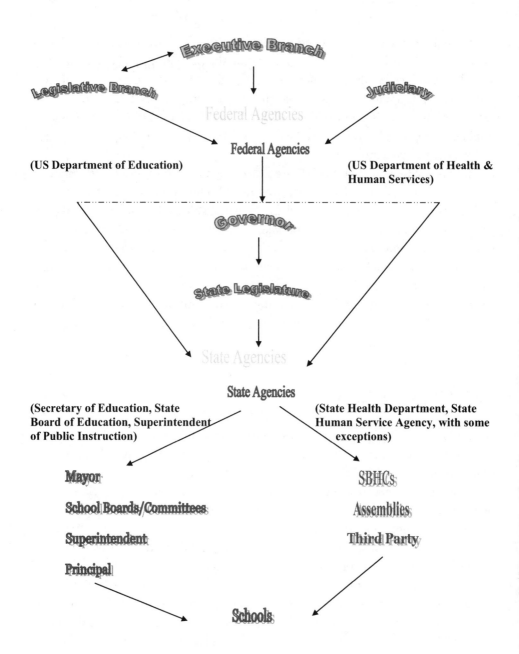

Figure 11.1—Education and health policymaking.

bodies and agencies do, however, influence schools through incentive programs that tie funding to certain programs or practices.

Some federal funds are available only to schools in compliance with various legislated acts, such as the Civil Rights Act of 1964, the Individuals with Disabilities

Education Act (IDEA), and NCLB. In this way, Congress can directly impact aspects of school operations. Federal agencies such as the Department of Education are charged with ensuring the enforcement of legislated mandates through the establishment of regulations.[24]

Governors, like the President of the United States, exert an indirect influence on schools. Their power is tied to their approval or veto of bills and the appointments that they make to policymaking bodies as provided in their state's constitution. State legislatures have the broadest prerogative to pass laws or delegate power to other bodies, such as state departments of education or boards of education. They pass education laws that distribute funds, govern state licensure of teachers and administrators, delineate school districts, and prescribe and evaluate curricula. State boards of education are called upon to implement and enforce the mandates set forth by the state legislature or its designees. While the specificity of language differs from state to state, the general premise is the same: states have formally assumed the responsibility of providing public K–12 education to their citizens. Consequently, the most influential bodies relative to schools are found at the state level.[10]

Local school boards and educational agencies interpret the state mandates and manage the operating funds, and in some cases physical capital resources coming from federal, state, and local sources. School districts tend to be headed by a superintendent who serves as a chief executive officer. Schools—with their administrators, faculty, and support staff—are in turn charged with the implementation of directives from federal, state, and local authoritative bodies.[10]

Native American education systems are complex in different ways than state public educational systems because tribes have the right to enter into self-determination contracts with the federal government (as per the Indian Self-Determination and Education Assistance Act of 1975) as it relates to the role of the Bureau of Indian Affairs, and federal mandates such as IDEA and NCLB place accountability standards on schools.[6]

In addition to learning about governance structure, the principle policy with which grantees needed to become familiar was NCLB because it had a direct impact on virtually all K–12 policies and decisions. The NCLB Act of 2001 represented an unprecedented increase in the scope of federal mandates complete with punitive consequences for noncompliance.

Governors and the National Conference of State Legislatures have decried the pressures of NCLB compliance on state budgets because of spiraling Medicaid and other health care expenses, which deplete funds required to comply with public education mandates, particularly the NCLB-driven testing costs.[25,26] For example, it has been estimated that 5.5% to 14% of every dollar spent for public schools is now being spent on testing and test administration services.[27] Understanding that health and education budget allocations tend to represent the two largest expenditures of every state's budget helped grantees grasp the significance of seeking health–education partnerships that were not founded on financial support requests.

For purposes of the SBHCPP, the most important aspect of NCLB was this: school districts and states are preoccupied with meeting the statutory criteria because failure to do so places 6–10% of school budgets at risk. Furthermore, in order to comply, states and municipalities have had to divert funding from other programs that might have been successful in order to meet NCLB standards. In light of the significance of NCLB to potential education collaborators, grantees were provided information about the law that was directly related to their work. As one example, grantees were provided guidance as to the SBHC services that would be supportive of their school's NCLB accountability (see Table 11.1). Once a basic understanding of education policy was mastered, attention turned to actively engaging schools in SBHC advocacy.

INTEGRATING EDUCATORS INTO SCHOOL-BASED HEALTH CENTER ADVOCACY

As it relates to the SBHCPP intended impacts, the WKKF created an expectation of grantees that educational policy and engagement of the educational community would be integrated as strategic and valued in the sustainability and vitality of SBHCs. Figure 11.2 on the education policy adoption continuum displays bench-

TABLE 11.1 — ALIGNING SCHOOL-BASED HEALTH CENTER (SBHC) SERVICES WITH NO CHILD LEFT BEHIND (NCLB) ACT MANDATES

NCLB Criteria	SBHC Contribution
Title I — Part C Education of Migratory Children	Immunizations and health records of migrant children served are required to be supplied to the national database. As SBHCs treat clients, data could be provided to the schools to input.
Title I — Part D Prevention and Intervention Programs for Children and Youth Who Are Neglected, Delinquent, or At-Risk	Prevention and intervention services, information, screening, and treatment of affected students could be performed at SBHCs.
Title IV — 21st Century Schools	Drug and alcohol prevention education, testing, screening, counseling, and treatment options might already be provided in SBHCs.

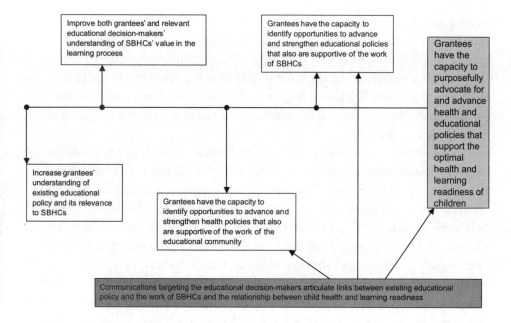

Note. SBHC=school-based health center.

Figure 11.2 — School-based health care policy program educational policy learning curve and policy development continuum.

marks of progression toward health and educational policy integrations. Throughout the tenure of the SBHCPP, the continuum served to help the Foundation measure the progress of grantees toward the goal of integrating the educational community into their work as though the "silos" no longer existed.

"Tell, Show, Do" was the mantra of SBHCPP technical support. As the terms reflect, before expecting a transformation of practice (e.g., embracing educators as advocacy partners), grantees needed to be told why partnerships were relevant and how to begin a shift from their disciplinary "silo"-ed paradigm. Then, they needed coaching on how to integrate education representatives and educational policies into their work. Finally, armed with the tools of "tell" and "show" they were equipped to "do" the work necessary to meet the WKKF's expectations.

Documents provided to grantees described federal, state, and local educational governance ("tell"). Presentations at conferences with other members of the SBHC community were used to provide evidence of the benefits of actively engaging educators ("show"). Workshops were hosted by grantees during which the Foundation provided technical assistance demonstrating the value of engagement, providing practical tips for engaging school personnel, and identifying policy targets that bridged health and educational priorities ("show"). Gradually, given the combination of the explicit expectation to engage the educational community and ample technical support that included grantees' forums wherein the resource team[a] provided specific examples of how to take advantage of opportunities that existed in each state, grantees began to reap the benefits of their new appreciation of educators as advocacy partners. Educators were invited to serve on state assembly boards, participate in advocacy events, and advocate for mutually relevant education and health policies ("do").

An example of terminology that improved grantees' understanding was the framing of educators as a "community" with its own language, priorities, governance, and political pressures. This concept was presented at the Learning Forum conducted approximately midway through the grant tenure. The proverbial light bulb came on at least in part due to the widespread attention the resource team had placed on community engagement, the need to engage populations different than oneself sensitively, and strategic use of communications tools to do so. Having experienced the importance of honoring the idiosyncratic dimensions of the communities they served provided an intellectual framework for viewing educators in a new way. This process affirmed the power of language not only in terms of advocacy but also relative to encouraging changes in perspective.

The WKKF program leadership also supported educational policy integration in the psyche and advocacy efforts of grantees. The WKKF program director consistently insisted that work plans, annual reports, and evaluation reports demonstrate inclusion of the educational community. Thus, annual feedback to grantees included acknowledgment of advances in integrating educators and educational policy as part of the program's overarching goal, as well as missed opportunities. This annual reinforcement demonstrated adherence to the "Tell, Show, Do" paradigm.

One demonstration of integration of education was the selection of school dropouts as an issue of great significance to both the health and education communities. Using Nicholas Freudenberg and Jessica Ruglis's article as a basis for discussion, an American Public Health Association (APHA) session was co-sponsored by the WKKF where representatives from each of the SBHCPP disciplines[b] discussed how their areas of expertise could inform the role SBHCs could play in reducing and recovering dropouts.[18]

The years of nudging grantees to become savvy about educational policy took consistent support and time, but, as the SBHCPP final assessment can assert, the results were impressive. During the early days of the Obama Administration,

---

[a] The resource team was the SBHCPP name given to the group of experts providing technical assistance to grantees.

[b] Education and Health Policy, Strategic Communications, Community Engagement, Multicultural Lens, and Evaluation.

educational initiatives such as Race to the Top[c] and the release of the *ESEA Blueprint for Reform* propelled SBHC advocates into action in ways that they would not have prior to participation in SBHCPP. Webinars on how to be supportive of state Race to the Top applications were jointly hosted by the National Assembly on School Based Health Care and the California School–Health Centers Association and included experts informing partnership building. As another example, the Coalition for Community Schools became a valued partner particularly well positioned given the high visibility of community schools[d] in both the federal Departments of Health and Human Services and Education.

SCHOOL-BASED HEALTH CARE POLICY PROGRAM EDUCATION AND HEALTH POLICY SYNERGY

Despite the multidisciplinary jargon about addressing barriers to education, re-engaging students who have become disconnected and unmotivated, and creating "successful safe and healthy students," little is directly coming from the educational community that is supportive of preventative health interventions, early detection, and health maintenance critical to healthy students ready to learn.[28] This, as was noted earlier, is at least in part due to the overwhelming accountability demands on educators.

Restated, advancing health is not part of the fundamental mission of schools nor has it been integrated into public consciousness as a fundamental pillar of learning. Because schools serving students with the greatest needs also tend to command the fewest resources, it seems that a public health ecological-oriented strategy of comprehensive partnerships targeting prevention and early intervention would be prudent.[5] If there is to be movement from rhetorical acknowledgment that health disparities and achievement gaps interact, it appears the impetus will have to come from the public health community.

Synergy has been defined as the simultaneous action of separate agencies that together have a greater impact than the sum of their individual contributions. The many successes of collaborations of SBHCPP grantees and the educational community discussed throughout both this chapter and volume support the value of

---

[c] The American Recovery and Reinvestment Act of 2009 provided $4.35 billion for the Race to the Top Fund, a competitive grant program designed to encourage and reward states that are creating the conditions for education innovation and reform.

[d] A comprehensive education model where schools are the site of a cadre of social support services, including the provision of health and dental services, and community-defined programming during and after traditional school hours designed for students and their families.

continued efforts in this regard for the school-based health care movement. As such, there are five useful tenets used in the SBHCPP that can influence the replication of the program's success: embrace the mindset, map existing relationships, seek opportunities to collaborate, optimize opportunities and interactions, and build on existing tools and resources.

Embrace the mindset refers to engaging educational partners and pursuing educational policy that is not an "add on" but rather a strategic decision to be more efficient and effective in the policy work that ultimately will help sustain your organization and the school-based health care movement. There is potential advocacy reciprocity in School–SBHC collaborations that can positively impact youth. **Mapping existing relationships** with educators is a good place to begin to cultivate "champions" and make in-roads into the educational policy arena. **Seeking opportunities to collaborate** calls for an examination of existing or new education policies, as well as those policies in the process of reauthorization that have health implications and provide opportunities to collaborate. **Optimizing opportunities and interactions** requires advocates to familiarize themselves with the "world" of educators in order to optimize interactions, e.g., timing of visits in the school year cycle, NCLB linkages, and local education issues, such as district consolidation. And finally, becoming an active stakeholder contributing to the advocacy movement can be augmented by **taking advantage of "tools" available** to make presentations and gather data, anecdotes, and stories rather than starting from scratch. For example, school-based health care state association websites and the NASBHC have many free resources available.

For the purposes of advocating for the neediest of America's children, knowing who to target and when is paramount not only for the SBHCPP grantees but also for those fueling the school-based health care movement. In the final analysis, what matters most to vulnerable children is a comprehensive integrated intervention approach to health and educational success. The words of former Surgeon General Joycelyn Elders ring true when she said,

> If I could make any changes at all to the current health care system, you know I would start with education, education, education. You can't educate people that are not healthy. But you certainly can't keep them healthy if they're not educated.[29]

REFERENCES

1. World Resources Institute. *Linking Environment and Health: Poverty, Health and the Environment*. Washington, DC: World Resource Institute; 1999.

2. Fiscella K, Kitzman H. Disparities in academic achievement and health: the intersection of child education and health policy. *Pediatrics.* 2009;123(3):1073–1080.

3. Richardson JW. The health and cognitive consequences of international child poverty. In: Yeakey CC, Richardson JW, Buck JB, editors. *Suffer the Little Children: National and International Dimensions of Child Poverty.* Amsterdam, The Netherlands: Elsevier Press JAI; 2006:335–358.

4. Seith D, Isakson E. *Who Are America's Poor Children? Examining Health Disparities Among Children in the United States.* New York, NY: National Center for Children in Poverty; 2011.

5. Basch CE. *Healthier Students Are Better Learners: A Missing Link in School Reforms to Close the Achievement Gap.* New York, NY: The Campaign for Educational Equity, Teachers College Columbia University; 2010.

6. Children's Defense Fund. *The State of America's Children 2004.* Washington, DC: Children's Defense Fund; 2004.

7. Guo G, Harris KM. The mechanisms mediating the effects of poverty on children's intellectual development. *Demography.* 2000;37(4):431–447.

8. US Department of Education National Center for Education Statistics. *The Condition of Education 2004.* NCES 2004-077. Washington, DC: US Government Printing Office; 2004.

9. Geierstanger SP, Amaral G. *School-Based Health Centers and Academic Performance: What Is the Intersection?* April 2004 Meeting Proceedings. White Paper. Washington, DC: National Assembly on School-Based Health Care; 2005.

10. Richardson JW. *Public K–12 Federal Educational Policy.* Battle Creek, MI: The W. K. Kellogg Foundation; 2006.

11. Richardson JW. *The Full-Service Community School Movement: Lessons From the James Adams Community School.* New York, NY: Palgrave MacMillan; 2009.

12. Juszczak L, Schlitt J, Odum M, Barangan C, Washington D. School-based health centers: a blueprint for healthy learners—data from the 2001–2002 School-Based Health Center Census. In: Lear JG, Isaacs SL, Knickman JR, eds. *School Health Services and Programs.* San Francisco, CA: Jossey-Bass; 2006:294–307.

13. Takanishi R. Leveling the playing field: supporting immigrant children from birth to eight. *The Future of Children.* 2004;14(2):61–79.

14. Massachusetts Department of Education. Dropouts in Massachusetts Public Schools: 2003–04. Malden: Massachusetts Department of Education; 2005.

15. Van Dorn RA, Bowen GL, Blau JR. The impact of community diversity and consolidated inequality on dropping out of high school. *Family Relations.* 2006;55(1):105–118.

16. Swanson CB. *Cities in Crisis: A Special Analytic Report on High School Graduation.* Bethesda, MD: America's Promise Alliance; 2008.

17. Bridgeland JM, DiIulio JJ Jr, Morison KB. *The Silent Epidemic: Perspectives of High School Dropouts.* Washington, DC: Bill & Melinda Gates Foundation; 2006.

18. Freudenberg N, Ruglis J. Reframing school dropout as a public health issue. *Prev Chronic Dis.* 2007;4(4):1–11. Available at: http://www.cdc.gov/pcd/issues/2007/oct/07_0063.htm. Accessed July 24, 2011.

19. Patterson JA, Hale D, Stessman M. Cultural contradictions and school leaving: a case study of an urban high school. *The High School Journal.* 2007;91(2):1–15.

20. Geierstanger SP, Amaral G, Mansour M, Walters SR. School-based health centers and academic performance: research, challenges, and recommendations. *J Sch Health.* 2004;74(9):347–352.

21. Hamm EM. Managing asthma in the classroom. *Childhood Education.* 2004;81(1):16–20.

22. Bireda S. Healthy students are better students: health reform bill gives a boost to school-based health centers. Center for American Progress. 2010. Available at: http://www.americanprogress.org/issues/2010/05/healthy_students.html. Accessed July 24, 2011.

23. Walker SC, Kerns SE, Lyon AR, Bruns EJ, Cosgrove TJ. Impact of school-based health center use on academic outcomes. *J Adolesc Health.* 2009;46(3):251–257.

24. Wirt FM, Kirst MW. *The Political Dynamics of American Education.* Second ed. Richmond, CA: McCutchan Publishing Corporation; 2001.

25. Odland J. NCLB—More Questions Than Answers. *Childhood Education.* 2005;81(3): 158b–158c.

26. Richard A, Davis MR. Governors seek help from federal officials on NCLB law, funds. *Education Week.* 2005;24(26):19.

27. Baines LA, Stanley GK. High-stakes hustle: public schools and the new billion dollar accountability. *Educ Forum.* 2004;69(1):8–16.

28. Center for Mental Health in Schools. *Turning Around, Transforming, and Continuously Improving Schools: Federal Proposals Are Still Based on a Two- Rather than a Three-Component Blueprint.* Los Angeles: University of California Los Angeles; 2010.

29. Great-Quotes.com website. Available at: http://www.great-quotes.com. 2011. Accessed August 29, 2011.

About the Authors

Jeanita W. Richardson, PhD, MEd – is an Associate Professor in the Department of Public Health Sciences at the University of Virginia School of Medicine. Her scholarship highlights the inextricable links between health and learning readiness, particularly for disenfranchised children and youth. Her work has been published and presented in numerous national and international journals and conferences. Her consulting energies (Turpeau Consulting Group, LLC) are devoted to supporting healthy children who are ready to learn through the creation of health and educational policy bridges and include five years as a consultant to the W. K. Kellogg Foundation's School-Based Health Care Policy Program. For more information, email TConsultingG@aol.com.

Terri D. Wright, MPH, ABD – is Director of the newly established Center for School, Health, and Education at the American Public Health Association. She provides leadership to the strategic development of school-based health programming and policy to avert school dropout. Formerly, she served for 12 years as a Program Director for Health Policy at the W. K. Kellogg Foundation and provided leadership for the Foundation's school-based health care policy program. Terri was Maternal and Child Health Director and Bureau Chief for Child and Family Services at the Michigan Department of Community Health where she managed policy, programs, and resources with the goal of reducing preventable maternal, infant, and child morbidity and mortality. She has a Bachelor's degree in Community and School Health and a Master's degree in Public Health. She is currently a doctoral candidate in Public Health at the University of Michigan. Terri takes an active leadership role in several professional and community organizations including the Institute of Medicine Roundtable on the Promotion of Health Equity and the Elimination of Health Disparities.

Bringing a Multicultural Approach to School-Based Health Care Policy Advocacy

Valerie Batts, John Capitman, and Douglas Weinstock

While school-based health centers (SBHCs) seek to be recognized through financing and regulation as essential community-based health care providers for children and families, there has been growing attention to local, state, and national policy advocacy. The W. K. Kellogg Foundation, building on other programmatic efforts to address health inequities, initiated a six-year program in 2004 to support nine state SBHC associations and the National Assembly on School-Based Health Care (NASBHC) in strengthening their capacity for policy advocacy and program improvement.[1,2] An essential aspect of this initiative to strengthen coalitions promoting the SBHC movement has been adoption of a multicultural/racial equity (MC/RE) lens on policy goals, advocacy, local access and engagement, and quality enhancement. Service provider organizations and clinicians have been core participants in school health advocacy, and many found themselves challenged to learn new skills around systems and policy change. Further, since most SBHC leaders are from historically included groups (i.e., Whites, formally educated, middle class, and so on) and many in the SBHC clientele, and natural allies and potential collaborators, are from historically excluded groups, school health movement leaders are recognizing the need to adopt a multicultural approach across their efforts. This chapter will explore the tenets that informed the integration of an MC/RE lens with the SBHC grantee's comprehensive development. Highlighted are key lessons learned regarding how to empower school health advocates to adopt an MC/RE lens in order to foster policy change.[3]

BUILDING A SCHOOL HEALTH MOVEMENT

The school-based health care movement started in the early 1970s with a handful of projects and reached a critical mass in the early 1980s. Currently, there are more than 1,900 SBHCs in 43 states serving over two million young people across the United States every year. A number of states are in the process of planning for and opening new centers. Approximately 40% of students served have no other medical home, due to limited health care for youth. A goal of the W. K. Kellogg School-Based Health Care Policy Program (SBHCPP) was to support the movement in creating and sustaining policy change to provide health care for young people from historically excluded groups. Technical assistance was provided to grantees in the areas of community engagement, strategic communications, leadership enhancement, organizational development, resource development, health and education policy change, and evaluation as an organization decision-making tool.

The W. K. Kellogg Foundation further sought to infuse a focus on MC/RE into each of these core areas. Figure 12.1 illustrates this dynamic.[4] W. K. Kellogg technical assistance providers, inspired by SBHC stakeholders, worked together to articulate the process. The figure illustrates an emerging vision for how SBHCs can be supported in helping to increase equity in youth outcomes. A critical aspect of this integrated approach to policy change that emerged was the need to ensure that educators' voices were included in the movement in the same way historically excluded groups were integrated into the work. This involved hearing educators' views and perspectives on the benefits of SBHCs currently and what educators saw as possibilities. Though released after the SBHCPP began, another critical reason for educators' inclusion was validated by the recent report from the Robert Wood Johnson Foundation in 2009 demonstrating that the single best way to support health is to create and sustain quality education.[5]

DEFINING KEY ELEMENTS OF A MULTICULTURAL/RACIAL EQUITY LENS

The initiative infuses an MC/RE lens into comprehensive development efforts with the SBHC grantees by using current thinking on the causes of health and education inequities as its theoretical framework. Both training and consultation materials and practices reflected this model. Growing literatures in both public health and education have sought for years to explain and manage the interacting roles of macro-individual (historical and socioeconomic context, public policies, service accessibility) and individual factors in shaping youth health and educational

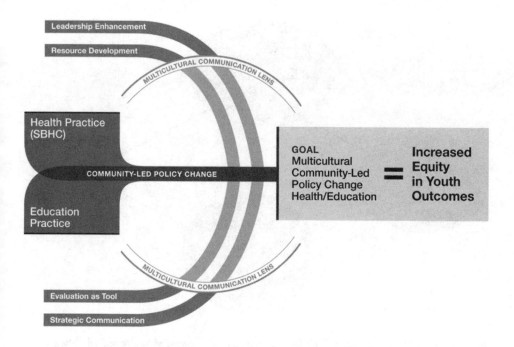

Note. Adapted from work by Capitman and Herrera.[4] This model was further informed by input from the School-Based Health Care Policy Program (SBHCPP) Resource Team, Maria Elena Campisteguy, The Metropolitan Group, Jeanita Richardson, Douglas Taylor, Southwest Community Research Center, and Terri Wright, Kellogg Foundation Program Director. The original model was developed by The Metropolitan Group for the W. K. Kellogg SBHCPP.

Figure 12.1 — Integrated model to increase equity in youth outcomes.

outcomes.[6–10] Figure 12.2 combines several of these approaches in a simplified theory of the causes of health and educational equities.

As summarized in Figure 12.2, three sets of factors are inter-related, and each has direct effects on health and educational inequities. In this context, we are using "inequity" interchangeably to reference sustained differences in life outcomes among socially defined groups (such as gender, social class or racial/ethnic groups) that are unfair. These differences are unfair in the sense that they are in addition to effects of individual differences in genetics, motivation, or behavior. The three factors that shape health and education inequities are **unequal social and environments** (groups with less economic and political power are exposed to less health-promoting environments and settings, such as differences across communities in access to after-school physical activity space or less access to computers), **unequal access to health care and education** (groups with less economic and political power are less likely to have the resources and support to acquire access to needed health

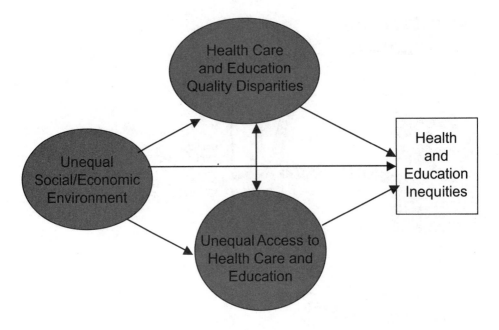

Figure 12.2 — A theoretical framework for understanding the causes of health and education inequities.

care and education resources on a timely basis, such as differences across communities in access to supports for lifelong adherence to prevention advice or the creation of a college-going culture), and **health care and education disparities** (groups with less economic and political power are exposed to lower quality, less individualized, and less responsive health care and education services). Using a simplified heuristic (Figure 12.2), this framework notes that past policies and practices have created disparate opportunity contexts for youth, exposing some to environments and programs that directly reduce their chances for positive health and educational outcomes. At the same time, historic and current inequities are also associated with (1) unequal access to health and educational services and (2) unequal quality of health and educational services. Each of these discrete inequities interacts with one another multiplying the disadvantage experienced by some groups.

The translation of this conceptual framework to building community-led policy development and advocacy is an ongoing educational process. It requires moving from a "monocultural"/time-bound approach to a multicultural approach that emphasizes taking the needed time to develop engagement, trust building, and so on. The current political climate in general and the specific debate on health care reform are key examples of how hard it is for our country to address with civility fundamental differences in worldview and circumstance. SBHC providers and advocates quickly recognized that given the differences in demographics between users, providers, and decision-makers, a shift in perspective among all was critical. Through the W. K. Kellogg initiative, SBHCPP grantees have begun to understand that recognizing, understanding, and changing this power dynamic is a critical contributor to effective SBHC clinical and advocacy efforts. In this context, SBHC advocates are joining with others in the growing commitment to address the role of racism/ethnocentrism, classism, and so on, in the continuation of health and education outcome inequities. Moving from an individual model of understanding illness and disease to a social, policy, and systems change approach is often challenging for parents, families, and educators.[11–13] Based on experiences in the SBHC initiatives, there appear to be at least five elements necessary for nurturing a movement that emphasizes culturally sensitive practice, inclusive engagement and organizing, and equity-focused advocacy.[14]

CONSIDER BOTH GROUP AND INDIVIDUAL IDENTITIES

Individual identity has become the US standard of care and of education. A key first step in the incorporation of a multicultural lens is being willing to and intentional about viewing all issues (i.e., relationships, communication, power dynamics, access, policy, practices), with attention given to both group and individual implications. For example, in considering how to move beyond its more traditional role of serving individuals, SBHCs are attending to their essential role of reaching historically excluded groups in order to reduce health inequities (e.g., Native Americans, Somali immigrants, migrant worker families). With one fairly recent immigrant group, it became clear that there was a need to understand the stigma around immunizations and to create a bridge between western medicine and beliefs within the community. Over time, the SBHCs most involved with this immigrant group realized that there was a need not only to address immunization stigma but also to understand the influence of native country demography on health decisions and intragroup interactions.

UNDERSTAND OPPRESSION AND CREATE CHANGE AT FOUR INTERLOCKING LEVELS

Analysis for policy change is strengthened by attention to four levels and their intersections: personal (attitudes, beliefs, values), interpersonal (behavior), institutional (rules, practices), and cultural (aesthetics, unwritten/covert rules).[15] Targeting of only similarities hampers building effective partnerships at any of these levels. For example, an SBHC association may have predominantly sought collaborations with individual leaders who share its political perspectives and thus missed chances to build partnerships with individuals and organizations that differ. In one state, given concerns of Republican legislators about reproductive health services, there was outreach that used messages to diffuse myths about such services, funding, and decision-making. In terms of the goal of building a "social movement" around SBHCs, another state association came to realize that using the term "social" created suspicion on the part of those who associated it with "socialist" or "social justice." Subsequently, they described the work as a "collaboration," which was a useful redefinition of the mission.

RECOGNIZE, UNDERSTAND, APPRECIATE, AND UTILIZE DIFFERENCES

A multicultural lens utilizes similarities and differences. This is important at the personal and interpersonal levels and in how we structure systems to allow for both of these dimensions. A helpful analogy might be to conceive of the goal as representing who is and who is not at the table, where the table is located, how it is "set," and what is "served." Akin to learning a new language, there is the need to immerse oneself and/or one's organization in the "new" approach, i.e. attention to differences and to the idea that if "we do not use it (in this case, the inclusive language), we lose it." One state association realized that they needed to change the time that meetings were held in order to get a wider range of people and stakeholders at the table. This led to examining other cultural practices, i.e., how meetings are held, where, and so on.

CREATE A HEALING ENVIRONMENT TO SUPPORT "VULNERABLE" POPULATIONS

Fostering effective systems requires organizational climates that support no "blame, shame, attack" and personal and organizational accountability for the incorporation of a multicultural approach. This is a lifelong process of uncovering our assumptions, beliefs, biases, and so on, based on lived experiences and messages both caught and taught, as well as on challenging historically and covertly exclusive systems. There will need to be ongoing formal and informal strategies for engaging new members who come into the environment. It is also critical to consider the strengths of all populations. A White state association board member, in an attempt to make a new African American board member feel more comfortable stepped outside her "comfort zone" to take time to chat with her outside the meeting. This example of the importance for some of having personal connections beyond the "business" at hand has implications for building authentic and sustainable relationships with potential collaborators for policy change.

UNCOVER SUBTLE, UNINTENTIONAL POWER IMBALANCES

It is important to build in a process for examining and challenging "modern" subtle ways in which "isms" can play out in relationships, programming, policy analysis, and change.[16] Effective work includes naming and creating strategies for challenging often invisible power imbalances. Questions need to be asked, such as, "How does the process allow adequate contact with all relevant players and consider cultural sensitivities about policy advocacy? Does it provide help that is actually helpful?" Instead, it is common for well-intentioned people who are "in charge" to spend considerable time and effort trying to determine what will work best for "others." In the case of determining hours of operation for an SBHC, it was important that a process be established for obtaining genuine input (advocacy) from all potential users so that the center could be accessible to various populations in the community. Examination of times that parents and caregivers from historically excluded groups were available exposed one critical way that class and other barriers were operating at the systemic and structural policy level.

DEFINING A POLICY AND SYSTEM CHANGE FRAMEWORK

State as well as national SBHC associations and SBHCs have needed to become their own advocates and join with others to make changes at the local, state, regional, and national level.[17] It became clear early in this initiative that the majority of the active state players came from a background of experience as health service providers. Therefore, enhanced understanding of policy and advocacy skills became critical. It also seemed apparent that teaching stakeholders to understand and utilize a collaborative approach to policy and systems analysis for change would be key to effective collaborative building and systems change.

Further, such change efforts, to be transformative, must include ongoing relationship development with people and groups who are similar and different. Such work must support ongoing, meaningful multicultural community engagement. This process involves identifying values, objectives, and interests of the various collaborators and competitors and what policies are needed to support effective change. Participants found this process both challenging and rewarding.

Creating a policy and systems change framework for the SBHC movement also required naming power imbalances. Access to health care and other supports for healthy development have been more available to some groups than to others. Groups historically excluded and discounted by policies and culture include students and families of color, working and lower socioeconomic class members, young people, elders, and immigrants. Other groups, such as Whites, middle- and owning-class persons, and those who are US born historically have been empowered and advantaged by policies and culture. These historical inequities perpetuate disparities in access to care, appropriateness of care, financing, and other dimensions. Table 12.1 summarizes these power imbalances.

In light of these power imbalances, over time most collaborations use at least four arenas to guide their analyses:

1. Inclusion, power, and fairness—Who is at the table? What do they want?
2. Resources—How does the money flow?
3. Creating systems with equitable access—How is care delivered?
4. Opportunities for immediate and sustained change—How are short-term improvements and "root causes" addressed?[18]

These questions and subsequent processes to address responses invite both historically included and historically excluded group members to think about themselves and others as participants in the policy and advocacy process.

TABLE 12.1—POWER CONCEPTS OF HISTORICALLY EMPOWERED AND EXCLUDED GROUPS

Power Concepts	Historically Excluded and Discounted by Policies and Culture	Historically Empowered and Advantaged by Policies and Culture
Racism	African American, Latino, NHOPI, Native American, Asian American	Whites
Sexism Heterosexism	Women, transgender GLBT	Men heterosexual
Classism	Working and lower socioeconomic class	Middle/owning class
Ageism	Ages <25 and >55 years	Ages 25–55 years
Xenophobia	Immigrants and their children	US born
Ableism	Chronically ill/disabled	Temporarily able

Note. NHOPI=Native Hawaiian or Pacific Islander; GLBT=gay, lesbian, bisexual, transgender.

DESCRIBING THE PROCESS OF CHANGE

All participants in this initiative were asked to understand how an MC/RE lens works on a number of dimensions. To facilitate change, the framework first defined inequities in power and outcomes. Participants explored examples of the new behaviors they could adopt to promote change across a range of contexts—personal, interpersonal, systemic, and cultural. Participants then looked at those within their organizations and networks who filled various roles in the community. Identifying and building on relationships by understanding the motivations of potential collaborators and competitors was emphasized. Participants were taught that change comes from recognizing, understanding, and appreciating similarities as well as differences in each of these areas. Given this broad understanding, participants were provided education and technical assistance with respect to defining the key health and education policy issues most important to SBHCs.

Participants then began to identify multiple factors that needed to be considered to create system changes that reduce unfair outcomes. They were learning how to identify the problems to be addressed and how current policies created and sustained these problems.

Participants were encouraged to identify across different aspects of the social, economic, and physical environments (1) how unequal conditions and opportunities shape the well-being and healthy development of children, adolescents and communities and (2) the range of public and private policies that create and sustain these inequalities. Participants began to see how their concerns around school-based health care were interwoven with a broader range of policy factors and advocacy agendas. As participants continued to build their collaborative, they gained understanding of individual and group shared interests and began to define wants and needs. Three elements of the W. K. Kellogg approach to integrating an MC/RE lens in the SBHC movement are described below and key lessons are highlighted in Table 12.2.

MULTICULTURAL/RACIAL EQUITY LENS AS A CONDITION FOR PARTICIPATION

The W. K. Kellogg Foundation used an intentional process that required potential grantees to think about a multicultural lens as a condition of their selection, stating clearly from the beginning in 2004 that this was a "cross cutting" theme that was to permeate all of the grantees' work.[19] Participants in this initiative were

TABLE 12.2—KEY ELEMENTS IN CREATING A MULTICULTURAL/RACIAL EQUITY (MC/RE) LENS AND IMPLEMENTATION CONSIDERATIONS

Key Element	Implementation Considerations
MC/RE lens as a condition for participation	• Assess level of readiness of potential grantees to adopt MC/RE lens given their resources and community dynamics • For many grantees, MC/RE lens will create unforeseen interpersonal and organizational dynamics • Know that most in this movement think first of service delivery • Provide education on applying a multicultural lens related to organizational development and policy and systems change
Awareness and skill-building training for key stakeholders	• Establish ongoing assessment across multiple knowledge and skill areas (cultural/emotional literacy, organizational development, policy analysis, advocacy) • Provide tools for applying MC/RE lens to organizational development and policy advocacy • Be prepared for staff and board turnover; provide new members with MC/RE lens and other training • Integrate MC/RE lens into work of all members of the technical assistance/resource team supporting initiative
Ongoing technical assistance	• Be clear what is negotiable and what is not with respect to how grantees work with the integrated approach • Continue to deepen participants' understanding and lessons learned from working in collaboratively run multicultural teams • Continue to help them refine policy targets and systemic changes needed • Reward successes and persistence

in very different places with respect to their readiness to engage, often because they did not know this "language" or "weren't aware of what they didn't know" in this regard. For example, most of the state SBHC assemblies and associations were founded by dedicated health care professionals who were volunteering their time, and the organizations were being "governed" by Executive Boards comprised of these mostly White "founding mothers." For some, it took a while to understand the importance and necessity of expanding Board membership to incorporate more diversity in terms of background (similar to users of the centers) and experience. In some situations, this presented the challenge of replacing current White female Board members with new members from more diverse backgrounds and of determining ways to value and use what these members had to offer.

AWARENESS AND SKILL-BUILDING TRAINING FOR KEY STAKEHOLDERS

Key stakeholders, in intensive four-day experiences, began and/or enhanced their ability to use a common language to uncover how racism and other forms of oppression play out in their work. Efforts were made over time to integrate the MC/RE lens into all facets of the program to ensure that the ongoing application would occur. For example, a situation arose in the four-day training for 12 staff and board members (some SBHC practitioners) from one of the grantees. The racially mixed group (four Black, eight White, one of whom was a gay father) differed from prior compositions of the organization. The group arrived to start day two with some tension and hard feelings. For dinner the previous evening, the well-meaning White Executive Director had hoped to arrange for their whole "delegation" to dine together. As it turned out, the Black members of the group opted to dine on their own (in this very White, New England seaside town) and the Executive Director was distressed. It turned out to be an excellent opportunity for the group to become more cohesive, by coming to understand the dynamics in this situation as well as lingering prior resentments, all using a MC/RE lens.

ONGOING TECHNICAL ASSISTANCE FOR EFFECTIVE IMPLEMENTATION

A key challenge is managing the competing needs that grantees are addressing. It is important to establish flexible and revisable time lines that allow grantees to explore thoroughly what they want that is new versus what they think they should want. For instance, many of the grantees have become committed to engaging youth in meaningful ways, with at least one having created a Youth Board. This has created a need for adults to enhance their "multicultural lens" by looking at issues of "adultism" as they provide youth with increasing power. Training was provided by an adult and youth multicultural consultation team for staff and youth Board members in order to enhance the working relationship between these groups. Staff and Board had already made some changes to their meetings as a result of new meeting methods learned from youth Board members.

CONCLUSION

It is too early to know how the adoption of the MC/RE lens has influenced the effectiveness of the SBHC movement in establishing its role in the health care system or promoting equitable outcomes for children and families. In light of the multiple variations in the contexts and strategies characterizing program participants, it may be difficult to disentangle the influence of the MC/RE lens from other elements in the initiative. One way to capture the multicultural lens "journey" of both individuals and organizations is to consider the progression from "unconscious incompetence" (we don't know what we don't know) to "unconscious competence" (naturally incorporating the perspective into ways of being and doing work). As shown through the examples in this chapter, there is evidence of such progression. Whatever the final assessment, our experiences indicate that the SBHC movement members are stretching and growing as they challenge often entrenched social systems. This initiative provides additional tools and an emerging model for navigating the road to equity that are relevant to ongoing efforts in many arenas.

REFERENCES

1. W. K. Kellogg Foundation. Brochure on Applying Policy Tools to Achieve Long-Term Change. 2003.

2. W. K. Kellogg Foundation. Brochure on Guidelines for Informing Public Policy. 2002.

3. W. K. Kellogg Foundation. School-based health care policy program. Available at: http://www.schoolbasedhealthcare.org/?page_id=156. Accessed October 29, 2009.

4. Capitman J, Herrera G. Binational Health Summit. Central Valley Health Policy Institute; California State University; October 25, 2006.

5. Egerter S, Braveman P, Sadegh-Nobari T, Grossman-Kahn R, Dekker M. Education matters for health. *Issue Brief 6: Education and Health*. Princeton, NJ: Robert Wood Johnson Foundation, Commission to Build a Healthier America; 2009.

6. Krieger N. Does racism harm health? Did child abuse exist before 1962? On explicit questions, critical science, and current controversies: an ecosocial perspective. *Am J Public Health*. 2008;98(Suppl 1):S20–S25.

7. Capitman JA, Bhalotra S, Ruwe M. *Cancer and Elders of Color: Opportunities for Reducing Health Disparities*. Hampshire, England: Ashgate; 2005.

8. Betancourt JR, Green AR, Carrillo JE, Park ER. Cultural competence and health care disparities: key perspectives and trends. *Health Aff (Milwood)*. 2005;24(2):499–505.

9. Evans T, Whitehead M, Diderichsen F, Bhuiya A, Wirth M. *Challenging Inequities in Health: From Ethics to Action*. Oxford, UK: Oxford University Press; 2001.

10. Mays VM, Cochran SD, Barnes NW. Race, race-based discrimination, and health outcomes among African Americans. *Annu Rev Psychol.* 2007;58:201–225.

11. Sue DW, Capodilupo CM, Torino GC, et al. Racial microaggressions in everyday life: implications for clinical practice. *Am Psychol.* 2007;62(4):271–286.

12. Trujillo MA, Bowland SY, Myers LJ, Richards PM, Roy B. *Re-Centering Culture and Knowledge in Conflict Resolution Practice.* Syracuse, NY: Syracuse University Press; 2008.

13. Tervalon M, Murray-García J. Cultural humility versus cultural competence: a critical distinction in defining physician training outcomes in multicultural education. *J Health Care Poor Underserved.* 1998;9(2):117–125.

14. Jones CP. Confronting institutionalized racism. *Phylon (1960–).* 2002;50(1/2):7–22.

15. Camara PJ. Levels of racism: a theoretic framework and a gardener's tale. *Am J Public Health.* 2000;90(8):1212–1215.

16. Batts V. Is reconciliation possible? Lessons from combating modern racism. In: Douglas IT, ed. *Waging Reconciliation.* Syracuse, NY: Church Publishing; 2002.

17. National Assembly on School-Based Health Care. National Assembly on School-Based Health Care website. Available at: http://www.nasbhc.org/site/c.jsJPKWPFJrH/b.2554077/k.BEE7/Home.htm. Accesssed November 5, 2010.

18. Tesh SN. *Hidden Arguments: Political Ideology and Disease Prevention Policy.* New Brunswick, NJ: Rutgers University Press; 1988.

19. Shapiro I. *Training for Racial Equity and Inclusion: A Guide to Selected Programs.* Washington, DC: The Aspen Institute; 2002.

About the Authors

Valerie Batts, PhD – is the Executive Director of VISIONS, Inc, which supports healing and empowerment in health and education settings while addressing institutional, structural/cultural, and personal barriers. Author of *Modern Racism: New Melody for the Same Old Tune* and *Is Reconciliation Possible: Lessons From Combating Modern Racism*, Dr. Batts has written extensively on strategies for creating racial equity. Since 1976, she has provided change strategies to service providers, educators, community leaders, philanthropists, and managers, both nationally and internationally. Dr. Batts helped conceptualize a multicultural approach to the W. K. Kellogg's school-based health center (SBHC) project and helped all technical assistance providers seek use of a multicultural lens.

John Capitman, PhD – a cofounder of VISIONS, Inc, is a social psychologist specializing in racial/ethnic, age, and class inequities in health and well-being. Dr. Capitman helped to develop the modern racism theory and its application to policy and systems change highlighted in VISIONS workshops and consultations. He earned his Doctorate from Duke University. From 1986 to 2005, he was Director of Long-Term Care Studies and Coordinator of the Inequalities Concentration at the Heller School, Brandeis University. Currently Dr. Capitman is Executive Director of the Central Valley Health Policy Institute (CVHPI) and Nickerson Professor of Public Health at California State University, Fresno. A model developed at CVHPI provided the template for the "Multicultural Approach to Policy and Systems Change Strategy" document that grew out of the W. K. Kellogg SBHC Initiative.

Douglas Weinstock, Med – has been a multicultural consultant with VISIONS, Inc, since 2001. In that capacity, he provided multicultural training and consultation to grantees of the W. K. Kellogg Foundation's School-Based Health Care Policy Program from 2005 to 2010, including state SBHC association staff, board members, youth, and direct service providers. His involvement was informed by many years of experience as a public school administrator, along with his commitment to meaningful inclusion and empowerment of the full range of stakeholders in the SBHC movement.

Application of a Multicultural Lens to Policy Work in Native American Communities

Maria Elena Campisteguy

Every day, thousands of advocacy organizations encounter the challenges of working in an increasingly multicultural society. Few organizations, however, authentically engage diverse communities in their advocacy for policy work, often by rationalizing that these communities have been unresponsive to their particular issue. This is a missed opportunity to unlock new resources and bring additional perspectives and talents to the table to develop innovative and sustainable solutions to our most challenging social, environmental, and economic issues. As the demographics of this country change, communities of color are increasing as proportions of the national population and are quickly becoming the voters, members, volunteers, donors, and stewards of tomorrow. Consequently, engaging diverse communities in advocacy for policy is an absolute necessity for organizational success and for building healthy communities.[1]

To engage in any meaningful discourse, and to create ownership of an issue, requires a deep understanding of a person's or group's cultural context—the norms, ideas, beliefs, and totality of meaning shared by a cultural group.[1] It is important for community organizers to understand the dynamics of power, language, relationships, values, traditions, world view, decision-making, and historic experiences with the issue and with political engagement overall.[2] Ultimately, for advocacy efforts to be truly sustainable, the people most impacted by an issue need to willingly take leadership roles and become intimately engaged as decision-makers and owners of strategy.[2]

In the multiyear School-Based Health Care Policy Program (SBHCPP) launched by the W. K. Kellogg Foundation (WKKF) to advance this model of care, this deep analysis of cultural context in advocacy for policy work was referred to as the "*application of a multicultural lens.*" At its core, this term refers to the intentional and continuous application of a perspective that recognizes, understands, and appreciates one's own cultural background and the cultural backgrounds of others.[3] This chapter describes the lessons faced and learned by "4 Youth" in leading policy work in Indian Country as captured by the youth and community organizers leading the work. The name of the group "4 Youth" is both a play on words (for youth) and a reference to significant Native cultural symbols (the four seasons, the four directions).

SBHCPP was guided by the vision that local communities most impacted by school-based health centers (SBHCs), especially young people, should be actively engaged in shaping the content, quality, delivery, and financing of health care in their communities. SBHCs are typically located in communities that include disproportionate numbers of vulnerable populations comprised of diverse racial and ethnic groups. The most recent census by the National Assembly of School-Based Health Care indicates that 70% of the student bodies in schools that have SBHCs are non-White. They include youth from Latino (36.8%), Black (non-Latino; 26.2%), Asian/Pacific Islander (4.4%), Native American/Alaskan Native (1.7%), and "other" (1.4%) communities.[3]

The WKKF awarded funds to nine state associations and 40 community partners with established SBHCs, including three sovereign nations in New Mexico: Navajo, Laguna Pueblo, and Acoma Pueblo. Each grantee, in turn, developed partnerships with youth and local groups to engage in advocacy campaigns at the local, tribal, state, and federal levels.[4] The diversity of constituents within SBHCs, combined with the unique geographic, political, and economic factors facing each participating state, made it a necessity to recognize that a "one size fits all" approach to advocacy work would be ineffective. Thus, multicultural development in all policy work was not just a strategy advanced by the WKKF and program; it was a core expectation.

Throughout the life of the program, state associations and their community partners experienced a multicultural process of change at four levels:

- Personal—the beliefs, feelings, attitudes, values, and prejudices about issues of diversity, inclusion, and multiculturalism;
- Interpersonal—behavior, interactions, and communication styles that maintain or enhance a multicultural environment within their organizations, particularly across race, ethnicity, and class;
- Institutional/Systemic—examining how policies, procedures, practices, and rules succeed or fail to support multicultural populations within their organizations; and
- Cultural—currently valued norms, customs, unwritten rules, symbols, rituals and expectations for professionalism and success that contribute to a sense of respect for diverse cultural backgrounds and feeling of inclusion within an organization.[4]

SBHCPP state association grantees applied a multicultural lens to all aspects of their advocacy work—from volunteer leadership and staff recruitment to community engagement, resource development, and communication. Further, the program recognized that the strength of policy advocacy hinged on applying a multicultural lens not only when engaging the youth most impacted by the centers but also when collaborating with diverse professional groups and partners. The most important professional partners were the historically distinct health and education communities, in light of the obvious intersection of both sectors within the world of school-based health care.[4]

LESSONS LEARNED IN INDIAN COUNTRY POLICY WORK

There were multiple lessons learned with respect to the application of a multicultural lens to policy work that emerged from this six-year journey of the SBHCPP. Some of the most profound learning took place in the advocacy work led by 4 Youth through "Reaching Native American Youth Through School-Based Health Care," a project of the New Mexico Alliance for School-Based Health Care.

Funded as a grantee of the SBHCPP, 4 Youth focused on achieving changes in the federal and tribal systems that deliver health services for Native youth. One of their major state policy goals was to reduce the health disparities of Native youth in New Mexico, specifically the highest rate of youth suicide in the nation.

Eight distinct lessons emerged from observations and experiences and present valuable learning opportunities for other advocacy organizations planning to work within Indian Country, especially for those from outside Native communities.

1. Policy Work in Indian Country Requires a Long-Term Perspective and Approach

Key to implementing any advocacy for a policy campaign will be the recognition that it will take a more extended period of time to conduct organizing with Native communities.[5] What can be done in five years in a non-Native community takes seven or more years in Indian Country. For example, the University of New Mexico has a seven-year rule for accepting grants in Indian country.[6]

2. The Community Organizing Process Should Be Based on Informed Research of Local Tribal Governance

Tribal communities and sovereign nations each have a unique and distinct culture, governmental structure, process, demographics, and geography. Their histories with state and federal policies differ from tribe to tribe and must be acknowledged when designing an advocacy campaign.[6] This requires detailed advance planning prior to engaging tribal members and active input and feedback from tribal members. To understand political relationships, ask questions such as: "Who are the traditional and nontraditional tribal members with familial or clan ties to a specific stakeholder?"[5] Then assess whether respondents are positive, negative, or neutral to the target issue.

3. The Unique and Distinct Culture and Traditions of Each Tribe Must Be Recognized in All Aspects of Policy Work

Integrating multiculturalism into policy work includes the acknowledgment that there is great diversity among Native tribes and advocacy strategies that need to be adapted to each tribe's customs and traditions.[6] The same strategies may not be effective in all cultures and bureaucracies in Indian Country. Similar to the research needed on tribal governance just described is the need to fully understand and integrate cultural traditions into the planning and organizing process.

When contextualizing the planning process to reflect tribal traditions and values, one should consider ceremonial or religious considerations, institutional review board processes, religious and governmental hierarchies, tribal connections, cultural methods, and tribal historical considerations (such as historical trauma, tribal relationships with state and federal governments, and so on). For example, honoring tribal traditions, such as opening a meeting with a prayer by an elder in his or her native tongue, will help set the right tone for the meeting.[5]

Facilitators must create space and opportunity in meetings for participants to comment and provide feedback. Silence does not necessarily indicate that people are in agreement about what is being said. In addition, the decision-making process should be well paced by allowing ample time (even weeks) for issues to settle and become local priorities (Aaron Carr, former program director of 4 Youth, interview, 2007).

4. Partner Advocacy Efforts With a Native American Facilitator and/or Community Organizers Who Are Knowledgeable About Tribal Customs and Values

As previously noted, every sovereign nation and tribal community has its own set of values, traditions, and beliefs. Non–Native American facilitators should partner with a tribal facilitator who is knowledgeable about the cultural norms in that community and, ideally, who is also familiar with federal Indian Law. The Native American facilitator will provide the cultural and political context unique to his or her tribal affiliation. One example is the distinction that is made between financial poverty and cultural poverty (loss of language and culture) in many Native American communities. A facilitator without local knowledge of this philosophy could risk placing a focus on "poverty levels" that could be considered as disrespectful by not acknowledging cultural values.[5]

In the case of direct organizing efforts, community organizers and others who work and live in the community are often the best to help design programs that work, particularly if they are not part of the state or tribal bureaucracies and are free to "organize."[6]

5. When Utilizing Non-Native Organizing Models, Ensure Careful Review of the Curriculum and All Terminology for Maximum Sensitivity

Language can be helpful in bridging the gap between the traditional values of a community and the benefits and resources offered through non-Native organizing models.[6] However, the application of a multicultural lens for Native policy advocacy must include the recognition that some strategies that work well in non–Native communities may not be appropriate to Native communities.[6]

The work requires cultural respect and avoidance of language that could be misinterpreted as confrontational. Examples of terminology from the model that may need to be examined with tribal members and possibly replaced include terms like "targets," "demands," and "altering the relations of power." There may be an opportunity to replace inappropriate terms with tribal lexicon or traditional language.[5]

6. Engage Tribal Elders and Native American Organizations

Once research has been conducted and thoughtful reflection has been applied to adapting the organizing process, it is crucial to meet with tribal elders prior to initiating any organizing activities. The engagement of elders to solicit support and guidance will help alleviate any potential tensions and conflicts in moving forward. Depending on the tribal nation or community, elders may require varying levels of involvement.[5]

It is critical to remember that due to historical experiences, some tribal members can be distrustful or skeptical.[6] Collaboration with Native American organizations as trusted allies, influencers, and pathways in the community is also helpful.[3]

7. Work on Health and Education Policy in Indian Country Is Complex and Multilayered

Health and education issues in Indian Country necessitate an understanding of multiple issues, jurisdictions, and systems that are interwoven within the fabric of Native American communities as sovereign nations and as distinct political groups that each have a special relationship with the federal government. Advocacy work requires a respect for tribal sovereignty and the understanding that each tribal government has an inherent authority to govern its own internal affairs, including the development of programs and implementation of budgets, policies, regulations, and other activities through government-to-government consultations with federal and state agencies. In the context of the SBHCPP, it is the tribal leaders who determine how they design centers in their own tribal communities.[6] Therefore, each community required a separate and customized strategy.

8. Native Voices Telling Their Own Stories Are the Most Effective With Policymakers

The organizing process in Indian country is slow and requires extreme patience and perseverance. But the end results can be rewarding and impactful. In the case of the 4 Youth project, for the first time in New Mexico Native American communities, youth took the leadership role in policy advocacy and successfully advocated for the establishment of a Native American peer-to-peer teen suicide prevention program.[7]

The young advocates not only identified the policy priority, researched the issue, and identified a sponsor for a bill at the state legislature, they also provided extensive testimony at legislative hearings and maintained a direct relationship with Governor Bill Richardson's office to ensure he did not exercise a line item veto. Once funding was secured, the youth collaborated with the New Mexico Department of Health to identify a suicide prevention program that would best meet the needs of Native youth.[6]

CONCLUSION

Any time we work with individuals from a culture whose values, perspectives, and expectations are different from our own, we must keep an open mind and acknowledge that there is much to learn. Part of this learning may present us with mental and emotional challenges on many different levels; our norms and what we know in our culture may be completely questioned by another culture.

As this chapter demonstrates, there is not a specific "one-size-fits-all" approach to working with and authentically engaging diverse constituents in policy work. Instead, the unique norms, values, traditions, and needs of each cultural group—whether Native Americans, other racial or ethnic groups, or even youth—must be carefully considered prior to engaging in the work.

REFERENCES

1. Campisteguy ME, Lee Dellinger LK, Friedenwald-Fishman E, Detman B, Gilstrap Hearn J. *Increasing Relevance, Relationships and Results: Principles and Practices for Effective Multicultural Communication.* Washington, DC: Metropolitan Group; 2008.

2. Friedenwald-Fishman E, Lee Dellinger LK, Gilstrap Hearn J, Pai-Esponsa J. *Building Public Will: Five-Phase Communication Approach to Sustainable Change.* Washington, DC: Metropolitan Group; 2009.

3. Zimmerman JB, Campisteguy ME, Parks L, Richardson JW. The School-Based Health Care Policy Program Capstone Evaluation. Battle Creek, MI: W. K. Kellogg Foundation; 2011.

4. Zimmerman JB, Campisteguy ME, Mandel L, Weymouth J. School-Based Health Care Policy Program: The Journey from 2004 to 2008. Program Evaluation. Battle Creek, MI: W. K. Kellogg Foundation; 2009.

5. W. K. Kellogg Foundation. Direct Action Organizing Model with Native American Communities Requires Cultural Adaptations. Battle Creek, MI: W. K. Kellogg Foundation; 2011.

6. New Mexico Alliance for School-Based Health Care. Capstone Report. Battle Creek, MI: W. K. Kellogg Foundation; 2010.

7. Campisteguy ME. Native American Youth Organize to Impact Health Policy. Battle Creek, MI: W. K. Kellogg Foundation; 2008.

About the Author

Maria Elena Campisteguy–is a Principal/Executive Vice President of The Metropolitan Group, a social marketing firm, where she leads the firm's Multicultural Communication practice. She has more than 25 years experience helping nonprofit organizations develop powerful brands and messages, develop strategies to engage new constituents, expand programmatic and service reach, advance policy, and increase their base of support. For five years, she was a consultant to the W. K. Kellogg Foundation's School-Based Health Care Policy Program, providing technical assistance to participating state associations and community partners. For additional communication resources, visit http://www.metgroup.com.

Using Strategic Communication to Advance Behavioral, Attitudinal, and Systems Change

Maria Elena Campisteguy and
Karen L. Saverino

Communication that fuels lasting change and creates staying power for an issue, idea, or point of view is a powerful tool for social change. For advocacy organizations, communication is an especially vital element of their work, whether aimed at influencing decision-makers, altering behavior patterns of private citizens, or triggering a change in the economic, political, or social expectations of society.[1]

Advocacy organizations require expertise in communication strategies within the policy arena; within their own organization, membership, and volunteer base; and across organizational partners. Communication with members and with policymakers is considered one of eight key indicators of capacity for state associations to effectively advance policy.[2]

This chapter describes the six-part strategic approach that Metropolitan Group uses to help clients craft effective communication. We have applied the approach to public health initiatives, including tobacco cessation and prevention among urban and rural populations; increasing HIV/AIDS testing and results retrieval among young males in cities across the country; lowering infant mortality and the incidence of low-birth-weight babies among Somali, Latino, and low-income White women; and helping to prevent fetal alcohol syndrome among the children of college-age women. (More examples are available at http//:www.metgroup.com.) For the past four years, we have used this approach while working with state associations affiliated with the W. K. Kellogg Foundation's School-Based Health Care Policy Program (SBHCPP).

A PRACTICAL AND NECESSARY ART: INTEGRATING COMMUNICATION WITH SCHOOL-BASED HEALTH CARE POLICY

In the SBHCPP, strategic communication has been used to help advance local, state, tribal, and federal policies that support school-based health care and to promote behavioral changes. In building support for the idea or issue, the art of communication is practical and necessary. If audiences don't value an idea or an issue, it won't gain traction or the support required to sustain it. Communication includes four elements: speaker, listener, message, and occasion/channel. The ultimate purpose of all communication is audience response.[3] Taking a multicultural approach increases the relevance and impact of the organization's communication by recognizing, respecting, and engaging the cultural backgrounds of all audiences and framing the communication in ways that invite real participation and dialogue.[1]

Strategic communication has successfully persuaded students to visit their school-based health center (SBHC), and it helped to support local advocacy efforts to persuade school districts to change their policies about serving fattening and sugary foods or about offering reproductive health services in an SBHC. Strategic communication in such vehicles as websites, news articles, and direct mail helped raise awareness about the need for the passage of legislation for state-level funding and reimbursement from Medicaid and managed care.

Examples of the role that strategic communication played in advancing policy include an effort to bring healthier milk to the nation's largest school district, New York City. Following media coverage of advocacy efforts by the city in the media, including news stories and editorials addressing the high-fat milk being served to students, the Department of Education decided to replace whole milk with 1% milk and to ban low-fat chocolate milk with chocolate skim milk in all public school lunchrooms. The policy change was featured in a front-page article of the *New York Times*.[4] And, in a small, primarily Hispanic community in Massachusetts, whose residents are often uninsured and experience high rates of poverty, high school students launched a campaign that included writing letters to their school board and speaking publicly for healthier choices in the school district's food service. As a result, school meals were changed to include nutritional information and a daily "healthy meal of the day" option that includes fresh fruit. In addition, the food services program established an after-school culinary club to teach students how to cook nutritiously.[5]

In addition to advancing policy targets and goals, state associations have used strategic communication to raise awareness about the effectiveness of SBHCs in meeting primary care and other health needs such as mental and oral health.

Strategic communication has helped associations to leverage public and private resources, attract donors, reach out to and engage diverse community members, and increase membership. Essential to the program has been increasing the capacities of state associations and local community partners (most often SBHCs) to identify audiences, formulate relevant messages, establish evidence and stories in support of these messages, and identify the appropriate delivery mechanism through selection of the right messengers and communication tools.

Affirming the importance of this approach, Terri D. Wright, Program Director of W. K. Kellogg Foundation's School-Based Health Care Policy Program, said,

> Strategic communication was vital to this program from the outset. We needed to advance this model of health care for children and adolescents and to show the value of school-based health centers in supporting school wellness and preventing issues such as school violence and school dropouts. Of critical importance was using a multicultural perspective so that our work could reach each audience with messages and messengers that resonated for them as individuals and therefore helped move them to action (Terri D. Wright, personal communication, February 3, 2009).

SIX STEPS TO CREATING STRATEGIC COMMUNICATION

There are six steps to creating strategic communication: identify the audience, develop the message, select the messengers, pick effective channels and tools, implement communication, and measure results.

Step 1. Identify the "Audience"

Many organizations that are new to communication mistakenly think that the "general public" or the persons they are currently reaching are their audience. Strategic communication requires going beyond the so-called "usual suspects" and identifying the individuals and organizations that are fundamental to achieving organizational and policy goals. By closely considering the priority audiences, limited human and financial resources can be targeted most effectively.

To help organizations select priority audiences and design specific communication messages and strategies to reach those audiences effectively, we use an audience identification map as indicated in Table 14.1. This tool facilitates thinking about priority audiences and how to connect the organization's issue with the needs, values, and motivators of those audiences, thereby causing them to act.

TABLE 14.1—AUDIENCE IDENTIFICATION MAP: EXAMPLE FOR SECURING A BILL TO CREATE A STATE-FUNDED NATIVE AMERICAN PEER-TO-PEER TEEN SUICIDE PREVENTION PROGRAM

Audience	What Do They Need and Value?	Pathway[a] and Messenger[b]	Channels/ Tools[c]	Call to Action[d]/ Message	Opposition Messaging[e]
New Mexico Native American State Representative	Healthy kids. Addressing health disparities (Representative formerly ran a youth center).	Policy director has relationship and can introduce members of the youth advisory group to tell their story.	Personal stories by youth. Bring toolkit to show video, share fact sheet developed by youth about health disparities for Native American youth suicide.	Sponsor bill; "Healthy kids do better in school."	How much is the state already investing in tribal suicide programs/ health programs? Bring data that shows very little investment and reinforces need.

[a] Who can help connect the organizations?
[b] Who is the right person to relay the message?
[c] Where and how do they get information?
[d] Where and how do they get information?
[e] What can we anticipate?

Specific to the SBHCPP, state associations worked to determine which "audiences" should be engaged in their advocacy work and who should be persuaded to take some form of action. For most of the associations, these audiences included local, state, and federal policymakers; youth and parents from diverse cultural communities; representatives of health and education communities; and strategic partners such as organizations that share a similar vision.

Working with staff, board members, and local partners, the audience identification map was adapted to guide each state association's outreach to particular audience groups. In some instances, additional columns, such as the desired action from that audience and content for messages, were included. In situations where the issue might be controversial, we also anticipated what the opposition would say and developed messages and data to respond.

The New Mexico Assembly on School-Based Health Care serves as an example of the value of the audience identification map in action. Their community partners included three sovereign tribes, and they determined that it was important to reach tribal leaders in New Mexico, as well as state policymakers, to advance this model of health care to serve the needs of Native American children in rural communities. "The audience mapping process made our team think more strategically about whom we needed to approach in order to raise awareness about school-based health care. It also helped us see where we needed to gather new alliances and partnerships," said Regina Begay-Roanhorse, program director for 4 Youth, a community partner-led project of the New Mexico Assembly on School-Based Health Care (Regina Begay-Roanhorse, personal communication, October 21, 2009).

A critical piece of policy work that 4 Youth worked on, primarily supporting the advocacy work of youth, was a teen peer-to-peer suicide prevention program. The audience mapping was helpful in reaching and securing support for a bill and appropriate funding. As the example in Table 14.1 indicates, a key audience was a Native American Representative of the New Mexico legislature who had formerly been a youth center director. He valued healthy kids and was committed to addressing health disparities. The project director was identified as the best pathway. She had worked with the Representative on other policy work. Knowing his passion for young people, the youth themselves were determined to be the most effective messengers. The channel was a direct meeting to share their personal stories and a preview of a video showing the impact of SBHCs on students, particularly those dealing with serious issues like suicide. The call to action was a request for the Representative to sponsor the bill. The opposition anticipated was the Representative's interest in data about existing state and tribal investments in suicide prevention programs, so as to avoid duplication of funding and efforts. Thus, data were researched ahead of time in conjunction with facts about disparities impacting Native American youth suicide.

Step 2. Develop the Message

Having effective messages is central to the success of any communication effort. Messages should be culturally relevant and based on having researched the audience's knowledge of and attitudes toward the issue. Various cultural groups have unique ways of perceiving, organizing, and relating to information. They may have different needs, values, motivators, and behaviors. The norm for one group may not necessarily be relevant or appropriate for another group. The message must fit the cultural context (the norms, ideas, beliefs, and totality of meaning shared by a cultural group) of the desired audiences. The more advocacy organizations learn about the specific communities they want to engage, the more strategic, specific, and effective their communication and outreach strategies can be.

Effective messages define the issue in clear terms (why there's a need for action), convey the relevance of the issue to the specific audience (why the audience should care about the issue), and provide a clear call to action (what the messenger is asking the decision-maker or audience to do). Values trump data when it comes to decision-making. People make decisions consciously and unconsciously based on their values, and then they utilize data to rationalize and support their choice. For individuals to maintain a lasting commitment to an issue as a personal priority and to hold a conviction that leads to action, the issue must connect to closely held personal values. Individual choices to speak out or take action on an issue flow from resonance between the issue and a person's core value system.[6]

Strategic messages are most often based on the gathering of data and evidence to support the messages and address potential resistance or opposition to an issue. The messages are brought to life by compelling stories. The stories help to magnify the values and to balance out the data so there is still emotional appeal.

To ensure that a consistent set of compelling messages was being used to help create awareness and unify communication across the field of school-based health, the WKKF retained a national research firm to poll voters on their likelihood to support SBHCs. The foundation hired a team of communication consultants, including the authors, to apply the data to create a set of messages that clearly describe school-based health.

The national polling results showed that two thirds of voters supported school-based health care once they learned more about it. Data also showed that getting into too much detail about the long list of services offered by SBHCs made voters less likely to support them. In addition, the research showed that voters liked that SBHCs made health care more accessible, kept children in school and learning, and provided mental health services to address issues like bullying and depression.[7]

Armed with this information, a set of overarching messages was drafted. The primary message was the result of the research itself: two thirds of voters support the concept of school-based health care. Knowing that keeping the message simple was key, the team came up with a brief analogy, "like a doctor's office in a school," to explain SBHCs. Users of the message were encouraged to select local stories and to include polling data from their states to further customize the messages for their audiences.

The importance of crafting and customizing messages for specific audiences was reinforced when the New Mexico Assembly noted that the analogy of the doctor's office in the school did not bring up a positive experience for Native American community members. The message describing school-based health care was then adapted to "The best way to make sure students are getting the medical care they need to grow up strong and healthy is to bring quality health care services to them—right inside their school buildings."

The consistent application of messages describing school-based health facilitated advocacy efforts. The data supporting the messages added credibility and changed the nature of conversations on Capitol Hill. Brooke Lehmann, a policy consultant advocating for school-based health care on behalf of the National Assembly on School-Based Health Care, said,

> Washington responds to numbers—it's just part of the legislative process. Members who were unsure how to proceed with our requests for support were given security in the numbers of constituents who supported the model, and members who were already supportive were made to feel that their support was justified.

She added:

> Was this responsible for changing the mind of these more oppositional members of Congress? Not in and of itself, but the information was definitely a critical tool in our arsenal and, if nothing else, offered these members something to think about before unilaterally rejecting our requests. (Brooke Lehmann, personal communication, October 19, 2009).

Step 3. Select the Messengers

As with other forms of persuasive communication, presenting a compelling case depends heavily on the messengers chosen to deliver it. Generally, there are two types of messengers: those considered experts in their fields and those who represent an authentic voice as it relates to the issue of concern, most often individuals directly affected by the issue. Identifying the most effective voice to deliver the message can be as important as the message itself.

One way to determine the best selection of messengers, particularly as it relates to reaching policymakers, is to conduct "influence mapping," a technique that identifies the most powerful links to activate individuals, institutions, and communities. At the grassroots level, influence mapping seeks to identify groups of individuals and organizations with influence over the intended audience. For example, parents have influence over schools, and constituents have influence over their elected officials. Individual representatives within these groups, recruited as ambassadors, advocates, and endorsers, can encourage greater participation among their peers or mobilize their members of Congress.

At the individual level, sometimes referred to as the "grass tops" level, influence mapping identifies the sphere of influence for each individual audience member (such as a specific elected official or decision-maker). Often this will include individuals or organizations that have some sort of relationship with that person or are recognized as formal or informal community leaders. These "champions" can carry the messages directly or act as pathways to help introduce others to that individual.

In the SBHCPP, the most effective voices are often those of youth and parents. For example, state associations in California, Oregon, Michigan, and New Mexico found that students from youth advisory boards of local centers were the most effective messengers to reach legislators in support of SBHCs. In New Mexico, youth-driven policy work led to $100,000 in special funding from the state for a teen peer-to-peer suicide prevention program.[8]

Step 4. Pick Effective Channels and Tools

Sometimes face-to-face communication works best. Other times, newsletters, websites, direct mail, stories placed in the media, or messages delivered through social networking sites are most effective. Strategic communication requires delivery of the right message through the channel that is most appealing to the desired audience.

In the New Mexico example, they identified the need to develop a specific set of communication tools that would resonate with tribal leaders and state policymakers (convening of Native American tribal leaders and health leaders, Albuquerque, New Mexico, 2007). It was also determined that in order to engage these audiences in understanding the school-based health model, the most powerful voices were those of the youth served by the centers. Because the long distances in New Mexico make regular in-person visits by students difficult to schedule, the New Mexico Assembly turned to a video and written stories featuring young people as the channel to deliver their message.

The decision to let the youth tell their story proved to be the right one. "The Native American legislators were grateful that we showed the geographic, social, and environmental issues faced by Native youth. The non-Native legislators finally understood the barriers that Native youth have to overcome in order to access health care," said Regina Begay-Roanhorse. She added, "Legislators and others were emotional hearing young people talking about issues of suicide and poverty and were moved to help" (Regina Begay-Roanhorse, personal communication, October 21, 2009).

Step 5. Implement Communication

Once the messages have been developed and the channels and methods of communication have been identified, the communication strategy is ready for implementation. Most important in this step is to consider the audiences and what will resonate with them. As previously noted, in order to truly connect with diverse cultural audiences, it is critical to apply a multicultural frame to communication. This is especially important during the development and implementation of strategies and tools. The process requires embracing the social nuances of diverse cultural groups and actively engaging them in the creation of relevant communication strategies, tools, and messages that have the best opportunity to achieve the desired action.

The process of adaptation for new audiences is much broader than the words on a page. In fact, ensuring that the content resonates with the culture and identity of the desired audiences is more important than the language to use in communication materials.

Effective multicultural communication takes into account how people from a unique cultural, ethnic, or racial group will interpret the verbal or nonverbal messages. It entails appropriate interpersonal communication dynamics, the right context, and appropriate usage of culturally relevant imagery, vocabulary, vernacular, metaphors, or slang.

When communicating to an audience whose language is not English, it is critical to remember that translation makes things readable but not necessarily relevant. A better approach is to make a conscious choice between translating existing concepts, relating existing concepts into new images and words that convey ideas more effectively, or developing a completely new message frame, copy, and imagery.[6]

In the New Mexico example, the video was produced by a Native American communication firm. The supporting materials, including a PowerPoint presentation, were developed by the primary author with regular and ongoing input and final approval from individuals representing four national Native American organizations, representatives from the staff and board of the New Mexico Assembly, and each of the young people featured in the video and materials.

In a final review, some of the music in the video, an important context setter, had to be changed so that it was inclusive of diverse tribes. This important point would not have been caught had members of the desired audience not been engaged in the final review and approval process.

Step 6. Measure Results

Measuring the impact of communication is critical for making adjustments to a communication program and ensuring the appropriation of the right level of resources to future communication. Too often, evaluating communication is viewed as impractical or too costly. Instead, organizations only look for anecdotal evidence of success.

Measuring the efficacy of a message, communication strategy, or tool does not have to be an expensive proposition. At Metropolitan Group, we divide change measures between those that measure *action* and those that measure *result*. Action measures are those that seek to quantify *inputs* ("what we put in") and *outputs*

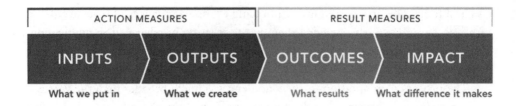

Figure 14.1—How to measure the return on investment of strategic communication to advance policy.

("what we create"), while result measures quantify the *outcomes* ("what results") and ultimately *impact* ("what difference it makes"), as reflected in Figure 14.1.

All four measures (*inputs, outputs, outcomes,* and *impact*) tell you something important. Measurement of action—as reflected in *input* and *output* measures—is by far the most common form of measurement. Action measures include quantification of the *input* associated with pursuit of social impact (e.g., time and resources invested) or the activities undertaken in this pursuit. Action measures also include the *output* of such activities, such as the partnerships and collaborations that are created, the community outreach that is conducted, the value of donated ad space or time, the number of direct mail pieces or news releases distributed, the number of visits to a website, the amount of time that audiences spend on a particular online page, or the "gross impressions" associated with potential exposure to a news story or advertisement. Such measures are generally acknowledged as "basics" that should be part of any measurement process.

Result measures are harder to obtain than *action* measures but are arguably more directly related to mission advancement. The most common forms of result measures are those associated with quantification of *outcomes* and *impact*. In general, *outcomes* are defined as the direct and intended result of having engaged in social change creation (e.g., the number of people who responded to a "call to action"), while *impact* is generally used to connect outcomes to the mission of the sponsoring organization (e.g., those who responded to the call to action engaged in a behavior that benefited them or their community, such as tobacco cessation or getting a flu shot).[9]

CONCLUSION

The SBHCPP is one illustration of how the application of strategic communication can support policy advocacy. Any organization seeking policy change or to make its communication more effective can apply the six-step process.

The identification of audiences will help focus resources so that they are most effectively applied. Once audiences are identified, messages that will resonate with them, based on their needs, values, and motivators, are developed. The selection of the right messenger and the right channel will help ensure that messages effectively reach the desired audience and will be perceived as credible. Finally, measuring the impact of the communication will allow for midcourse corrections to communication strategies so they are most effective, allow for continued learning, and maximize the organization's return on investment.

REFERENCES

1. Friedenwald-Fishman EM, Lee Dellinger LK, Gilstrap Hearn J, Pai-Espinosa J. *Building Public Will: 5-Phase Approach to Sustainable Change.* Washington, DC: Metropolitan Group; 2009.

2. National Council of Nonprofit Associations. *Toolkit: Building Capacity for Public Policy.* Washington, DC: National Council of Nonprofit Associations; 2004.

3. LaRusso DA. *The Shadows of Communication: Nonverbal Dimensions.* Dubuque, IA: Kendall/Hunt Publishing Company; 1977.

4. Herszenhorn DA. In New York schools, whole milk is cast from the menu. *New York Times.* February 2, 2006. Available at: http://www.nytimes.com/2006/02/02/nyregion/02milk.html. Accessed February 4, 2006.

5. Zimmerman JB, Campisteguy ME, Parks L, Richardson JW. *The School-Based Health Care Policy Program: Capstone Evaluation.* Battle Creek, MI: W. K. Kellogg Foundation; 2011.

6. Campisteguy ME, Friedenwald-Fishman EM, Lee Dellinger LK, Detman B, Gilstrap Hearn J. *Increasing Relevance, Relationships, and Results: Principles and Practices for Effective Multicultural Communication.* Washington, DC: Metropolitan Group; 2009.

7. National Assembly on School-Based Health Care. Capitol Hill briefing explains school-based health centers' roles as first responders to students in crisis. 2007. Available at: http://ww2.nasbhc.org/RoadMap/Public/PR_nationalrelease1.25.pdf. Accessed January 31, 2007.

8. W. K. Kellogg Foundation. *School-Based Health Care Policy Program Grantees Make Major Strides.* Battle Creek, MI: W. K. Kellogg Foundation; 2008.

9. Kirkpatrick KT, Friedenwald-Fishman E, Gilstrap Hearn J. *Measuring What Matters: The Challenge of Quantifying Social Change.* Washington, DC: Metropolitan Group; 2009.

About the Authors

Maria Elena Campisteguy—is a Principal/Executive Vice President of The Metropolitan Group, a social marketing firm. She leads the firm's Multicultural Communication practice. She has more than 25 years experience helping nonprofit organizations develop powerful brands and messages, develop strategies to engage new constituents, expand programmatic and service reach, advance policy, and increase their base of support. For five years, she was a consultant to the W. K. Kellogg Foundation's School-Based Health Care Policy Program, providing technical assistance to participating state associations and community partners. For additional communication resources, visit http://www.metgroup.com.

Karen Saverino, APR—is President of Eightfold Strategy, a branding, marketing, and communication firm that works with nonprofits, foundations, and socially conscious companies. As Vice President at The Metropolitan Group, Karen worked on the team that advised program officers and grantees of the W. K. Kellogg Foundation's School-Based Health Care Policy Program on communication to advance policy, resulting in the 2010 passage of federal legislation to authorize funding for school-based health centers. She earned a Bachelor's degree in English from The College of Notre Dame of Maryland and is accredited in public relations from the Public Relations Society of America. She lives in Washington, DC.

Messages Matter: Using Data to Inform School-Based Health Care Policy Advocacy

Jeanita W. Richardson and Terri D. Wright

RATIONALE

From its inception, the W. K. Kellogg Foundation deemed strategic communications and assessment of voter sentiment about school-based health centers (SBHCs) critical contributors to School-Based Health Care Policy Program (SBHCPP) advocacy success. At the time of the national polling initiative discussed in this chapter, there were approximately 1,709 SBHCs throughout the country. Forty-one percent of them were located in Title I schools, the federal designation for schools serving high numbers of economically disadvantaged students.[1] Their presence has been documented to improve childhood access to medical care, and, in addition, they have been touted as one solution to the pervasive dilemma of unserved or underserved youngsters relative to their health needs. Studies of the impact of SBHCs affirm their positive influence on reducing absenteeism and improved management of chronic disease such as asthma, for example. Despite these demonstrated contributions, SBHCs constantly struggled to secure a reliable funding base due at least in part to existing policies and voter perceptions that hampered their sustainability.[2–8]

In the policy decision-making process, polls have become vital tools of the political trade in the 21st century. Barely a day goes by without the dissemination of polling results. Commercials, news broadcasters, and newspapers regularly incorporate data gained from "surveying the public" to substantiate a preferred product, policy preference, or conclusion.[9–12]

Authors concur that one of the values of identifying the priorities of average persons in particular is the potential increased responsiveness of the democratic process. In the absence of data confirming average voter views, the louder voices of special interest groups can unduly influence the decision-making process.[13,14] Another value of polling can be the data compilation that helps elected officials avoid mistakes caused by misreading public opinion.[14] Thus, in an effort to support the advocacy work of the SBHCPP grantees and the school-based health care movement, the W. K. Kellogg Foundation commissioned a national survey conducted by Lake Research Partners.[15]

The six categories of questions guiding the study sought to shed light on: (1) existing support for SBHCs, (2) voter views of what support means and exploring how participants feel about services offered at SBHCs, (3) the outcomes of the centers that make voters more supportive, (4) funding issues, (5) the impact of opposition points, and (6) messages that elicit voter support. Though this particular survey was designed to support SBHC political activism, broader lessons about the value of national issue-specific polling and how to apply said data to messaging are of worth to the health policy community broadly.

METHODS

The purpose of this investigation was to assess attitudes, i.e., positive and negative orientations toward SBHCs, and to attempt to predict support or aversion. The term *poll* is generally used to reflect subject matter with some political significance; however, for methodological purposes, polls are surveys designed to collect qualitative and quantitative data.[10,16,17] Random-digit dialing (RDD) has been advanced as a preferred means of sampling the total population in telephone surveys that are grounded in statistical and probability theory.

Lake Research Partners (http://www.lakeresearch.com), a national public opinion and political strategy research firm known for their expertise on child-related political issues, was commissioned by the W. K. Kellogg Foundation to design, implement, and provide the findings of the aforementioned poll. The methodologies applied by Lake Research Partners were in compliance with generally accepted standards.[10,13,17]

Twelve focus groups were convened between February 13, 2006, and May 30, 2006. With the exception of the two groups of senior citizens, all other sessions, conducted in Maine, California, Oregon, Michigan, New York, and New Mexico, consisted of one half of a representative sample of the national population with school-age youngsters in their households and the second half of households without school-age children. Focus group findings were then used to fine-tune the survey instrument and check for understanding of key terms with various constituent groups that would participate in the national survey.

Telephone numbers for all surveys were drawn from an RDD sample and were administered by professional interviewers. All samples were stratified geographically based on the proportion of the voters in each universe and randomly assigned a designation of "A" or "B" (each totaling 50% of the total). Phone numbers were further sorted into "AC," "AD," "BC," or "BD" (each accounting for 25% of the total number of participants). Single and double letter designations of participants indicated to interviewers which questions should be asked. Responses to the 49 questions were solicited from nine regions: New England, the Mid-Atlantic, East-North Central, West-North Central, South Atlantic, East-South Central, West-South Central, Mountain, and Pacific and accounted for all 50 states.

The survey reached 2638 registered voters, ages 18 years or older nationwide between May 16 and June 11, 2006. This included a base sample of 1,294 and oversamples of 204 African Americans, 214 Hispanics, and 301 residents in Maine, 320 in Louisiana, and 305 in Massachusetts, which were weighted to reflect the actual population of registered voters, yielding a total sample of 1,294 participants. The data were additionally weighted slightly by age, education, party identification, and race to reflect the attributes of the actual population of registered voters. The margin of error for the base sample is ±2.8%. Participants responded to questions using a Likert-like scale.

The range of answer choices varied in some cases when the sample was split (e.g., AC, AD, BC, BD). For example, while questions or statements remained constant, e.g., "Mental health services including grief therapy, peer pressure, bullying and suicide prevention," participant AC's responses might range between "Very important," "Somewhat important," "A little important," "Not at all important," and "Don't know." Conversely, BC's choices tied to the same prompt were "Much more supportive," "Somewhat more supportive," "Somewhat less supportive," "Much less supportive," and "Don't know." In a few cases, statements (e.g., "Students will get health care who might otherwise not seek care") were rated on a scale of 1 to 10 with 1 representing one of the worst things that could happen and 10 meaning one of the best things that could happen if SBHCs are located in schools. In addition, one half of the sample was queried about how SBHCs should be funded. Questions were prefaced with information about the current nature of funding, which often requires annual searches for fiscal support from various sources.

RESULTS

In the aggregate, 66% of respondents favor offering health services in schools (21% oppose and 13% don't know). Respondents found it quite problematic that so many children do not have access to health care because they were uninsured, underinsured, or located in areas with scant availability of services.

Differences between subgroups identify nuances relative to the range of support. African Americans and Hispanics tended to be more in favor of the proposed health delivery concept than were Whites (87%, 79%, and 63%, respectively). Overall, women (55%) were more supportive than were men (46%). Groups more likely to strongly favor services delivered in schools, in addition to the groups already noted, were single mothers, unmarried women, those under 30 years old, college women, single and divorced voters, those in the East, persons who were uninsured, and those with high school diplomas or less. Republican men were the group least enthusiastic about health services in schools. Though the majority of total responders agreed that SBHCs were a beneficial institution, and they were concerned about children who did not have health coverage, the theme of competing priorities (financial and social) lowered SBHC support as it had in the focus groups.

In the main, voters believe some action is merited to ensure childhood health, with certain services yielding more or less support (Table 15.1). Health education, mental health, acute illness/ trauma, and chronic illness secured sufficient affirmation, placing them in the first tier of services (56%, 51%, 44%, and 43%, respectively), and also were associated with high levels of total support (82%, 78%, 70%, and 71%, respectively). The second tier of favored services included sports physicals, with 41% much more supportive; comprehensive physicals (37%) and dental services (36%) followed next. The least popular services among the choices were sexually transmitted disease (STD) screening and treatment (33%), reproductive health services (30%), dispensing of medication (21%), and prescribing medication (20%).

The first time services were mentioned in the survey, they were contextualized in terms of whether they were deemed important to offer. The second time the same services were mentioned in the survey, some services shifted between tiers two and three. In tier one the same four categories remained very important though changing in priority. Mental health was rated most often as "very important" (63%) followed by health education (62%), acute illness/trauma (61%), and chronic illness (54%). Tier two included in descending order, STD screening and treatments, sport physicals, reproductive health, and comprehensive physicals (48%, 42%, 41%, and 38%, respectively). Services deemed "very important" included dental services and dispensing and prescribing medication (35%, 35%, and 29%, respectively).

In this second scenario, STD screening and treatment and reproductive health moved from the third to second tier, whereas dental services dropped from the second to the third tier. White women in particular were very disposed to negative opinions of SBHCs when services traditionally under parental control were read,

TABLE 15.1—SERVICES OFFERED BY SCHOOL-BASED HEALTH CENTERS, BY SUPPORT TIER

	Much More Supportive, %	Somewhat More Supportive, %	Combined Support, %	Less Supportive, Not Supportive, or Don't Know, %
Tier 1				
Health education	56	26	82	18
Mental health	51	27	78	22
Acute illness/Trauma	44	26	70	30
Chronic illness	43	28	71	29
Tier 2				
Sports physicals	41	32	73	27
Comprehensive physicals	37	28	65	35
Dental services	36	25	61	39
Tier 3				
STD screening and treatment	33	23	56	44
Reproductive health services	30	22	52	48
Dispense medication	21	28	49	51
Prescribe medication	20	24	44	56

Note. STD=sexually transmitted disease.

e.g. "My major concern is that parents are not involved in this, and there is no telling what the children are going in there for, and, I am sorry, I just can't go along with it." Responses were most adamantly opposed to medication prescriptions. As one Portland, Oregon, participant said, "I wouldn't (want) someone just writing my son a prescription. I would not be happy at all."

Other gauges of support were the potential outcomes of having an SBHC available to children. The prompt was, "Now let me read you some things that some people have said may happen if school-based health centers are located in school." The categories offered were:

- Students will get health care who might otherwise not seek care;
- Uninsured and underinsured children will have better and easier access to health care;

- Chronic health conditions, like asthma and diabetes, can be caught early through screening and possibly prevented;
- More access to mental health services so children with emotional and psychological problems will be identified and treated;
- SBHCs will help children stay healthy and give all students an equal chance to succeed in school;
- Health care access will be increased in rural areas;
- Parents will not have to take time off from work to get children the care they need; and
- High-quality comprehensive care will be provided to students who need it.

A clear majority (80%) of participants believed getting health care, easier access, and management and screening of chronic conditions would be a "very likely" or "somewhat likely" outcome of having an SBHC in a school. Getting health care, easier access, and screening and management of chronic illness all exceeded 50% as "very likely" if an SBHC was operational in a school. SBHCs as an appropriate vehicle to increase access to mental health services, staying healthy, supporting success in school, and improving rural access ranged from 45% to 41% (in the category of "very likely"). The final two categories, parents not taking time off from work and SBHCs offering a high quality of care, had significantly weaker support (39% and 35%, respectively).

Relative to resources (See Table 15.2), one half of participants were asked to identify preferred funding sources for SBHCs, which could range from one to all of the options posed. A majority of respondents believed the federal government (65%), insurance companies (64%), state governments (65%), and schools (58%) should sustain SBHCs. When queried about a willingness to personally support the SBHC model of care (that virtually all respondents deemed appropriate and valuable in previous responses), most were not strongly in favor of increasing their federal tax burden. Only 38% strongly favored a $10 increase, and 28% strongly favored a $50 increase annually.

Opposition points were explored to test the sensitivity of supporters. It is important to note that the opposition messages used were not grounded in fact, but rather were arguments commonly used to discourage support in policy discourse (see Table 15.3). Responses confirmed that participants were suspect of SBHCs' ability to support the primary role of schools (63%). In addition, SBHCs were deemed potentially problematic relative to the parameters of parental controls (56%), and there were doubts that the quality of service that might be available in a school setting would rival traditional venues (48%). Even the most ardent support was found to be sensitive to opposition messages, particularly as it relates

TABLE 15.2—FUNDING POSSIBILITIES FOR SCHOOL-BASED HEALTH CENTERS, BY SUPPORT RECEIVED

Funding Source	Strongly Favor, %	Not so Strongly Favor, %	Total in Favor, %	Do Not Favor or Do Not Know, %
Federal money set aside	50	15	65	35
Insurance company requirement	48	16	64	36
State money set aside	47	18	65	35
School money set aside	41	17	58	42
Medicaid reimbursement requirement	39	16	55	45
Require taxpayers to pay $10 more per year in federal taxes	38	15	53	47
Require taxpayers to pay $50 more per year in federal taxes	28	16	44	56

to the quality of care. Demographic groups most sensitive to opposition messages were Republicans, widowed voters, and men.

Voters tended to think that SBHCs were a good idea; however, themes confirmed descriptions containing more in-depth information eroded support. It should be noted that while a majority of participants were convinced of the value of SBHCs when hearing the standardized script, different regions of the country

TABLE 15.3—SCHOOL-BASED HEALTH CENTER OPPOSITION MESSAGE SENSITIVITY

Opposition Message	Very Likely, %	Somewhat Likely, %	Total Likely, %	Not Likely or Don't Know, %
Money and attention will be taken away from more important education priorities	33	30	63	37
Students will get health care without their parents' consent	28	28	56	44
The quality of health care will not be good	16	32	48	52

and different demographic groups varied in their responsiveness to messages. For example, women found the "Provide care"[a] (41% vs. 33%) and "Disaster support"[b] (36% vs. 31%) message more convincing than did men. For those in the Northeast and Midwest, "Provide care" was rated very convincing (38%), while in the South "Disaster support" (41%) was most convincing. In the West, unlike any other region, the "Studies"[c] script was most convincing (38%), followed by "Provide care" (36%).

DISCUSSION

This study sought to inform the advocacy efforts of grantees in the SBHCPP by seeking to understand voter perceptions. There were, however, several limitations to the study. Polling data are not a panacea-type tool for groups attempting to understand voter behavior because depending upon the type of poll and purpose of the survey, methodologies and interpretations of data can vary widely.[13,14,18] Shortcomings notwithstanding, standards advanced by learned societies provide some benchmarks for data interpretation that has been applied in this case. The reality is that consumers and politicians seem to have an insatiable thirst for predictions, and, as such, polling's utility seems to outweigh its insufficiencies, as evidenced by their prevalent use. Given the interrelationship between voter behaviors and the interest in predicting their behavior, polls have become one means of expeditiously securing reliable information, particularly for politicians.[19] Advocacy efforts in the SBHC movement context can benefit from an assessment of public sentiment in the framing of messages aimed at solidifying support.

---

[a] The script for "Provide care" was: "There are still many children whose parents cannot afford health insurance. Unfortunately, too often this means that some kids go without the health services they need. Nearly forty percent of students served by school-based health centers have no other health care and cannot access any other health care options. These centers provide care to students who need it and give them the support and guidance that they cannot get elsewhere."

[b] The script for "Disaster support" was: "School-based health centers are a vital resource in our communities and should be a critical part of any preparedness plan. These facilities can be our first line of defense against outbreaks of infectious disease like the mumps or Avian flu or they can be a vital medical resource when dealing with natural calamities, like hurricanes. Obviously, we hope we never have to use the centers in this way, but school-based health centers can strengthen the public health system by providing additional first responders and medical supplies in times of emergency. Additionally, the centers are in the locations that communities would most likely use as emergency shelters in the event of a natural disaster or a terrorist attack."

[c] The script for "Studies" was "Studies by John Hopkins University, Emory University, and other respected institutions show that school-based health centers decrease absenteeism, tardiness, and school discipline or behavior problems. Additionally, they show that centers save money by reducing the number of visits people make to the emergency room for the wrong reasons. These centers deserve stable financial support to continue their mission of providing care to all who need it."

What emerged from this study was substantiation that messages used to increase an understanding of SBHCs as a way to garner voter affirmation require careful verbiage crafting. A majority of the voters polled support offering health care service in schools. Support for SBHCs, particularly when the numbers of uninsured children are revealed, was positive. Access to care that might not otherwise be available and management of chronic illnesses were also viewed favorably by voters. On the other hand, as specificity increased relative to claims that are documented by SBHCs, such as decreased time parents have to take off from work and that they offer a high quality of care, voters were less convinced.

Results also showed that as groups seek to bolster voter support for SBHCs, it is best to avoid a litany of services. Core services such as health education, mental health services, treating acute illness, treating sudden trauma, and managing chronic illnesses tend to be least controversial. However, voters also recognized that financial resources were limited and were reluctant to add any new burdens to what they perceived to be an overburdened budget and overly taxed citizens. Thus, even though rhetorical support for services exists, any advocacy for additional funds for SBHCs will have to compete with a myriad of issues that voters already believe are urgent.

To build a strong advocacy base, findings allude to the need to frame conversations around preventative and acute care. Focusing on specific interventions is critical to shoring up support because, while initially voters believe the concept of school-based health care is a good idea, their perceptions of it run the gamut from the beleaguered school nurse to full-service clinics. In defining school-based health care, less detail is more effective in bolstering support.

Reservations uncovered in this poll confirm that complex explanations of services and school-based health care concepts lead to more questions. Sticking to the basics (core messages and first-tier services) should guide strategic communications. Mental health services, for example, are positively viewed and should be advanced in the context of grief, peer pressure, bullying, and suicide prevention counseling in order to prevent voters from focusing on their concerns about labeling, misdiagnosing, and unnecessarily overmedicating active children. It is equally critical to avoid talking about prescribing and dispensing medication, as these services proved controversial and increased voters' opposition to school-based health care.

Parental consent, fiscal feasibility, and attention being taken away from education priorities are points that the opposition can seize upon to reduce public support for school-based health care. To mitigate the impact of counterarguments, reminding voters that, for the most part, parental consent is required before service delivery yields positive responses. Voters concerned about parental consent and funding also fueled our recommendations not to put reproductive services in the forefront of messaging (if at all). As one example, there was conflict between the theoretical support of offering reproductive health service in schools and concerns about imposing on parental consent territory. Participants tended to reject claims that parental consent will be obtained for this service because they draw upon perceptions of family planning clinics where consent is not always required. Voters also questioned assertions that the quality of care provided in SBHCs matched traditional medical offices.

Several positive SBHC outcomes should be emphasized, and these points tend to cluster. Key messages that increase support are:

- SBHCs provide health services to children who might not otherwise seek care;
- SBHCs provide better and easier access to health care for uninsured and underinsured children;
- Forty percent of students served by the centers have no other health care options;
- SBHCs promote prevention and early intervention in cases of chronic conditions, as well as mental health; and
- SBHCs will help children stay healthy and give all children an equal chance to succeed in school.

The top message, "Provide Care," taps into voters' concern about children whose parents cannot afford to provide insurance and have no other health care options. As is the case with many social programs, there is a bit of schizophrenic support of SBHCs. Even when services or outcomes were deemed very important to provide, respondents wavered around who should pay for services, and voters were sensitive to opposition messages and the text of messages, both positive and negative. This would appear to support Wolf and Holian's[20] premise that individuals do not easily evaluate new information in isolation of their established belief about an issue. For example, even in light of support for federal money set aside for SBHCs (65%), just over 38% would be willing ("strongly favor") to pay an extra $10 in federal taxes.

Message parameters supported by this study's findings are:

- Keep it simple. Message discipline is paramount.
- Highlight health education, mental health (with modifiers such as depression and bullying), and acute and chronic illness.
- Constantly remind voters that parental consent is a prerequisite to access to services.
- Focus on the children that will be helped and the 40% that are being currently helped and have no other health care option.
- Focus on giving children a chance to stay healthy and have an equal chance to succeed in school.

- Dispensing and prescribing medication in messaging dilutes support.
- Avoid leading with the benefit to parents who work.
- Important services, benefits, and outcomes fostered by SBHCs solidify support (using recommended language).
- Make sure you are using the strongest wording in your message, and repetition matters.
- Talk about the need for support and that these centers don't have guaranteed stable funding sources.

There are additional lessons that are applicable to the general policy community. Advocates shouldn't assume they know what people think. Accumulating a body of evidence about trends in public opinion can be a tool to prompt policy change.[10–12,21] Polls are valuable; however, they should be considered with their shortcomings in mind, e.g., they are specific to the topical focus and as such they represent just one tool at one point in time in the arsenal of those seeking to advance policy change.[14]

One of the most significant findings of the poll on SBHCs seems on the surface to be quite simplistic. Those desiring to influence policy change need to frame their issue with communications that inform voters and garner support proactively, or the issue will be framed by opposition messages, uninformed, or underinformed opinions.[10,21] Stated another way: messages matter.

REFERENCES

1. National Assembly on School-Based Health Care. *School-Based Health Centers: A National Definition*. Washington, DC: National Assembly on School-Based Health Care; 2002.

2. Geierstanger SP, Amaral G, Mansour M, Walters SR. School-based health centers and academic performance: research, challenges, and recommendations. *J Sch Health*. 2004;74(9):347–352.

3. Guo JJ, Wade TJ, Keller KN. Impact of school-based health centers on students with mental health problems. *Public Health Rep*. 2008;123(6):768–780.

4. Juszczak L, Schlitt J, Odum M, Barangan C, Washington D. School-based health centers: a blueprint for healthy learners—data from the 2001–2002 School-Based Health Center Census. In: Lear JG, Isaacs SL, Knickman JR, eds. *School Health Services and Programs*. San Francisco, CA: Jossey-Bass; 2006:294–307.

5. Mansour ME, Rose B, Toole K, Luzader CP, Atherton HD. Pursuing perfection: an asthma quality improvement initiative in school-based health centers with community partners. *Public Health Rep*. 2008;123(6):717–729.

6. Richardson JW. From risk to resilience: promoting school-health partnerships for children. *IJER*. 2008;17(1):19–36.

7. Richardson JW, Juszczak LJ. Schools as sites for health-care delivery. *Public Health Rep*. 2008;123(6):692–693.

8. Wade TJ, Mansour ME, Guo JJ, Huentelman T, Line K, Keller KN. Access and utilization patterns of school-based health centers at urban and rural elementary and middle schools. *Public Health Rep*. 2008;123(6):739–750.

9. Mann TE, Dionne EJ Jr. Polling and public opinion: the good, the bad, and the ugly. *Brookings Rev*. 2003;21(3):2–3.

10. Weisberg HF, Krosnick JA, Bowen BD. *An Introduction to Survey Research, Polling, and Data Analysis*. 3rd ed. Thousand Oaks, CA: Sage Publications; 1996.

11. Druckman JN, Jacobs LR. Lumpers and splitters: the public opinion information that politicians collect and use. *Public Opin Q*. 2006;70(4):453–476.

12. Greenwald HP, Beery WL, Pearson D, et al. Polling and policy analysis as resources for advocacy. *J Public Adm Res Theory*. 2003;13(2):177–191.

13. Costello M. Public opinion polling. *Editor Res Rep*. 1976;1(5):167–184.

14. Altman D, Brodie M. Opinion on public opinion polling. *Health Aff*. 2002:W276–279.

15. W. K. Kellogg Foundation. *School-Based Health Care Policy Program*. Battle Creek, MI: W. K. Kellogg Foundation; 2008.

16. Igo SE. "A gold mine and a tool for democracy": George Gallup, Elmo Roper, and the business of scientific polling, 1935–1955. *J Hist Behav Sci*. 2006;42(2):109–134.

17. Scheuren F. *What Is a Survey?* Washington, DC: American Statistical Association; 2004.

18. Scammon RM, Wattenberg BJ. *The Real Majority*. New York, NY: Coward-McCann; 1970.

19. Fried A. The forgotten Lindsay Rogers and the development of American political science. *Am Polit Sci Rev*. 2006;100(4):555–562.

20. Wolf MR, Holian DB. Polls, elite opinion, and the President: how information and issue saliency affect approval. *Pres Stud Q*. 2006;36(4):584–606.

21. Haider-Markel DP, Delehanty W, Beverlin M. Media framing and racial attitudes in the aftermath of Katrina. *Pol Stud J*. 2007;35(4):587–605.

About the Authors

Jeanita W. Richardson, PhD, MEd – is an Associate Professor in the Department of Public Health Sciences at the University of Virginia School of Medicine. Her scholarship highlights the inextricable links between health and learning readiness, particularly for disenfranchised children and youth. Her work has been published and presented in numerous national and international journals and conferences. Her consulting energies (Turpeau Consulting Group, LLC) are devoted to supporting healthy children who are ready to learn through the creation of health and educational policy bridges and include five years as a consultant to the W. K. Kellogg Foundation's School-Based Health Care Policy Program. For more information, email TConsultingG@aol.com.

Terri D. Wright, MPH, ABD – is Director of the newly established Center for School, Health and Education at the American Public Health Association. She provides leadership to the strategic development of school-based health programming and policy to avert school dropout. Formerly, she served for 12 years as a Program Director for Health Policy at the W. K. Kellogg Foundation and provided leadership for the Foundation's school-based health care policy program. Terri was Maternal and Child Health Director and Bureau Chief for Child and Family Services at the Michigan Department of Community Health where she managed policy, programs, and resources with the goal of reducing preventable maternal, infant, and child morbidity and mortality. She has a Bachelor's degree in Community and School Health and a Master's degree in Public Health. She is currently a doctoral candidate in Public Health at the University of Michigan. Terri takes an active leadership role in several professional and community organizations including the Institute of Medicine Roundtable on the Promotion of Health Equity and the Elimination of Health Disparities.

How State Policies Can Support School-Based Health Care

Joshua Rovner, Linda Juszczak,
and John Schlitt

More than 1,900 school-based health centers (SBHCs) provide a vital piece of the nation's health care safety net. The number of SBHCs has increased from a few dozen in the 1980s to nearly 2,000 today—largely without federal support. The growth has been remarkable. SBHCs historically were located mostly in the Northeastern and Atlantic states, mostly in urban areas, and mostly in high schools. Today, there are SBHCs in 44 states and the District of Columbia. Despite a history that stretches back to the 1970s, SBHCs were defined in federal law for the first time in 2009 through the reauthorization of the Children's Health Insurance Program in 2009.[1] As shown in this chapter, the growth of SBHCs has been driven by financial support and policy at the state level, not federal policy or funding.

There is little uniformity in the ways that state policies are used to support SBHCs. Instead, states have blended various ingredients to support school-based health care within their borders. This chapter shows how some states' policies have buttressed their existence through widely varying levels of financial support, technical assistance and training to their SBHCs, and use of public insurance programs to reimburse care.

GROWTH OF SCHOOL-BASED HEALTH CENTERS

The raw numbers show a steady rate of increase for SBHCs. In 1986, there were 74 known SBHCs[2] (see Figure 16.1); the National Assembly on School-Based Health Care's (NASBHC's) 2007 Census identified 1,909 SBHCs.[3] After a period of accelerated growth that lasted most of the 1990s, the growth rate has slowed by roughly

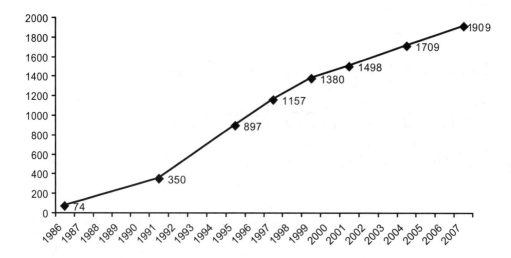

Figure 16.1—Number of school-based health centers, by school year.

50% since 1999. The strongest growth period occurred while the national economy was at its peak. A stronger economy matters a great deal to states, whose revenues are highly dependent on income, sales, and property taxes. Conversely, a weaker economy during the first decade of this century meant less revenue for states available to support their SBHCs (along with many other priorities; see Figure 16.2).

Since 2000 to 2001, the largest states have been home to the largest number of SBHCs, but still, the distribution of SBHCs has changed over time. SBHCs were once disproportionally located in a handful of northeastern states, and today, the presence of SBHCs is not a regional phenomenon. In 1999, Lear et al.[4] noted the rapid increase in SBHCs in the Midwest, Southwest, and Rocky Mountain states, a trend that continues today.[a]

A question worth asking is: Why have states been willing to support health care in schools even as public investments in other areas dried up? Comprehensive health care reform failed under the Clinton Administration for a variety of reasons, but the lack of action on a national level may have motivated states to fill a void.[b]

---

[a] The 12 states with the largest number of SBHCs in 1999 were New York, Arizona, California, Florida, Texas, Maryland, Connecticut, Massachusetts, Oregon, Illinois, Michigan, and North Carolina. Some of these states are politically conservative (Arizona, Texas, and North Carolina), some are moderate (Florida, Connecticut, Michigan), and some are liberal (New York, California, Maryland, Massachusetts, Oregon, and Illinois). Two years later, North Carolina and Oregon were no longer in the top 12, replaced by Louisiana and New Mexico. By 2007, Indiana had replaced Illinois as a top 12 state.
[b] The data in this chapter don't include any years after the passage of the Patient Protection and Affordable Care Act in 2009.

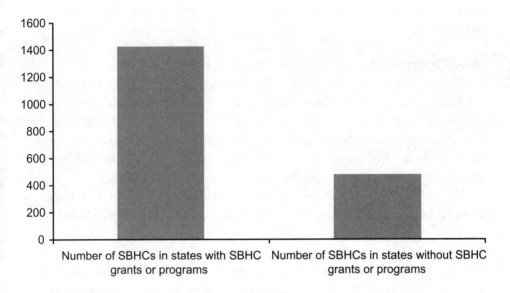

Figure 16.2—Relationship of school-based health centers (SBHCs) and state support.

Writing in 1996, Lear noted that despite broad disagreements over the federal role in health care, states were willing to adopt SBHCs as a targeted approach to providing health care—neither too costly in the short term nor creating an open-ended entitlement.[5] Another possible reason states support SBHCs is that they address a state's public health agenda, e.g., tobacco cessation, prevention of teen pregnancy and transmitted infections, asthma management, and obesity and bullying reduction. As will be discussed later in this chapter, reproductive health care at SBHCs is limited in some states.

HOW STATES SUPPORT THEIR SCHOOL-BASED HEALTH CENTERS

States have found many ways to support their SBHCs. Twenty states and the District of Columbia fund or sponsor a grant program specifically dedicated to SBHCs, using state general funds, block grants provided to states under Title V of the Social Security Act, and tobacco-settlement dollars as the largest sources of support. Twenty-one states provide technical assistance from a state program office. Eighteen states have operating standards for their SBHCs, offering quality assurance. A more complex comparison is how states address SBHCs under the two public insurance programs, Medicaid and the Children's Health Insurance Program.[c]

State Programs and Grants

Total state-directed funding for SBHCs varies widely, ranging from $12,000 in Alaska to $22.8 million in New York. In total, 18 states and the District of Columbia provide nearly $74 million (a 32% increase from 2004 when 20 states provided $56 million in funding).[d] Clearly, having a state program matters; these 20 states and the District of Columbia are home to 75% of the nation's 1,909 SBHCs. Only three states without a state grant program have more than 30 SBHCs.[e]

As noted earlier, there are four major sources of state-based SBHC funding. Table 16.1 reveals the funding sources for 20 states and the District of Columbia.

Direct State Support

State governments can raise revenue through user fees (such as fees charged when renewing a driver's license), sales taxes, property taxes (such as personal property and real estate taxes), and income taxes (individual and corporate). These revenues are used to support the many functions of a state government, and they are often used to support school-based health care, as well. Among states that provide direct financial support to their SBHCs, the state general fund is the sole source of state-directed funding in eight states; three states and the District of Columbia provide no direct support from state dollars. Seven states use a mixture that includes local revenues.

As seen during the most recent recession, state revenues are not stable. During economic downturns, consumers buy less, reducing sales tax revenues. Real estate property taxes are sensitive to fluctuating property values, and the contemporary bursting of the "housing bubble" has negatively impacted state budgets. Combined, the aforementioned dilemmas and high rates of unemployment that are increasing the pool of individuals in need of safety net payments are all important concerns for SBHCs.

Title V

Title V of the Social Security Act supports state and local efforts to extend health services for mothers and children. Allocated to all states as a block grant,

---

[c] This chapter is based on previous unpublished results from a survey mailed to public health departments in all 50 states, as well as those of the District of Columbia and Puerto Rico in 2009. NASBHC's prior State Policy Survey was conducted in 2005.
[d] The list in 2004 and 2008 is not the same. In 2004, Arizona, Kansas, and Rhode Island had grant programs for their SBHCs that no longer exist. New programs have emerged in Alaska, the District of Columbia, Indiana, and Washington State.
[e] Mississippi, Arizona, and California.

TABLE 16.1—MAJOR SOURCES OF STATE-DIRECTED FUNDING FOR SCHOOL-BASED HEALTH CENTERS

State	Total State-Directed Funding in 2008, $	State Revenues, % of Total Funding	Title V, % of Total Funding	Tobacco Settlement, % of Total Funding
AK	$12,000	0%	100%	0%
CO	$2,187,993	68%	9%	0%
CT	$9,168,186	100%	0%	0%
DC	$1,800,000	0%	17%	83%
DE	$5,400,000	100%	0%	0%
FL	$367,149	100%	0%	0%
IL	$4,234,400	22%	31%	46%
IN	$271,000	0%	100%	0%
LA	$10,249,813	27%	29%	70%
MA	$3,893,559	100%	0%	0%
MD	$2,731,206	100%	0%	0%
ME	$745,300	29%	0%	71%
MI	Not reported	-	-	-
NC	$1,627,000	100%	0%	0%
NJ	$624,000	100%	0%	0%
NM	$3,870,000	91%	0%	0%
NY	$22,800,000	89%	11%	0%
OR	$2,838,000	100%	0%	0%
TX	$1,000,000	50%	50%	0%
WA	$125,000	0%	100%	0%
WV	Not reported	-	-	-
TOTAL	$73,944,606	MEDIAN: 89%	MEDIAN: 0%	MEDIAN: 0%

Note. Columns may not add up to 100% due to other funds not listed. Michigan and West Virginia did not respond to survey.

many states use these dollars to support SBHCs as a means to provide health care for children and adolescents. For several states and the District of Columbia, Title V funding provides support for SBHCs.[f] In Illinois and New York, Title V provides more than $1 million each year. Title V dollars can be affected by Congressional

---

[f] Alaska, Colorado, the District of Columbia, Illinois, Indiana, Louisiana, New York, Texas, and Washington state.

actions: For example, a bill passed in March 2011 by the House of Representatives[6] cut $50 million from Title V. That Title V can be used to support SBHCs does mean that increases in Title V will invariably benefit SBHCs; decisions on how to spend those dollars are made by state governments. However, the expansion of SBHCs in the 1990s was largely driven by Title V dollars.[5(p183)] In 1994, states allocated $12 million of their Title V block grant funds to their SBHCs and $22.3 million in general funds. Today, that ratio has shifted away from Title V dollars and toward state support from general funds.

Tobacco Settlement Funds

In 1998, 46 states signed an agreement with the four largest tobacco manufacturers to settle lawsuits over the billions of dollars of damages caused by the toll of tobacco in their states.[7] Signed in the wake of the notorious "Joe Camel" advertising campaign directed at children, the Master Settlement Agreement (MSA) created a broad array of restrictions on the advertising, marketing, and promotion of cigarettes. The central purpose of the MSA was to reduce smoking, particularly youth smoking, in the United States. States are expected to spend their tobacco settlement dollars on programs that reduce youth smoking, though some have used the dollars to balance their budgets.[8]

Only a handful of states are using the MSA as a major source of support for SBHCs. The question is why others are not. SBHCs are a part of many states' public health strategy, and as such their performance measures can include reductions in alcohol use, asthma care, depression, and so forth. Prevention of tobacco use is another specific performance indicator in seven states.[g] Consequently, it could make sense for each of those states to use the MSA to fund their SBHCs. However, the tobacco settlement is a one-time funding source. This year (2011) marks the halfway point in the 25-year settlement. As such, dependence on the fund may have to be made up through other sources as the MSA expires. For the District of Columbia, the tobacco settlement provides 83% of direct public support to SBHCs. Thus, the dependence on tobacco settlement funds means that the funding for SBHCs in at least four jurisdictions is not sustainable.

STATE INFLUENCE ON THE SCOPE OF SERVICE AND QUALITY OF CARE AT SCHOOL-BASED HEALTH CENTERS

States can support their SBHCs in ways other than direct funding. Many states offer technical assistance to their SBHCs. As noted in the previous section discussing

---

[g] Delaware, Florida, Louisiana, Maine, North Carolina, New York, and West Virginia.

the MSA, states see school-based health care as a way to advance a public health agenda. State standards provide detailed requirements that school-based or school-linked health centers must meet in order to receive state funding for their programs. Eighteen state program offices have established operating standards for their SBHC grantees, which are monitored by the state program office via site visits (3 states and the District of Columbia), or a combination of paper surveys and office visits (12 states). Eight states license SBHCs as health care facilities.

Twenty-one states provide development technical assistance to their SBHCs and to communities. California, Nebraska, and Pennsylvania are the only states reporting they provide this assistance without offering grants to SBHCs. The size of the office providing assistance can be as large as eight or ten staff (in Louisiana and New Mexico, respectively). Table 16.2 identifies the type of technical assistance that states report providing to their SBHCs. The most common forms of assistance are planning and implementing an SBHC, facilitating interagency coordination (presumably, helping SBHCs navigate the government bureaucracy), program evaluation, and quality assurance. Less common services are assistance with managed care contracting and assistance with accreditation. Some states offer a comprehensive range of services to their SBHCs, and more staffing allows for more comprehensive assistance. However, in states like Illinois, Michigan, and North Carolina, fewer than three full-time equivalent state employees work to assist SBHCs. Thus, it is possible for states to provide a wide range of technical assistance to SBHCs even if states do not have a large staff to provide this support.

State policies and funding impact how certain health care services are provided, such as mental health, reproductive health, and oral health. Examples of how state policy can influence these services include:

- In Connecticut, the state's operating standards for SBHCs[9] require a clinically trained master's level social worker (MSW) be on staff (with a licensed clinical social worker [LCSW] preferred).
- Sixty percent of SBHCs report that they cannot distribute contraceptives.[3(p5)] Clinics report that just 10% of the time, state law has taken the decision out of the hands of the SBHC medical staff. Such laws exist in many states—not just Alabama and Louisiana, but also Delaware, Michigan, and New Jersey, among others.
- State laws in Michigan and Louisiana explicitly limit the ability of medical staff to comprehensively care for students who are pregnant. "The adolescent health center shall not, as part of the services offered, provide abortion counseling, services, or make referrals for abortion services," according to Michigan's state standards for adolescent and elementary health care centers.[10] In Louisiana, "Centers are prohibited by State law from distributing

TABLE 16.2—TYPES OF TECHNICAL ASSISTANCE OFFERED BY STATES

	Planning	Interagency Coordination	Training for SBHC Staff	Program Evaluation	Financial Sustainability	Quality Assurance	Clinical Guidelines	Coding and Billing	Managed Care Contracting/ Credentialing	Certification, Licensing, and Accreditation	Information Systems
CA	X	X						X			
CO											
CT	X	X		X	X	X	X			X	X
DC	X	X		X		X	X				
DE	X	X	X	X	X	X	X		X		X
IL	X		X	X	X	X	X	X		X	X
LA	X	X	X	X	X	X	X	X		X	X
MA		X	X	X		X	X				X
MD	X	X			X	X					
ME	X	X		X		X					
MI	X	X	X	X	X	X	X	X	X	X	X
NC	X	X	X	X	X	X	X	X	X		X
NE											
NJ		X		X							
NM	X	X	X	X	X	X	X	X	X	X	X
NY		X	X	X	X	X		X			
OR	X	X	X	X	X	X	X	X		X	X
PA	X	X									
TX	X			X	X	X	X				
WA	X										
WV	X	X	X	X	X	X	X	X			
TOTAL	16	16	10	15	12	15	12	9	4	6	9

contraceptives or abortifacient drugs or devices, and from counseling or advocating abortion, or referring any student to an organization for counseling or advocating abortion." Moreover, this statement must be posted in the SBHC.[11]

- Colorado's state standards[12] consider oral care to be part of the list of core elements that all centers ought to provide. In New York,[13] oral health assessments are expected to be a part of the routine care provided by an SBHC. SBHCs in Maryland[14] must include oral health services either on-site or by referral.

REIMBURSEMENT FOR CARE PROVIDED AT SCHOOL-BASED HEALTH CENTERS

Public Insurance

As per the Kaiser Family Foundation, Medicaid covers one in three children—roughly 30 million, most of who live below the federal poverty line—in the United States,[15] making it the largest source of health coverage for children. It is one of the anchors of the health care safety net, particularly with regard to families living at or near poverty. (It also covers very poor adults who are too young for Medicare.) Medicaid also pays for nursing home and community-based long-term care. Because Medicaid is an entitlement, coverage is available for anyone who is eligible to participate. However, states are given great latitude to determine the reimbursement rates paid to doctors, nurse practitioners, and other medical professionals. The majority of SBHCs bill Medicaid (81%), but strong barriers exist to reimbursement at many centers.

In 2008, Schlitt et al. noted that the growth of state SBHC investments in the 1990s corresponded with the growth of Medicaid managed care. However, Morone et al.[16] noted that SBHCs have challenged the managed care organization (MCO) model. The rationale for the success of MCOs depends on the assumption that patients tend to "consume" too much health care at too high a cost. They noted:

[SBHCs] are organized on the reverse assumption: that adolescents underuse health care services. SBHC culture encourages repeat visits, active outreach, and leisurely paced visits, where children are encouraged to discuss anxieties or high-risk behavior that may be masked by their health complaints. The centers fill gaps in health education, counseling, and mental health care.[16(p134)]

Lear, writing about an SBHC in Far Rockaway High School in Queens, New York, found that most visits there were high-intensity visits—only 19% lasted less than 10 minutes, 38% lasted 10 to 20 minutes, and 43% lasted more than 20 minutes.[5(p183)] Although considered pivotal to long–term sustainability, according to Schlitt et al., "reimbursement to SBHCs from Medicaid—and later, SCHIP—historically has been challenging for a host of reasons (both policy and capacity related)."[2(p736)] Several states have established policies to mandate or enable (but not always guarantee) reimbursement for services delivered in SBHCs to Medicaid and State Children's Health Insurance Program (SCHIP) enrollees.

Patient revenue is the cornerstone of sustainability for any health care operation. For SBHCs, that means collecting from Medicaid and SCHIP. Because states dictate how these public insurance revenues are accessed—defining who gets paid, for what services, and at what rate—they have the power to ensure an SBHC's solvency by entitling it to reasonable reimbursement for services delivered to enrolled children (as is afforded to other safety net providers). The utility of meticulous billing, at best, has not resulted in adequate reimbursements between SBHCs and these federal–state funded patient care revenue streams, giving SBHCs little incentive to bill and collect.

Explicit recognition—or preferential treatment—of SBHCs by a state Medicaid program is becoming increasingly more common (see Table 16.3). Eleven states reported to NASBHC that they define SBHCs as a specific Medicaid-eligible provider or service (see Boxes 1 and 2). Three states have created a distinct payment methodology specific to SBHCs. A handful of states have taken steps to ensure reimbursement to SBHCs within managed care systems: twelve states reported that prior authorization requirements for billing Medicaid are waived for SBHCs, enabling SBHCs to see and bill for Medicaid enrollees irrespective of the child's managed care home. Four states mandate contracts between SBHCs and Medicaid managed care plans.

TABLE 16.3—HOW STATES DEFINE SCHOOL-BASED HEALTH CENTERS (SBHCs) AS A PROVIDER TYPE

Policy	States
States define SBHCs as Medicaid provider type in code or regulations	IL, IN, LA, MD, ME, MI, MS, NC, NJ, NM, RI
Reimbursement for SBHCs is created uniquely for state-defined SBHC provider type	DE, ME, NM
State waives prior authorization policy for SBHCs to bill Medicaid	CT, IN, IL, LA, ME, MI, MS, NM, NY, NC, OR, RI
State mandates contract between SBHCs and managed care network	CT, MI, NM, RI

BOX 1—STATE SNAPSHOT: MICHIGAN

State funded school-based health centers (SBHCs) in Michigan are required to bill for their services and have been since 2003. SBHCs are reimbursed by both public insurance programs and private insurance carriers. This model has served SBHCs well in Michigan—there are 90 in the state, with relatively stable funding even as Michigan's economy struggles.

Michigan's Medicaid program covers a yearly preventive exam, immunization administration, and problem and acute care office visits. Medicaid also reimburses for Clinical Laboratory Improvement Amendments (CLIA) waived lab procedures and many in-office procedures such as wart removal, inhalation treatments, EKG services, burn dressings, and so on. In Michigan, mental health services are covered by many of the Medicaid health plans, but they may require contracting with an outsourced behavioral health organization.

Medicaid reimbursements are calculated on a fee-for-service basis; providers must be enrolled within a billing group for such reimbursement. Groups are enrolled with a specialty of "Child and Adolescent Health Center" (SBHC designation) when they are certified as an SBHC by the state. This certification allows for centers to bill Medicaid Health Plans and receive fee-for-service reimbursement without prior authorization from a primary care provider and without a contract.

The state Medicaid office allows centers to become certified SBHCs when certain requirements are met. In order to become certified, SBHCs must provide immunization screening, primary care services for common and acute illnesses, and be able to refer to other clinics for services not provided at the SBHC. They must also meet administrative requirements, have a quality assurance plan, and follow parental consent and confidentiality guidelines.

Once the center is certified, it has the ability to bill Medicaid Health Plans without prior authorization or contract for medical services, and it is reimbursed at a minimum of Medicaid's published fee-for-service rates.

BOX 2—STATE SNAPSHOT: NORTH CAROLINA

School-Based Health Centers (SBHCs) in North Carolina are reimbursed by public health insurance programs and private insurers, but the recent recession will cause some health centers in the state, funded by local governments, to close their doors ("Asheville, Erwin school-based health centers to close." *Ashville Citizen-Times*. March 23, 2011).

As of 2011, there were 54 SBHCs in North Carolina; about half of them receive state funding. Medicaid carves out special payments for credentialed SBHCs. Once credentialed, SBHCs get their own Medicaid billing number and receive fee-for-service payments. (SBHCs that are not credentialed can still get Medicaid reimbursement, but they must get prior approval from the patient's primary care physician.)

North Carolina law requires that physicians must be on site when the services are being provided in order to get the full rate of reimbursement. Recognizing that most SBHCs in North Carolina are staffed by nurse practitioners, the state has exempted SBHCs sponsored by the state health department from this rule.

Private Insurance

Few SBHCs are contracting with private insurance to reimburse the cost of care for children and adolescents enrolled with those insurers. As a result, the cost of some visits are never reimbursed, leaving significant unrecovered expenditures of time and resources.

Connecticut has provided a model for how SBHCs can be guaranteed reimbursement by private insurance instead of focusing solely on public insurance. A report prepared by the state government found that of students seen at that state's SBHCs in 2006 and 2007, almost half were covered by Medicaid and another quarter were covered by private insurance.[17] Connecticut's SBHC nurse practitioners were found to be providing care to privately insured children for roughly 39,000 visits annually. These visits were not reimbursed, as they had not been deemed primary care providers. A visit by these same children at a Walgreens "Minute Clinic" was reimbursable.[18]

In June 2010, the Connecticut statute was changed to require that individual and group health insurance policies provide coverage for services received at SBHCs to the extent that such services are a covered benefit under the policy.[19] Connecticut's legislation provides an example of how other states could support their SBHCs through regulation of their private insurers. Given the political clout of the insurance industry in Connecticut, there is no reason to believe that other states cannot follow this example.

CONCLUSIONS

Focusing on state SBHC funding strategies has not exempted states from the overlapping influence of federal policy. SBHCs, found at the crossroads of education and health policy, also must navigate the difficulties of the state–federal relationship. Recent support for SBHCs in the Patient Protection and Affordable Care Act could provide an opportunity to return to the rate of growth of the 1990s. Even if this is the case, the essential pieces of public-sector support for SBHCs will likely remain in the hands of state governments.

The question of sustainability lurks over most of the funding sources: states' revenues fluctuate with the economy; the tobacco settlement will last 25 years, and it has reached its halfway point; Title V can be cut by Washington politicians. Thus, the best remedy for states is to make use of each of these funding sources but not to become too dependent on any one of them. That many more states are offering technical assistance and training for their SBHCs than offer direct financial support at least demonstrates that state governments value the contribution that SBHCs are making to the health and well-being of children in their state.

In the midst of fiscal uncertainty, the SBHC model thrives because it fills a gap left by traditional health care: children and adolescents. This is most poignantly the case for low wealth and minority youth who otherwise would be "left behind" in the for-profit health care sectors. State policymakers have an opportunity, as well as a challenge, to ensure the alignment of direct financial support and equitable reimbursement. If the history of SBHCs provides any lesson, it is that SBHCs will continue to flourish when direct state support is paired with a federal investment and fair reimbursement policies.

REFERENCES

1. Pub. Law 111-003; Section 505.

2. Schlitt JJ, Juszczak LJ, Eichner NH. Current status of state policies that support school-based health centers. *Public Health Rep*. 2008;123(6):731–738.

3. Strozer J, Juszczak L, Ammerman A. *2007–2008 National School-Based Health Care Census.* Washington, DC: National Assembly on School-Based Health Care; 2010.

4. Lear JG, Eichner N, Koppelman J. The growth of school-based health centers and the role of state policies: results of a national survey. *Arch Pediatr Adolesc Med.* 1999;153(11):1177–1180.

5. Lear JG. Health care goes to school. In: Garfinkel I, Hochschild JL, McLanahan SS, eds. *Social Policies for Children.* Washington, DC: The Brookings Institution; 1996:177–180.

6. H.R. 1, 112th Congress.

7. Levin P. Tobacco. National Association of Attorneys General. Available at: http://www.naag.org/tobacco.php. Accessed April 6, 2011.

8. Campaign for Tobacco-Free Kids. *Broken Promise to Our Children: The 1998 State Tobacco Settlement Twelve Years Later.* Washington, DC: Campaign for Tobacco-Free Kids; 2010.

9. Connecticut Public Act 06-195.

10. National Assembly on School-Based Health Care. Michigan: minimum program requirements for child and adolescent health centers. 2008. Available at: http://www.nasbhc.org/atf/cf/%7Bcd9949f2-2761-42fb-bc7a-cee165c701d9%7D/MICHIGAN%20STANDARDS.PDF. Accessed April 8, 2011.

11. Louisiana Department of Health and Hospitals, Office of Public Health, and Louisiana Assembly on School-Based Health Care. Principles, standards, and guidelines for school-based health centers in Louisiana. 2008. Available at: http://www.nasbhc.org/atf/cf/%7BCD9949F2-2761-42FB-BC7A-CEE165C701D9%7D/Basics_sbhcstandardsLA.pdf. Accessed April 8, 2011.

12. Colorado Department of Public Health and Environment. Quality standards for Colorado school-based health centers. 2009. Available at: http://www.nasbhc.org/atf/cf/%7Bcd9949f2-2761-42fb-bc7a-cee165c701d9%7D/QUALITY%20STANDARDS%20FOR%20CO%20SBHCS%20MARCH%202011.PDF. Accessed April 8, 2011.

13. Principles and guidelines for school-based health centers in New York State. 2006. Available at: http://www.nasbhc.org/atf/cf/%7BCD9949F2-2761-42FB-BC7A-CEE165C701D9%7D/Basics_sbhcstandardsNY.pdf. Accessed April 8, 2011.

14. Maryland School-Based Health Center Policy Advisory Council. Maryland school-based health center standards. Available at: http://www.nasbhc.org/atf/cf/%7BCD9949F2-2761-42FB-BC7A-CEE165C701D9%7D/Basics_sbhcstandardsMD.pdf. Accessed April 8, 2011.

15. Kaiser Commission on Key Facts. Medicaid matters: understanding Medicaid's role in our health care system. Kaiser Family Foundation. 2011. Available at: http://www.kff.org/medicaid/upload/8165.pdf. Accessed April 8, 2011.

16. Morone JA, Kilbreth EH, Langwell KM. Back to school: a health care strategy for youth. *Health Aff (Millwood).* 2001;20(1):122–136.

17. Connecticut Department of Public Health. Connecticut school-based health centers: healthy students make better learners: 2006–2007 annual report. 2009. Available at: http://www.ct.gov/dph/lib/dph/family_health/adlocents_and_school/annual_report_0607_final_5-06-09_pdf.pdf. Accessed April 8, 2011.

18. Testimony of Jesse White-Frese, Executive Director of the Connecticut Association of School Based Health Centers, before the Connecticut Public Health Committee. March 12, 2010.

19. Connecticut Public Act No. 10-118.

About the Authors

Joshua Rovner, MPP – is the Director of Policy and Advocacy for the National Assembly on School-Based Health Care where he is responsible for designing and implementing the National Assembly on School-Based Health Care's federal policy agenda. He has also served as Manager of Policy and Advocacy for Metro TeenAIDS, Associate Director of Federal Relations for the Campaign for Tobacco-Free Kids, and Policy Director for the Committee on Public Services for the Council of the District of Columbia. Rovner holds a Master's degree in Public Policy from George Washington University and a Bachelor's degree in Political Science from the University of Rochester.

Linda Juszczak, DNSc, MPH, CPNP – is President of the National Assembly on School-Based Health Care (NASBHC). Her 35 years of professional experience includes work as a nurse practitioner and a director for hospital, community, and school-based programs for adolescents. She has also held responsibilities as a faculty member and for developing policies impacting adolescents and school-based health centers. She was the founding President of the New York Coalition for School-Based Primary Care and is a founding member of the NASBHC. Linda's faculty appointments have been at Yale University, New York University, Cornell University, and Albert Einstein College of Medicine. She received her undergraduate degree from Skidmore College, a Master's in Nursing at the University of Colorado, a Pediatric Nurse Associate certificate and Master's in Public Health from the University of Minnesota, and a Doctorate in Nursing from Yale University. Linda has published extensively on adolescent health and school-based health care. She continues to maintain a practice as a pediatric nurse practitioner in adolescent medicine.

John Schlitt, MSW – is Director of Policy to Practice for the National Assembly on School-Based Health Care. From 1997 to 2008, Schlitt served as NASBHC's first executive director and rejoined NASBHC in 2011. Schlitt's 25-year career spans maternal, infant, and child health policy, practice, and advocacy arenas. He is a national authority on school-based health care financing, organization, and delivery and has authored several articles on school-based health care and teen pregnancy prevention. Schlitt received his Bachelor of Science degree in Psychology from the University of Florida and his Master of Social Work degree from Florida State University.

SECTION III

Strategic Partnerships for Fiscal and Policy Advocacy

OVERVIEW

Voices from the school-based health care field provide authentic, practical, and beneficial instruction. Chapters included in this section focus on initiatives or targeted partnerships, all of which were designed to influence institutional, local, state, or federal policy.

In Chapter 17, Murdock et al. discuss one of the most stubborn challenges facing school-based health centers (SBHCs): unstable funding. One grantee, the School Community Health Alliance of Michigan pursued an unprecedented strategy, securing a Centers for Medicare and Medicaid Services (formerly Health Care Financing Administration) waiver utilizing Michigan's network of SBHCs (also known in Michigan as Child and Adolescent Health Centers) to provide outreach and prevention services to Medicaid-qualified and Medicaid-eligible children. The federal Medicaid match was approved, providing valuable instruction to associations wishing to replicate securing a similar waiver.

Commitment to encouraging the political acumen of communities served by SBHCs has proven to be a powerful advocacy tool with spillover benefits to children and youth. Blinn, Carpenter, and Mandel, in Chapter 18, describe the unique way fourth and fifth graders were engaged to advance health and promote change in their elementary school. Elementary-age students are not often considered savvy enough to create and pursue their own policy agendas. However, as is pointed out in this chapter, elementary children possess the drive to make their school a better, healthier community when provided the opportunity.

In Chapter 19, Zorrilla, Baxter, and Heater deconstruct one California-based Youth Advisory Board (YAB) and how students promoted youth empowerment and policy change within the San Francisco Unified School District (SFUSD). In conjunction with clinic staff, the YAB conducted a needs assessment to assess youths' perspectives and knowledge regarding health care access and minor consent law, presented their findings at community meetings, and successfully advocated for policy change within the SFUSD. Application of what was learned from both this chapter and the one that precedes it can inform efforts to develop meaningful youth–adult collaborations, positive youth development, and school-based policy change.

In Chapter 20, the authors show how aligning SBHCs with the contemporary full-service community school movement demonstrates the specific advantages of partnerships as a model for educational delivery and community support and as a model for SBHCs. Adherence to the pure community school model requires inclusion of health providers and other safety net services as seamlessly integrated into the school environment. However, the expertise to identify health-related needs of students inherent in the community school model is beyond the capacity of most educators, which highlights the value of an SBHC collaboration.

There are times when serendipity lends a hand. This was the case when a well-publicized article by Nicholas Freudenberg and Jessica Ruglis[1] drew national attention to the public health consequences of high school dropouts. Carpenter, Blinn and Richardson, in Chapter 21, articulate the Massachusetts Coalition of School-Based Health Centers' multidisciplinary forums that sought to bring attention to the role that school-based health services can play in reducing school dropout rates by promoting interagency and multidisciplinary interventions for youth. They argue that SBHCs, given their ability to play a pivotal role in early identification and interventions on behalf of students entering a dropout danger zone, are a largely untapped resource.

Chance and preparation played a role in the ways SBHCs became an active recovery agent after Hurricanes Katrina and Rita in New Orleans. Lessons proposed by Broussard in Chapter 22 apply not only to post-disaster undertakings but also to consideration of SBHCs as a vital resource for emergency preparedness.

Finally, it is difficult for large-scale policy advocacy to take place without benefactors. Section II described with detail the W. K. Kellogg Foundation (WKKF) initiative, and, in Chapter 23, Villanueva reveals how a state-based foundation made an impact on the stability and the growth in the numbers of SBHCs in North Carolina. The Kate B. Reynolds Charitable Trust has been a champion in providing fiscal support for local safety net organizations that provide a medical home and increase access to primary care. In recent years they have sought to sustain their multimillion dollar investment by supporting the statewide school-based health association to provide technical assistance to clinics and to champion advocacy efforts. The Trust also leveraged a partnership with WKKF that resulted in an ongoing relationship, technical assistance, and additional dollars to the state.

REFERENCE

1. Freudenberg N, Ruglis J. Reframing school dropout as a public health issue. *Prev Chronic Dis.* 2007;4(4):A107.

Michigan's Medicaid Matching Initiative: Lessons Learned

Rick Murdock, Carrie Tarry, Kyle Guerrant,
Debbie Brinson, Brenda McLean,
and Jeanita W. Richardson

Contributions of school-based and school-linked health centers particularly for Medicaid-enrolled and Medicaid-eligible youth are in part a function of the communities they serve. Forty-one percent of school-based health centers (SBHCs) are located in Title I schools, a designation given to schools with high numbers of economically disadvantaged and otherwise at-risk students. Most SBHCs are located in urban communities (59%); however, their presence is increasing in rural schools (27%).[1,2] Though the scope of services is community specific, the range of services most consistently offered are comprehensive primary care, health promotion and disease prevention, early intervention and risk reduction, and limited mental health and counseling support.[1]

Evidence substantiating the cost–benefit and improved health care access associated with school-based and school-linked centers has done little, unfortunately, to mitigate the significant barrier to securing long-term sustainable funding streams.[2–5] For example, in Michigan most SBHCs receive state funding, but all of them must augment support with grants, community support, and other sources of revenue, including billing third-party payers.[1,2] Of significant note to this discussion, these centers struggle to remain viable not because there is a question of their value, but most often because of insufficient financial backing.

Clinicians in SBHCs have little time to seek funding because their time is consumed with caring for students and the associated recordkeeping. From this need, state associations have emerged with missions to advocate for school-based and school-linked health services for children and youth, stable funding sources, and educating political leadership and communities about the value of SBHCs as contributors to the continuum of care for children and youth. State assembly formation notwithstanding, the dilemma of undependable SBHC fiscal resources has persisted. The W. K. Kellogg Foundation's School-Based Health Care Policy Program (SBHCPP) sought to remediate this challenge by charging state assembly grantees with envisioning and advocating for formal and informal policies that would secure a more reliable fiscal foundation for centers while increasing access to health care and prevention services for vulnerable children and youth.

One grantee, the School Community Health Alliance of Michigan (SCHA-MI) partnered with Medicaid and the Michigan Association of Health Plans to pursue an unprecedented strategy, securing a Centers for Medicare and Medicaid Services (CMS, formerly Health Care Financing Administration) waiver utilizing Michigan's network of SBHCs (more commonly known in Michigan as Child and Adolescent Health Centers) to provide outreach and prevention services to Medicaid-qualified and Medicaid-eligible children. The federal Medicaid match was approved, allowing stable funding to Michigan's network of SBHCs.

This chapter describing SCHA-MI's initiative is informative to the field in several ways. First, it articulates fiscal and unanticipated benefits associated with this policy change that accrued to the state's SBHCs. Second, it reveals the steps taken to secure a formal policy change beneficial to sustainability while supporting the work of increased outreach for Medicaid-eligible children and youth. Third, as the waiver is the first of its kind, the process can inform others interested in replication.

BENEFITS OF SECURING A MEDICAID MATCH

State associations seeking more predictable funding for their SBHC members should consider the benefits and some of the challenges associated with pursuing a Medicaid match because for every state dollar allocation there is approximately an additional dollar disbursed from the federal government. As budgets increase (state plus federal allocations) so can the services for more Medicaid-enrolled and Medicaid-eligible children. It is possible, as was the case in Michigan, to use the additional resources to increase significantly the number of SBHCs in operation, thus mitigating barriers to traditional care and Medicaid enrollment by providing services to children in or near their schools. More funding to support economically disadvantaged children, improved stability of funding for existing SBHCs, increased predictability of dollars available for SBHCs (given the federal dollars are associated with state-appropriated line items), and potentially increasing the numbers of SBHCs all represent benefits of pursuing the Medicaid Match.

Benefits are also linked to challenges and barriers associated with the Medicaid match. For example, each state has its own memorandum of understanding (MOU) with CMS dictating the use of federal Medicaid dollars. Waivers are required when there are requests to change the scope of services specified in the prevailing MOU. Additionally, SBHCs are supported by different funding models (e.g., public, private, or varying combinations of public and private dollars). If an SBHC is not supported by a state budget line item allocation, a Medicaid match as described here may not be a possibility. Even if SBHCs are formal beneficiaries of state appropriations, securing the match requires a long-term commitment from the state association because, as was revealed in Michigan, even after the Medicaid match is approved, it is only available as long as states retain state fiscal support of SBHCs. Particularly in times of budget crises, time-consuming and labor-intensive advocacy will be required to protect the line item. All of that said, the benefits of securing the waiver and subsequent match in Michigan's case have outweighed the challenges.

MICHIGAN'S MEDICAID MATCH

The State of Michigan through the Michigan Department of Community Health (MDCH) had an appropriations commitment for SBHCs until November 3, 2001, when a gubernatorial order eliminated state funding for SBHCs. Through the extensive efforts of SCHA-MI and its members, the deleted level of funding was restored not to the health budget where it had been since its inception, but to the K–12 education budget. Despite its fiscal relegation to the Department of Education, oversight of SBHCs remained with MDCH, creating a new multiagency accountability paradigm.

To ensure long-term funding stability, SCHA-MI targeted agencies and organizations familiar with the role of SBHCs, the Michigan Medicaid MOU, and those to whom SBHCs were accountable. The team of representatives included the Michigan Association of Health Plans, the state Medicaid Office, Department of Community Health (the umbrella agency that also includes the Medicaid Office), the Department of Education, Michigan State University, and the Michigan Primary Care Association, and advanced the goal of exploring alternative funding opportunities to help sustain SBHCs. Creativity and extensive knowledge of the state and federal Medicaid systems yielded a proposal that acknowledged the unique role that SBHCs could play in delivering outreach services, which would qualify for a federal match of Medicaid dollars.[6]

Ultimately, the aforementioned group decided to target federal Medicaid outreach opportunities because Michigan's network of SBHCs provides prevention services to significant populations of Medicaid or Medicaid-eligible children, because outreach services were not at that time being reimbursed under the MOU, and because SBHCs are uniquely suited to help youth and families enroll in Medicaid. The consensus was that, if the state allocation could be used as a match for federal Medicaid dollars, the funding stream for SBHCs would be more predictable and protected. For this to be accomplished, the MDCH was required to submit an official waiver request as per consultation with CMS. To our knowledge, this was an unprecedented request.

As background, Medicaid-reimbursable services are articulated in state-specific agreements. Medicaid, per federal guidelines, can reimburse qualified providers for covered health services, such as outreach to ensure eligible children are enrolled in Medicaid and early and periodic screening, diagnostic, and treatment services (EPSDT). These services can be reimbursed if they have been administered by school personnel, other qualified practitioners with whom the school contracts (e.g., SBHCs), or a combined approach. [7,8] However, not all states take advantage of this provision to support SBHCs even though they technically qualify for reimbursement given their services.

The Michigan waiver was needed for two reasons. First, the source of the "new" federal money was underwritten by an adjustment in the capitation rates for children in Michigan. Capitation rates are billable costs associated with services that tend to be lower than physician private fee-for-services rates.[9] The capitation rate articulated in the Michigan MOU needed adjustment to include outreach services that included ensuring qualified children were enrolled in Medicaid.[a] Second, the waiver request would allow managed care health plans through agreement with the MDCH to contract with Michigan's network of SBHCs for said services.

SBHCs within the state had been strategically located to serve the highest need communities and had proven their worth as a valuable health care safety net for youth while also addressing critical public health and social concerns. At the time, Michigan funded 31 SBHCs that delivered services to 10- to 21-year-olds in urban, rural, and suburban districts. Michigan's Medicaid health insurance coverage of the nonelderly is predominantly allocated to children (58.2%), yet there were many low-income school-age children who qualified for Medicaid, were concentrated in predictable school districts, but were uninsured. For example, in 2007, 23% of the children in Michigan lived in families who met the poverty income benchmarks, and at least 13% of the state's children were uninsured and likely qualified for services. The state's school-age child health care utilization rates among Medicaid-eligible youngsters were also low and accounted for 15% of state Medicaid spending as opposed to the average child-utilization rate expenditures in the United States of

---

[a] Outreach is a significant goal of Medicaid given approximately two-thirds of uninsured children and youth are eligible for publicly funded insurance coverage, and in periods of economic downturns are often the only health insurance option for those under 18.[10]

approximately 19%.[10,11] By virtue of the aforementioned coverage rates and the concentrations of said population in certain school districts, the match team agreed that increasing the number of SBHCs could improve both utilization and outreach rates.

CMS had to affirm the proposal and increase the capitated payment rate that Medicaid-managed care plans received for providing outreach services to eligible Medicaid populations in Michigan. As per federal Medicaid authorities, a concept paper detailing proposed changes from historical practice was required. The concept paper proposed that the $3.74 million of state general funds should be appropriated as the match base. These state funds, then, would be used to access approximately $5.5 million in federal dollars to support expanded outreach services.[6] Proposed funds would first travel through the state's Medicaid-managed care plans and a fiduciary (the Michigan Primary Care Association) before arriving at SBHCs. The paper emphasized that the waiver would support Michigan's efforts to restore outreach services to Medicaid-eligible students and improve EPSDT[12,b] and rates of immunizations, screenings, and well-child visits. Most of this additional waiver-related money would in effect be turned over by the managed care plans to SBHCs for the purpose of delivering outreach and prevention services to Medicaid-eligible or Medicaid-enrolled students.[6]

Strengths of the Michigan proposal were the interagency support for the initiative, demonstrated population need, the existing infrastructure to implement the proposed plan, and MDCH's reporting and evaluation protocols for SBHCs. Additionally, the request was built on a tested service delivery model with a track record of serving high-need children, and permission for the match supported increased access and utilization of prevention and early intervention services that were below targeted performance levels. CMS' waiver became effective the summer of 2004.

HOW THE MEDICAID MATCH WORKS IN MICHIGAN

CMS is notified of the state allocation and remits the federal match back to the state Medicaid office, which then forwards the total (state and federal funds) to Michigan Medicaid health plans. All funding decisions for this program continue to be made jointly by the Michigan Departments of Community Health and Education. The additional federal match funds have made it possible to double the network of SBHCs throughout the state from 31 at its onset to 63 sites, increasing the number of children and adolescents served each year to over 100,000.[13]

---

b EPSDT services are both comprehensive and preventative child health interventions. They include but are not limited to physical examinations, vision and dental services, immunizations, laboratory tests, and other necessary health care.

Benefits of the federal match accrued immediately and continue to do so for SCHA-MI, SBHCs, MDCH, and CMS. CMS benefits because enrollment numbers have increased, in part because additional SBHCs funded by the federal match reach greater numbers of targeted children. Also, Michigan's state-mandated five-year review cycles of SBHCs and the regular MDCH reporting protocols provide a level of systematic accountability recommended by CMS.

Anticipated and unanticipated benefits to MDCH include a strengthening of inter- and intra-agency relationships. The federal match increased the dollars available to support a high-need population (80% of the children serviced at SBHCs in Michigan are Medicaid-enrolled or Medicaid-eligible) and to date has provided a stable funding mechanism for SBHCs. One unanticipated benefit was the interagency collaborative grant writing and advocacy reciprocity that have thus far ensured retention of the state Medicaid allocation for SBHCs. Another unanticipated value of pursuing the match has been an MDCH strategy to seek opportunities for consistent support of publicly funded programs with federal match dollars.

Michigan Medicaid health plans have a new appreciation for the ways SBHCs compliment their own mission. For example, services that historically raised concerns of being duplicative (e.g., primary care and immunizations) largely have been ameliorated. Additionally, the reporting criteria of SBHCs have tangibly aided health plans when compliance with mandated service targets (EPSDT, immunizations, and so on) must be demonstrated. Also, SBHC services tend to be those that are more cost-effective for Medicaid plans than are private fee-for-service interventions because the focus of SBHC service is preventative care, and providing early identification of at-risk health behaviors and prices are determined by the capitation rates.

Michigan has faced difficult state budget decisions given declining revenue and the recession. Passage of the federal stimulus package (also known as the American Recovery and Reinvestment Act of 2009) helped bridge budget shortfalls in Michigan in 2009, but were not enough to meet budget shortfalls in 2009, 2010, or 2011.[14,15] The current administration, led by Governor Snyder, passed a budget that cut $1.4 billion from general fund spending by imposing a stricter 48-month limit on welfare benefits, cutting clothing allowances for poor children, cutting state police resources, and cutting resources for local bus systems.[16] It is in this climate that the Medicaid match has revealed its insulation value. SBHCs are beneficiaries of the match because they are linked to a stable funding stream. As was noted earlier, the match has thus far been protective against cuts to SBHCs because of reminders that deletion of a $1 state investment would net an approximate $2 loss in federal dollars, which is significant given the extreme budget crises experienced by the state.

LIMITATIONS

As was noted earlier, centers receiving the Medicaid match are limited to either SBHCs having state line-item support or SBHCs that are funded in practice through state agencies with state dollars. SBHC state assemblies would need to assemble the requisite state agencies already affiliated with CMS to agree to pursue the federal match and implement necessary procedural changes. Finally, state-based agencies would need to affirm that increasing the SBHC network would be a worthy strategy to meet the state's childhood health and outreach service needs.

REPLICATING THE MICHIGAN MEDICAID MATCH

There are transferrable lessons for state associations interested in pursuing a Medicaid match to support their SBHC network. The bullets below summarize key points:

- Determine which decision-makers are critical to obtaining CMS permission;
- Ensure SBHC state assembly staff understand current and proposed inter- and intra-agency collaborations necessary for the match;
- Cultivate partnerships for securing the match and beyond; and
- Ensure continuation of the match once approved via long-term planning, including perpetual education of partner agency staff and legislators.

Prior to launching a similar strategy, assessments should be made regarding which decision-makers are needed to secure the federal match and ensure effective and efficient implementation. To accomplish this, it is critical to have staff with a full complement of skills, including familiarity with the education and health communities, Medicaid, SBHC contributions, and state governance.

The state SBHC assembly team should also familiarize themselves with the priorities, missions, and challenges of the organizations and agencies that are pivotal to the effort. For example, in Michigan's case the state match is in the K–12 appropriations. As a result, it was important to engage the Department of Education, as well as the various health agencies (e.g., MDCH, the Medicaid Office, the Michigan Association of Health Plans, and so on) that were directly accountable for SBHCs. In other states, the line item might be found elsewhere; however, the larger lesson here is that those who stand to gain or potentially lose in the federal match should be part of early discussions.

Partnerships for purposes of the match should include those empowered to make decisions for their respective organizations or agencies. SCHA-MI found that these collaborators are not only critical to crafting the state-specific match process but also essential to ensuring the agreed upon process is adopted within their organizations. Though the value of matched dollars seems a rational reason to retain the appropriation, it is not necessarily enough to insulate the Medicaid match from shifting governmental priorities and fiscal allocations. SCHA-MI also found empowered partners to be effective voices in legislative budget sessions relative to the multiplier effect of the match, particularly when it appeared the appropriation line item might be redistributed.

Education of managed care providers, legislators, and agency heads is not a one-time investment. Because of the turnover of individuals in these positions, validating the efficacy of this match to the state is ongoing, particularly in times of fiscal distress.

At this writing, it is not clear whether the Medicaid match will protect SBHCs from being cut from state appropriations partially or completely in the current budget cycle. However, it is undeniable (as confirmed by members of the state legislature) that the only reason fiscal support for SBHCs has lasted since 2004 in the face of perpetual budget constraints is because of the Medicaid Match Initiative. Thus, perhaps the greatest lesson of all is that proactive policy change, as the W. K. Kellogg Foundation anticipated, is a viable strategy to undergird SBHC sustainability.

REFERENCES

1. Juszczak L, Schlitt J, Moore A. *School-Based Health Centers: National Census School Year 2004–05*. Washington, DC: National Assembly on School-based Health Care; 2007.

2. Wade TJ, Mansour ME, Guo JJ, Huentelman T, Line K, Keller KN. Access and utilization patterns of school-based health centers at urban and rural elementary and middle schools. *Public Health Rep*. 2008;123(6):739–750.

3. Geierstanger SP, Amaral G, Mansour M, Walters SR. School-based health centers and academic performance: research, challenges, and recommendations. *J Sch Health*. 2004;74(9):347–352.

4. Richardson JW. Building bridges between school-based health clinics and schools. *J Sch Health*. 2007;77(7):337–343.

5. Schlitt JJ, Juszczak LJ, Eichner NH. Current status of state policies that support school-based health centers. *Public Health Rep*. 2008;123(6):731–738.

6. Brinson D, Murdock R, Reinhart P. *Effective Practices: Michigan's Medicaid Matching Initiative*. Battle Creek, MI: W. K. Kellogg Foundation; 2005.

7. Ryan J. *Medicaid: The Basics*. Washington, DC: National Health Policy Forum; 2009.

8. Scanlon WJ. *Medicaid: Questionable Practices Boost Federal Payments for School-Based Services*. Washington, DC: US General Accounting Office; 1999. Report No: GAO/T-HEHS-99-148.

9. Holahan J, Rangarajan S, Schirmer M. *Medicaid Managed Care Payment Methods and Capitation Rates: Results of a National Survey*. Washington, DC: The Urban Institute; 2009.

10. Kaiser Commission on Medicaid and the Uninsured. *State Medicaid Fact Sheets: Michigan*. Menlo Park, CA: Kaiser Family Foundation; 2006.

11. Kaiser Commission on Medicaid Facts. *Enrolling Uninsured Low-Income Children in Medicaid and SCHIP*. Washington, DC: Kaiser Family Foundation; 2005.

12. Centers for Medicare & Medicaid Services. *EPSDT Benefits*. Baltimore, MD: Centers for Medicare & Medicaid Services; 2005.

13. School-Community Health Alliance of Michigan. *School-Based Health Centers—Fact Sheet*. Lansing, MI: School–Community Alliance of Michigan; 2007.

14. Hornbeck M. Michigan's budget deficit gets deeper. *The Detroit News*. April 14, 2009. Available at: http://detnews.com/article/20090414/POLITICS02/904140348. Accessed June 14, 2011.

15. Luke P. Budget forecast: Michigan faces $1.58 billion deficit, $263 per student funding cut in 2011. Mlive.com. January 11, 2010. Available at: http://www.mlive.com/politics/index.ssf/2010/01/post_16.html. Accessed June 14, 2011.

16. Christoff C. Michigan budget cuts cops, aid to poor, and the arts. *Detroit Free Press*. May 5, 2011. Available at: http://www.ongo.com/v/871438/-1/C844497968CC0BAB/michigan-house-budget-cuts-cops-aid-to-poor-and-the-arts. Accessed June 14, 2011.

About the Authors

Rick Murdock's – Thirty-four years of work experience has been entirely in the health policy and finance area. Mr. Murdock earned a Bachelor of Science degree from Eastern Michigan University and a Master of Health Services Administration degree from the University of Michigan School of Public Health. He has been with the Michigan Association of Health Plans (MAHP) since 2002 and as Executive Director since 2004. Prior to joining MAHP in July of 2002, Mr. Murdock held several positions within Michigan State Government to include the Michigan Department of Community Health where he was responsible for direct administration of Michigan's Medicaid Managed Care; a financial specialist for the State Budget Office with focus in the Mental Health and Special Medicaid Financing areas; and a health policy specialist for the State Health Planning Office in areas of health professional training, preventive health practices, and health care cost analysis.

Carrie Tarry, MPH – has worked in the field of public health for over 15 years, including community-level experience in HIV/AIDS and state-level experience in adolescent health and development, school health services, and teen pregnancy prevention. Ms. Tarry is currently the Adolescent and School Health Manager for the Michigan Department of Community Health as well as the designated State Adolescent Health Coordinator for Michigan. In her present position, she supervises 14 public health consultants and contractual staff. She also manages multiple public health programs with an annual budget of over $22 million dollars that gets distributed across 100 contracted agencies and schools throughout the state. Ms. Tarry received her Master of Public Health from the University of Michigan in 1995 and a Bachelor of Arts in Communications from Michigan State University.

Kyle Guerrant, MSW, BA – received his BA in Psychology from Long Island University and his MSW from the University of Michigan. Mr. Guerrant has been a strong leader and advocate in youth health and safety issues in community-based nonprofits, local schools, and state government for the last 10 years. Currently, he is the Director of Coordinated School Health and Safety Programs unit at the Michigan Department of Education. For the past 5 years, Mr. Guerrant and his team have been charged with improving the health and educational outcomes of Michigan youth through the implementation of Coordinated School Health initiatives.

Debbie Brinson, MPA – is the CEO of the Ingham Community Health Center Network, a network of community health centers, including school-based health centers, serving vulnerable populations. Prior to that she served as the Executive Director for the School

Community Health Alliance of Michigan, an advocacy organization dedicated to ensuring that all children and youth have access to health care and prevention services. For more than 25 years, she has been working on behalf of children and youth.

Brenda McLean, MSA – is the Practice and Data Network Manager for the School-Community Health Alliance of Michigan. Brenda has worked in Billing for over 10 years, and her experience includes general practice, pediatrics, gynecological, and mental health billing and precertification. She has worked with Medicaid billing and Managed Care Organizations and has an understanding of the insurance industry related to billing practices. Brenda earned her Bachelor of Science in Business Administration with a major in Accounting and a minor in Finance from Central Michigan University and went on to obtain a Master of Science in Administration with a focus on Human Resources.

Jeanita W. Richardson, PhD, MEd – is an Associate Professor in the Department of Public Health Sciences at the University of Virginia School of Medicine. Her scholarship highlights the inextricable links between health and learning readiness, particularly for disenfranchised children and youth. Her work has been published and presented in numerous national and international journals and conferences. Her consulting energies (Turpeau Consulting Group, LLC) are devoted to supporting healthy children who are ready to learn through the creation of health and educational policy bridges and include five years as a consultant to the W. K. Kellogg Foundation's School-Based Health Care Policy Program. For more information, email TConsultingG@aol.com.

A Newfound Voice: Elementary-Age Student Engagement

Antonia M. Blinn, Nancy W. Carpenter, and Leslie A. Mandel

Youth civic engagement research and training tools have predominantly centered on high school– and college-age youth, and as a result, the elementary-age student either tends to be overlooked in advocacy efforts or approaches typically aimed at older students are utilized for these younger children.[1] Consequently, engaging, training, and mobilizing elementary school-age youth as part of an advocacy process to sustain and enhance school-based health centers (SBHCs) is unfamiliar advocacy territory. Mobilizing all groups affected by SBHCs is key to their sustainability because, notwithstanding documented success in improving health outcomes for children and adolescents,[2-5] SBHCs encounter challenges to their ongoing survival, such as (1) increased competition for funds, (2) inadequate third-party reimbursement, (3) limited awareness of the SBHC model, and (4) conflicting education policies and reform mandates.[6,7] In light of these contextual obstacles, SBHCs have struggled to be fully embraced by the fields of health and education.[8] SBHCs endure largely by tackling concerns through public education, community advocacy, collaboration, and support and participation of key SBHC stakeholders, including school-age children and youth.

Among the 1,909 SBHCs nationwide, 9.6% are in elementary schools, and another 33.7% are in combination schools that include elementary/middle schools and kindergarten through 12th grade schools.[9] The numbers of SBHCs in elementary schools provide opportunities to introduce health-promoting behaviors[10] and knowledge before at-risk behaviors become irrefutably ingrained. The prevalence of SBHCs in elementary schools also indicates that younger children should not be left out of the SBHC advocacy process. Elementary-age students, however, are not "little adolescents," and the approach to engaging them in advocacy requires a developmentally appropriate approach.

According to the National Council for the Social Studies, "Civic understanding in the elementary grades enables the development of responsible citizens."[11] Another study[12] confirmed that elementary school-age children were able to learn about the advocacy process, make and justify choices, identify leadership traits, and recognize and appreciate different opinions. Still, other researchers support the notion that early grades, particularly fourth and fifth grade, are uniquely suited for building civic action skills but require developmentally appropriate expectations such as responsible behavior and work habits, concern for others including groups and community, and initiative to help groups and schools make a positive difference.[1] To help meet civic expectations for elementary school youth, Chi, Jastrzab, and Melchior have advocated for a core foundation that includes knowledge and learning, thinking and participation skills, and disposition.[1]

Despite the challenges that SBHCs face, there are unique opportunities not afforded to more typical health care settings. Located in schools where students are readily accessible, SBHC health care providers have the potential to build relationships with students that extend beyond the conventional clinician–patient relationship that is often limited to an annual visit. SBHC clinicians not only see patients for health concerns and physicals but also deliver health promotion education either in the clinic setting and/or in collaboration with teachers, other school personnel, and community agencies. SBHC staff can also help children move beyond individual health concerns and learn to recognize, address, and improve schoolwide health issues. Further, as pediatric health care providers, they are trained to understand the developmental milestones and capacity of children and can incorporate this knowledge into health promotion and community advocacy activities.

PROGRAM DESCRIPTION

Since 2004, the Massachusetts Association for School-Based Health Care (the Association) has been part of the W. K. Kellogg Foundation's School-Based Health Care Policy Program (SBHCPP), a multiyear, national initiative designed to build and sustain SBHCs. A key component of the project has been civic engagement of youth who utilize SBHC services and/or attend a school in which there was an SBHC. At the inception of the SBHCPP in Massachusetts, the Association selected four state-based SBHCs to be community partners. Community partners were selected based upon geographic and demographic diversity within the state. The community partners were also generally reflective of the distribution of grade levels represented among SBHCs in the Commonwealth of Massachusetts. Based on the desire to change attitudes and strengthen relationships among young people and between young people and adults and also to support young people as an active force for change, a framework and curriculum were developmentally adapted from Youth on Board's[13] *15 Points: Successfully Involving Youth in Decision Making*, a comprehensive guide to youth involvement.[14] Worksheets, tips, resources, and fellow organizer experiences informed the training of the community organizers who guided students in discussions leading to a healthier school community.

The elementary school seeking to increase the advocacy acumen of its students is located in an inner-city school with 650 students in grades K to 5. Ninety percent of its students are eligible for free or reduced school lunches, a designation generally accepted as an indication of student economic need. The school population is culturally diverse with about 65% Hispanic, mostly recent immigrants from Guatemala,[15] as well as Cambodian, Russian, and Asian populations. Eighty-two percent of the students are enrolled to utilize the SBHC (Lorraine Murphy, RN, AP, MSN, MPH, SBHC Site Manager for the Lynn Community Health Center, unpublished data, 2008). The city hosting the elementary school is densely populated (89,050 residents), with nearly twice as many children living below 100% of the federal poverty level than the state average,[16] and the property crime and violent crime levels are higher than the state average.[17]

THE HEALTH CLUB IS BORN

A team consisting of the SBHC nurse practitioner, a community organizer, a college intern, and a school nurse led the group. This team worked with fourth and fifth graders over a four-year period in a Health Club meeting after school once a week for two hours. All fourth and fifth grade students enrolled in the school were eligible to participate in the Health Club. Each year, 25 to 35 students returned their bilingual English/Spanish consent forms to participate and met once a week after school in the elementary school library. Generally, students were involved in the Health Club for two consecutive school years.

Using an eight-step process (Figure 18.1), students identified issues that concerned them and affected their peers and then selected action items that were considered winnable.

The first year of the Health Club (2005) focused on creating a logo and identity for the Health Club, identifying health uses that concerned the student, and learning about the legislative budget and law-making process using the *School House Rocks* series. By 2006, Health Club members wanted to improve physical activity and

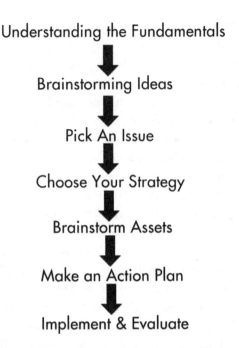

Understanding the Fundamentals

⬇

Brainstorming Ideas

⬇

Pick An Issue

⬇

Choose Your Strategy

⬇

Brainstorm Assets

⬇

Make an Action Plan

⬇

Implement & Evaluate

Figure 18.1 — Eight-step process for organizing and advocating for change.

targeted the playground. The playground was uninviting—a large, barren, open space with black asphalt and no equipment. Recess at the time consisted of 10 unstructured minutes, and fights among students were common during this period.

Working with a part-time community organizer, the students created a plan and met with the school vice principal to present options to improve recess. Though their initial ideas, such as planting trees and installing playground equipment, were not feasible due to space or cost, the students persevered and created a plan that was realistic for their budget and abilities. They adjusted their expectations to align with the resources available, an important early lesson in advocacy for these students.

The students developed a plan to paint the playground surface with games such as hopscotch. They planned the design and layout of the games on the black-top, and the nurse practitioner reached out to local high school student volunteers seeking community service hours to do the painting. A small grant supplied the paint, soft kick balls, and jump ropes. Once completed, there was more to do at recess, and the students knew they had been agents for positive change. Fueled by this success, they began thinking about health improvements that would result from prolonged recess time, eliminating greasy lunches, and strategies for being safe, including being careful around stray dogs encountered on the way to school.

CONCLUSION

Students learned important lessons about changing their school and their community from the experience, such as the value of being persistent even if initially denied what you want. At first, SBHC staff and students in the Health Club did not know how to conduct advocacy and awareness activities. Later, they saw themselves as model advocates. SBHC staff, including managers, commented that their own views of SBHCs also grew over time; they are now able to recognize that they do not just deliver primary care, they also have opportunities to actively engage children in their health care and in the health of the school and community. The principal feels that the Health Club has been a big help to her and to parents by engaging kids in a safe way in a nonsafe city. The school now sees the Health Club as advantageous on multiple levels. The students learned that they have the power to impact their world through their influence and advocacy. The SBHC is now seen as part of the fabric of the school, caring for both individuals and the greater school community.

The fourth and fifth graders were successful in their work because they were trained to understand what it means to be part of a community and participate in identifying and developing solutions for school and community issues. In addition, the guidance they received and expectations set were developmentally appropriate for their age. The students learned about identifying a local issue and thinking about possible solutions. They learned how to adapt expectations to fit realities. They also learned how to approach authority figures and to listen to and appreciate different ideas. These skills can be adapted and fostered for broader advocacy issues as long as they have meaning for the youth involved. While elementary-age children can work alongside older youth, they must be given activities and tasks that are in line with their understanding, intellectual capacity, and temperament. The great lesson of this initiative is that elementary-age students are not too young to be advocates. Instead, because of their unique energy, perspective, perseverance, and drive to make their school a better place, they too can contribute to healthier communities when provided the opportunity.

REFERENCES

1. Chi B, Jastrzab J, Melchior A. *Developing Indicators and Measures of Civic Outcomes for Elementary School Students.* Working Paper 47. College Park, MD: CIRCLE; 2006.

2. Pastore D, Juszczak L, Fisher M, Friedman SB. School-based health center utilization: a survey of users and nonusers. *Arch Pediatr Adolesc Med.* 1998;152(8):763–767.

3. Cohen DA, Nsuami M, Martin DH, Farley TA. Repeated school-based screening for sexually transmitted diseases: a feasible strategy for reaching adolescents. *Pediatrics.* 1999;104(6):1281–1285.

4. Kaplan DW, Brindis CD, Phibbs SL, Melinklovich P, Naylor K, Ahlstrand K. A comparison study of an elementary school-based health center: effects on health care access and use. *Arch Pediatr Adolesc Med.* 1999;153(3):235–243.

5. Guo J, Jang R, Keller K, McCracken AL, Pan W, Cluxton RJ. Impact of school-based health centers on children with asthma. *J Adolesc Health.* 2005;37(4):266–274.

6. Porter M, Kramer M. *Determining a Policy Agenda to Sustain School-Based Health Centers: NASBHC Assesses the Health Care Safety Net Environment.* Washington, DC: National Assembly on School-Based Health Centers; 2000. Available at: http://www. nasbhc.org. Accessed September 4, 2009.

7. Button J, Rienzo B. *The Politics of Youth, Sex, and Health Care in American Schools.* New York, NY: Haworth Press; 2002.

8. Lear J. *From the Margins to the Mainstream: Institutionalizing School-Based Health Centers.* Washington, DC: Making the Grade—Publications; 2000. Available at: http:// www.healthinschools.org/en/Model-Programs/From-the-margins-to-the-mainstream. aspx. Accessed April 21, 2009.

9. Strozer J, Juszczak L, Ammerman A. *Data of National Census of School-Based Health Centers—Draft Summary for School Year 2007–2008.* Washington, DC: National Assembly on School-Based Health Care; 2010. Available at: http://ww2.nasbhc.org/ NASBHCCensusReport07-08.pdf. Accessed April 18, 2011.

10. Stock S, Miranda C, Evans S, et al. Healthy buddies: a novel, peer-led health promotion program for the prevention of obesity and eating disorders in children in elementary school. *Pediatrics.* 2007;120(4):e1059–e1068.

11. NCSS Task Force on Early Childhood/Elementary Social Studies. *Social Studies for Early Childhood and Elementary School Children: Preparing for the 21st Century.* Alexandria, VA: National Council for the Social Studies; 1989.

12. Catapano S, Song KH. Let's collaborate and infuse citizenship education: kids voting in primary classrooms. *Soc Stud Res Pract.* 2006;1(1):55–66.

13. Youth on Board website. 2009. Available at: http://www.youthonboard.org/site/c. ihLUJ7PLKsG/b.2046673/k.C863/About_Us.htm. Accessed September 30, 2009.

14. Young KS, Sazama J. *15 Points: Successfully Involving Youth in Decision Making.* Somerville, MA: Youth on Board; 2006.

15. Massachusetts Department of Elementary and Secondary Education. School and District Profiles website. 2009. Available at: http://profiles.doe.mass.edu. Accessed September 30, 2009.

16. Hometown USA. Population and census data for Lynn, Massachusetts. 2011. Available at: http://www.hometownusa.com/ma/population/Lynn.html. Accessed September 30, 2009.

17. IDcide. Lynn, MA, Profile. 2011. Available at: http://www.idcide.com/citydata/ma/lynn.htm. Accessed September 30, 2009.

About the Authors

Antonia M. Blinn, CHES – is the Program Director for the Massachusetts Association for School-Based Health Care. Her career has focused on social justice and improving health services access for children and families who rely on publicly funded programs. Blinn utilizes policy, advocacy, outreach, and community engagement to expand collaborations and increase funding for school-based health services. Ms. Blinn has a Bachelor of Science in Community Health Education from the University of North Carolina at Greensboro and is a Certified Health Education Specialist. Blinn is an alumnus of the Blue Cross Blue Shield of Massachusetts Foundation, Massachusetts Institute for Community Health Leadership.

Nancy W. Carpenter – is Executive Director of the Massachusetts Association for School-Based Health Care. Carpenter has a background in public health policy, planning, and program development. During her 12-year tenure at the Massachusetts Department of Public Health, Carpenter was appointed as the first Director of the Health Resource Office, responsible for developing the state's policy, education, research, and service response during the initial years of the AIDS epidemic. Previously, Carpenter worked independently as a health care consultant on topics concerning the health care safety net, access for uninsured and vulnerable populations, and Medicaid managed care. She received Master's degrees in Public Health and Urban Affairs from Boston University.

Leslie A. Mandel, PhD, MA, MSM – is currently an independent program evaluator specializing in advocacy and policy change. She is also an instructor in the community health program at Pine Manor College. Dr. Mandel's dissertation explored organizational issues of partnerships between school-based health centers (SBHCs), health care systems, and public schools in Massachusetts. She is actively involved in national-level associations dedicated to evaluation and quality of SBHCs. She was one of the founders of the Massachusetts Association for School-Based Health Care. Finally, she was part of the management team at The Student Health Center at Boston High School.

Speaking Truth to Power: A Youth Advisory Board's Actions to Change School-Based Policy in San Francisco*

Marcia Zorrilla, Michael Baxter, and Heather Heater

Founded in 1928, Balboa High School in San Francisco, California, serves a diverse urban working class neighborhood. Today, 82% of the 1,000-person student body are Chinese, Latino, Filipino, or African American. The building itself is a designated historic landmark. Although the high school has experienced significant challenges in recent decades, it has made great progress since the entire faculty was dismissed in 1999. Most notably, the school was recognized in *Newsweek* magazine's list of "America's Top Public High Schools" in 2007 and 2008.

Reflecting its motto, "First on the Pacific," Balboa High School became the first high school in California to open a school-based health clinic in 1986. Operating out of what used to be the school's metal shop, it remains the only school-based health center in San Francisco to provide medical, mental health, and health education services. The Balboa Teen Health Center is a collaborative project of the San Francisco Department of Public Health, the Bayview Hunters Point Foundation, and the San Francisco Unified School District. It provides comprehensive medical and mental health care, including reproductive health services, and averages 6,000 visits annually.

The Balboa Teen Health Center is also a member of the California School Health Centers Association, the state's leading advocacy organization for bringing health services to schools. The California Association is one of nine recipients

---

* This chapter expands on an earlier report from Zorrilla M. *San Francisco Teens Educate Peers on Health Care Rights*. Battle Creek, MI: W. K. Kellogg Foundation; 2008.

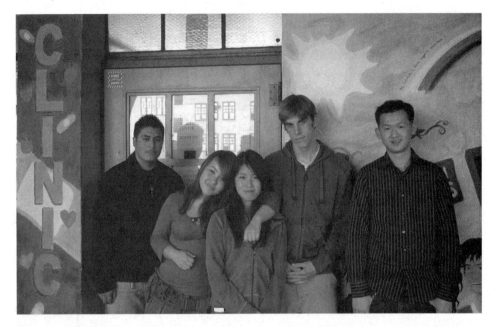

Figure 19.1—Five student leaders of the Youth Advisory Board at Balboa High School at the time it was pursuing a change in school board policy to educate students on their right to confidential medical services through their school-based health center. From left to right: Dario Zamudio, Rebecca Kaplow, Shirley Duong, Zach Dellé and Daniel Yim.

of multiyear funding from the W. K. Kellogg Foundation for its national School-Based Health Care Policy Program. Launched in 2004, the School-Based Health Care Policy Program aims to make quality care more accessible and sustainable for children and youth. A fundamental principle of the program is the promotion of a consumer-centered model of quality care—one in which local people, including youth, shape the content, quality, delivery, and financing of health care in their communities.

In 2004, the Balboa Teen Health Center was selected by the California School Health Centers Association to receive grant funds from the W. K. Kellogg Foundation's School-Based Health Care Policy Program. Consistent with the California School Health Centers Association's commitment to increasing youth engagement statewide to support school health centers, clinic staff used the funds to establish a Youth Advisory Board comprised of students from the high school. The Youth Advisory Board is funded by the Balboa Teen Health Center as well as by the Youth Advisory Board members writing grants themselves. Over the past few years, the Youth Advisory Board has been supported by teachers and administrators. It has integrated well in the school community and is viewed as a model of youth and community involvement. Returning Youth Advisory Board members sponsor a recruitment and application process in the fall of each year to replace members who graduated the prior spring. The Youth Advisory Board members receive a $250 stipend for their annual participation. Each week, the Balboa Teen Health Center Youth Advisory Board meets to discuss its projects and track progress toward its goals.

A DIVERSE STUDENT POPULATION AND A COMMON THEME

When it was formed, the Youth Advisory Board set two goals: to educate San Francisco youth about minor consent health rights and to provide information on how to access health care services. With guidance from Marcia Zorrilla, health educator at the Balboa Teen Health Center and staff liaison to the Youth Advisory Board, student members identified the activities they wanted to undertake in order to meet these goals.

Under California law, minors can provide consent for treatment for a variety of medical and reproductive services, including drug and alcohol-related problems, mental health, family planning, and sexual health. For teens, these services are confidential, i.e., information is not shared with their parents or providers without the teens' permission. "This can be a controversial topic," said Shirley Duong, a member of the Youth Advisory Board at the time. "The reason minor consent rights are so important is that they encourage students to seek out and receive the services they need without fear of repercussion from their parents."[1(p3)]

In undertaking its charge, the Youth Advisory Board conducted a needs assessment to assess students' awareness of California's minor consent law, the availability of confidential health services in San Francisco, preferences regarding health care access (e.g., type of provider, location, and so on), barriers to access (e.g., cost, transportation, confidentiality, and so on), and students' beliefs regarding the circumstances in which a clinic is required to obtain parental consent.

The needs assessment was piloted in the first year of the grant project, after which it was modified before being administered in seven public high schools in the San Francisco Unified School District. In coordination with the city's Student Advisory Council, the assessment was available in both English and Chinese. Responses to the assessment were anonymous, and a total of 1,617 completed assessments were collected and analyzed. Findings pointed toward a widespread lack of knowledge about access to confidential health services among San Francisco teens.

Despite the protections afforded teens by law, 28% of all respondents to the needs assessment survey believed incorrectly that parents must be notified prior to receiving birth control, 32% believed incorrectly that a clinic cannot perform an HIV test without parental consent, and 48% believed incorrectly that parental notification was required to obtain drug and alcohol counseling.

Students from Newcomer High School, a San Francisco school designed to serve teens who have recently arrived in the United States, showed the greatest lack of knowledge about services available to them. In particular, Chinese students at the school were the group least knowledgeable about their health care rights.

A local study on the health of Asian American, Native Hawaiian, and Pacific Islander youth conducted by the Asian & Pacific Islander American Health Forum in 2007 produced similar findings. The study found that none of the participants, aged 14 and 15 years, knew where to access reproductive health resources.[2] In a city where Asians represent 31.8% of the population,[3] it is clear that health care services need to be culturally and linguistically appropriate and accessible.

Nationally this need rings true as well. Eleven percent of Asian Americans and 13 percent of Native Hawaiian and other Pacific Islanders live in poverty, compared to eight percent of non-Hispanic whites.[4] These populations are extremely diverse and include groups that differ greatly in culture, language, religion, and history in the United States. Adding to this complexity is the fact that Asian and Pacific Islanders speak over 100 languages and dialects. The lack of culturally and linguistically appropriate care can be a major barrier to accessing preventive and primary care.[5]

"How you frame rights and services in a culturally appropriate manner is critical,"[1(p2)] said Marguerite Ro, deputy director at Asian & Pacific Islander American Health Forum, the national health advocacy organization for Asian Americans, Native Hawaiians and Pacific Islanders. The Forum is also a grantee of the W. K. Kellogg Foundation.

Despite the diversity of the student's surveyed, one common theme from the data was the value teens placed on confidentiality. "Youth seem to like to have confidential services regardless of their culture,"[1(p2)] said Zach Dellé, a Balboa High School student and member of the Youth Advisory Board at the time.

INFLUENCING STUDENT AWARENESS AND POLICY CHANGE

Having evaluated the data from the needs assessment, the Youth Advisory Board decided immediate action was needed to inform students about their consent rights as minors and encourage them to be more proactive about their health. The students designed a peer-to-peer education program that would especially resonate with new immigrant students at Newcomer High School. They identified the skills necessary to implement the project and then recruited other students with knowledge of Internet and DVD technology. They also recruited students with Chinese- and Spanish-language skills.

In developing the program, the students wrote and produced a skit that addressed the issues of teen pregnancy and alcohol dependency. Mindful of their audience and that the skit addressed issues that other students might have personally experienced or consider to be culturally taboo, the skit was designed to be sensitive, nonjudgmental, and (in parts) humorous, reflecting the speaking style of teens. "The humor takes the edge off," said Daniel Yim, then a senior at Balboa High School and member of the Youth Advisory Board. A sample of the dialogue is below.

> Girl: How do you expect me to go out there and get birth control when you weren't even smart enough to get a condom?
>
> Boy: I don't want my parents to know I needed condoms! You have no idea what they would have done to me.
>
> Girl: You drink too much. You think it'll solve all your problems. Maybe if you didn't spend all your money on alcohol, then you could have bought some condoms.
>
> Boy: I have too much to deal with at home. This is the only thing that calms me down, so give me a break.[1(p3)]

After the skit, the teens led a question and answer game, "Confidential or Not," that tested what audiences had learned from the performance. It was performed in Spanish and Chinese and followed by an informal discussion with students. The decision to perform the play in both languages was an easy one for the students. "We've been exposed to diverse cultures our entire lives," explains student Zach Dellé. "It's just something we live."[1(p3)]

In addition, the students determined that change could only be fully realized if policies affecting student health were reconsidered in the context of what they had learned from the needs assessment. Thus, they needed to find ways to "speak truth to power." The students developed a website and a PowerPoint presentation, which they presented to their school's Parent–Teacher Association. After attending a Policy Leadership Program on School Health,[a] the group realized that a more comprehensive approach to the challenge of correcting students' misunderstanding of their right to confidential health care was an appropriate goal.

---

[a] The Policy Leadership Program on School Health is a statewide program of the California Center for Civic Participation in collaboration with the California School Health Centers Association.

Thus, the students drafted and presented a position paper advocating for a change in district policy to include the following as part of routine health education curricula:

1. Explicitly describe California's minor consent law,
2. Inform high school students of their rights to receive confidential health services, and
3. Provide a list of confidential services available at clinics throughout San Francisco.

The resolution gained early support from the San Francisco Youth Commission, the Student Advisory Council of the San Francisco Unified School District Board of Education, and the San Francisco Health Commission. The resolution was also endorsed by the curriculum subcommittee of the San Francisco Unified School District.

On April 22, 2008, the Youth Advisory Board presented the Minor Consent Resolution to the San Francisco Unified School District Board of Education. The board agreed to pass the resolution, mandating the inclusion of minor consent law in the health education curriculum in all San Francisco public high schools, beginning in the 2008–2009 school year.

Following adoption of the new policy and prior to its implementation, Youth Advisory Board members trained teachers on the policy to broaden teen health education. The training reviewed California minor consent laws, and teachers participated in role play to make them aware of the obstacles youth encounter in accessing services.

In total, 66 faculty and staff were trained. In addition, the board authorized the training of teens who volunteer at the city's 15 high school wellness centers. Since the implementation of the new policy, high school health education classes in San Francisco high schools have specifically covered California's minor consent laws related to health care, including confidentiality on birth control, pregnancy, sexually transmitted infections and HIV testing, outpatient mental health treatment, alcohol and drug abuse treatment, rape and sexual assault, and mandated reporting.

To ensure the sustainability of the policy, the Youth Advisory Board asked the Board of Education to adopt the full resolution as a demonstration of its commitment to and support of the inclusion of minor consent rights in the public school health education curriculum, which the Board of Education did.

TACKLING TEEN HEALTH CHALLENGES ONE AT A TIME

Since the implementation of the new policy, the Youth Advisory Board at Balboa High School has continued to educate students on their health care rights and needs while addressing specific health challenges facing teens one at a time. The Youth Advisory Board is committed to the health and welfare of students by organizing in-class workshops, youth and adult trainings, and events on health issues and California minor consent rights. In 2010, the students developed and performed a play focusing on mental health and the stigma often surrounding the issue. In March 2011, the Balboa Teen Health Center's Youth Advisory Board performed a theater piece on teen pregnancy and male involvement. More than 1,000 students attended the performance of *One in a Million: Daisy's Story*, which tells the story of a 17-year-old girl with an unplanned pregnancy.

In this era of health care reform, school-based health centers will continue to be a critical site in the provision of health services to our nation's youth. As advocates *and* consumers of such centers, the Youth Advisory Board at Balboa High School demonstrates the power of the school-based health center user population. The Youth Advisory Board at Balboa understands that the youth voice must be heard in the process of developing and implementing health and education policies as they relate to teens. They exercised this "power" and sought to promote informed health decisions among their peers.

The process of ensuring that the youth voice is heard is not always easy. The students who served on the Youth Advisory Board found adult allies who were willing to listen to what the students had to say, were open to hearing their suggestions on how to resolve the challenges they identified, and were dedicated to committing their time to supporting youth-led initiatives. Their advocacy took them to regional, state, and local levels, including a meeting with the Chief of Staff for then Speaker of the House Nancy Pelosi. Of course, not all adults felt this way, and the bureaucracy involved in pursuit of the policy change was daunting.

Nevertheless, this experience demonstrates that an empowered Youth Advisory Board can be an effective strategy to engage youths on a peer-to-peer level and implement changes in school-based policy while simultaneously contributing to positive youth development.

REFERENCES

1. Zorrilla M. *San Francisco Teens Educate Peers on Health Care Rights*. Battle Creek, MI: W. K. Kellogg Foundation; 2008.

2. Asian and Pacific Islander Bay Area Health Council. *San Francisco Bay Area Asian American, Native Hawaiian, Pacific Islander Youth Health Status Report*. San Francisco, CA: Asian and Pacific Islander Health Forum; 2007.

3. US Census Bureau. *2006 American Community Survey*. Washington, DC: US Census Bureau; 2007.

4. DeNavas-Walt C, Proctor BD, Lee CH. *Income, Poverty, and Health Insurance Coverage in the United States: 2004*. Washington, DC: US Census Bureau; 2005.

5. W. K. Kellogg Foundation. *Asian American Pacific Islander Health Convening; Proceedings Summary. Chicago, IL, November 11, 2005*. Battle Creek, MI: W. K. Kellogg Foundation; 2005:8.

About the Authors

Marcia Zorrilla, MPH, CHES – is a health educator at the Balboa Teen Health Center where she has worked for the past 17 years. She has experience in designing, implementing, and evaluating health education programs ranging from nutrition to teen pregnancy prevention. Seven years ago, she created the Balboa Teen Health Center's Youth Advisory Board from the ground up to advocate for youth health care rights and school-based health centers. Marcia and the Youth Advisory Board received the Moving the Movement Award from the California School Health Centers Association for their role in furthering the school-based health centers movement.

Michael Baxter, MSW – has worked in adolescent health field for 25 years. He is currently employed by the San Francisco Department of Public Health as the Manager of Youth Programs and Development Services for its Community-Oriented Primary Care division and as the Director of Family Planning/Preconception Services for its Maternal, Child, and Adolescent Health division. Michael has implemented health education programs focusing on reproductive health for incarcerated youth, was instrumental in ensuring a continuum of HIV services for young people that continues to date, and has worked to increase school-based health services in San Francisco.

Heather Heater, MPH – lives and works in Portland, Oregon. She holds and Master's degree in Public Health from Portland State University. As a health educator at Multnomah County Health Department in Oregon, she is currently researching community- and policy-level approaches to Maternal Child and Adolescent Health as well as improving organizational infrastructure and capacity to implement best-practice strategies to improve population health. Her previous professional experience includes HIV prevention and sexuality education, with an emphasis on the social determinants of sexual and reproductive health.

Community Schools and School-Based Health Centers: A Partnership That Works for Children and Youth

Jeanita W. Richardson and
Amanda J. Richardson

> *A community school is established to perform a job of total educa-*
> *tion. . . . An integrated day and night program caters to all elements*
> *of the population and seeks to bridge cultural gaps which are largely*
> *the result of unfulfilled group needs. The ultimate objective of the*
> *programming is to develop good American citizens who will make*
> *positive contributions to society.*
>
> *—T. J. Anderson (1953)*[1]

The location of school-based health centers (SBHCs) in schools would seem to create an automatic kinship between the disciplines of health and education. Scholars and practitioners from both disciplines at least rhetorically agree that health is critical to educational achievement.[2-6] However, if an SBHC is located in a traditional, publicly funded school, the value of meaningful collaboration (the sharing of information and policy priorities) is not always obvious to educators. There is, however, an educational model that theoretically embraces the presence of SBHCs as partners on behalf of children and youth: community schools (also called full-service community schools [FSCSs]). This chapter seeks to inform the SBHC field about the FSCS model and its alignment with the existing goals and priorities of SBHCs.

As early as 1915, John Dewey, the famed educational philosopher, proposed the concept of community schools to address comprehensive community needs. Dewey's vision is now supported by decades of empirical literature concurring with the value of these institutions. Most notable among contemporary researchers, Joy

Dryfoos has contributed volumes that advocate for this model wherein a full range of social services are available to youth in the location they are most apt to spend significant time: their schools.[7-11]

One of the early adopters and funders of this educational approach is the Children's Aid Society, which defines a community school as a "public school that combines the best educational practices with a wide range of vital in-house health and social services to ensure that children are physically, emotionally, and socially prepared to learn."[12] Stated another way, the FSCS premise is well grounded in decades of research affirming the significance of holistic interventions for children and youth because disruptions in physical, social, psychological, and emotional maturation influenced by poverty and trauma, for example, potentially deter sensitive developmental sequences that impact learning.[13,14]

Community schools appear to have great potential to thwart otherwise predictable negative academic and health outcomes. For example, in a 2009 study comparing Children's Aid Society (CAS) community schools to other schools in New York City, CAS students scored significantly higher on math tests than in other city schools. In Chicago's community schools there is evidence of a steady narrowing of the achievement gap when compared to other Chicago schools. In Cincinnati, nine pilot community schools decreased behavior incidents by 10%, increased achievement tests by 10%, dental screening and treatment were received by 90% of students, attendance increased to 93% daily, and 95% of students were fully immunized during the 2007–2008 pilot year.[15]

Successes demonstrated by this educational approach borrow from the socio-ecological model of public health, i.e., FSCSs support the notion that concurrent spheres of influence impact youth and their ability to realize their potential (see Figure 20.1).

Community schools embrace the notion that individual, relationship, and community interactions must all be integrated into the school experience in constructive ways. This tends to be accomplished by soliciting partnerships that bring resources and expertise into the school building, such as those noted in Figure 20.1. This asset-based approach identifies existing resources within the community (e.g., clubs, faith-based organizations, local businesses) and pools them to facilitate the maximization of those resources. SBHCs provide a great example of critical support integral to FSCS health and well-being goals that positively impact communities. Furthermore, SBHC staff are an additional onsite source of trusted and caring adults with whom students can bond. Developing relationships with caring adults has been noted as one protective factor against education risk, such as dropping out of school.[16-19]

Configurations of community schools can vary widely because local challenges are idiosyncratic, thus community schools take on distinct characteristics

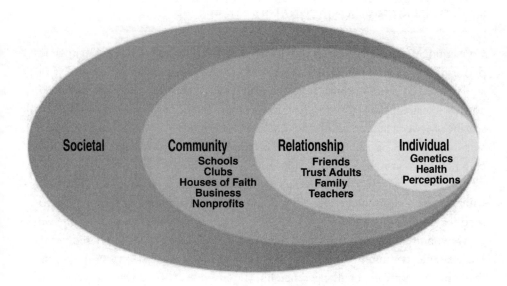

Figure 20.1 — Full-service community schools: an ecological approach.

not unlike the scope of SBHC services that are dictated by community norms and values. Community school programming can include but not be limited to health and social service agencies, SBHCs, family support groups, youth development organizations, government-sponsored programs, vocational and educational classes targeting adults, student tutoring and mentoring, and basic need services such as clothes closets and food pantries. Fundamentally, the myriad of activities and services are designed to support children and their families at the point of their need with a goal of optimizing economic, academic, and social potential. For disadvantaged youth in particular, a community school can be an oasis in the midst of an opportunity desert.

Common across descriptions of community and full-service schools are their capacity to adapt to the needs of the community and not vice versa. If the school is to be embraced by communities, it must be perceived as a problem-solving center and be available beyond traditional school hours. Also, the model prioritizes integrating everyday authentic values and problems into the curriculum and programming. For example, consider a neighborhood served by a school that has many undereducated adults whose low-wage jobs fail to provide basic insurance for their families. A vital function of the neighborhood community school would be to offer health services (such as those provided in SBHCs) and GED classes and job training for adults.[1]

FULL-SERVICE COMMUNITY SCHOOLS AND SCHOOL-BASED HEALTH CENTERS: A NATURAL PARTNERSHIP

Conventional public education settings are not ameliorating persistent academic performance gaps. This is especially the case for low-income and otherwise at-risk students.[20] The contemporary revival of interest in community schools rises from acknowledgment that ignoring the comprehensive needs of families facilitates dissonance between students, their school, and communities.[1,21] As a result, partnerships such as FSCSs and SBHCs could be considered a natural outgrowth of their common missions and impact.

However, as is the case with many traditional educators, SBHCs and their contributions to a community school's mission may not be immediately apparent to school administrators. FSCSs and SBHCS are natural partners because of the ways in which both have been proven to advance the well-being of children and youth. For example, community schools and SBHCs have the greatest impact on youth living in economically challenged neighborhoods.[2,6,11,15,23] Given the ability of each of these models to transform the health and well-being of youth, it is exciting to consider the impact of their partnership.

Both community schools and SBHCs are committed to supporting the resilience of youth by being protective factors against risk. Given the interaction between negative determinants of health and educational risk, there are clear opportunities for schools and their students to benefit from the presence of an SBHC. Consider integration of the health and education disciplines depicted in the "Community Schools: A Results-Based Logic Model" advanced by the Coalition for Community Schools (Figure 20.2). The comprehensive approach reflected in the model illustrates the need for health services in schools. The clear advantage of an SBHC collaboration is this health delivery model's specific expertise with children and youth issues, their demonstrated impacts, and the fact that their presence is not contingent on the particular school's budget. The proposed partnership is consistent with the elements of a highly functioning "results-based" community school.

Partnership is also consistent with the work that SBHCs are already doing. By virtue of an SBHC's presence, student attendance improves, the numbers of parents who otherwise might have to leave work to care for chronically ill students decreases, and hospital stays associated with chronic disease management also decrease.[6,22,24-28] Students' improved health and academic outcomes, continuity of and access to services, and more diverse learning opportunities have been proven to be associated with both FSCSs and SBHCs.[1,2,6,11,22,25-28] Furthermore, when adequate support services are available to students, educators can focus on teaching and learning.

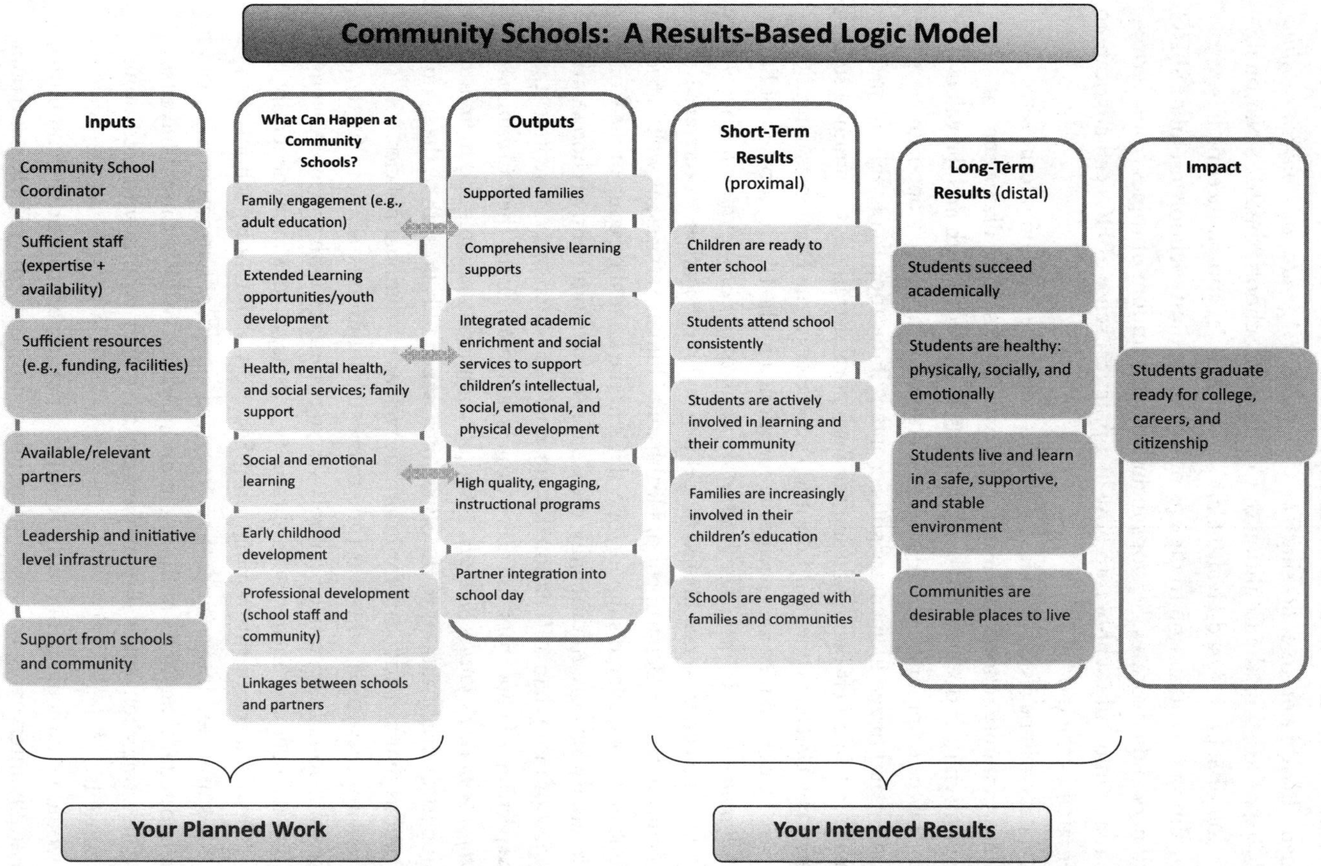

Community Schools: A Results-Based Logic Model

Inputs	What Can Happen at Community Schools?	Outputs	Short-Term Results (proximal)	Long-Term Results (distal)	Impact
Community School Coordinator	Family engagement (e.g., adult education)	Supported families	Children are ready to enter school	Students succeed academically	Students graduate ready for college, careers, and citizenship
Sufficient staff (expertise + availability)	Extended learning opportunities/youth development	Comprehensive learning supports	Students attend school consistently	Students are healthy: physically, socially, and emotionally	
Sufficient resources (e.g., funding, facilities)	Health, mental health, and social services; family support	Integrated academic enrichment and social services to support children's intellectual, social, emotional, and physical development	Students are actively involved in learning and their community	Students live and learn in a safe, supportive, and stable environment	
Available/relevant partners	Social and emotional learning	High quality, engaging, instructional programs	Families are increasingly involved in their children's education	Communities are desirable places to live	
Leadership and initiative level infrastructure	Early childhood development	Partner integration into school day	Schools are engaged with families and communities		
Support from schools and community	Professional development (school staff and community)				
	Linkages between schools and partners				

Your Planned Work — Your Intended Results

Figure 20.2 — Community schools: a results-based logic model.

The question of how to tap into the momentum surrounding the adoption of this educational model is already being explored by organizations in the SBHC movement. In addition to endorsing *The Community Agenda for America's Public Schools*[29] sponsored by the Coalition of Community Schools, the 2011 National Association of School-Based Health Care's (NASBHC's) annual meeting has devoted substantive attention to dimensions of community schools useful to SBHC practitioners and advocates. Sessions included a continuum of topics from clarifying what a community school is to how in a practical sense SBHCs can advocate to be integrated in the model.

Advocacy will be required to insert SBHCs into the education reform wave of which community schools are a part. However, SBHCs rightfully belong "at the table" given their documented contributions to student health and the values espoused by the community school model. A contemporary policy opportunity is the soon to be reauthorized Elementary and Secondary Education Act (ESEA; formerly known as No Child Left Behind during the Bush administration). Community schools are favored by US Department of Education's Secretary Arne Duncan as educational reform strategies, and they are specifically mentioned in the US Department of Education's *A Blueprint for Reform: The Reauthorization of the Elementary and Secondary Education Act* as an evidenced-based model worthy of replication.[30] Secretary Kathleen Sebelius of the US Department of Health and Human Services, as well as Secretary Duncan, have declared support for SBHCs at the annual meeting of the Coalition for Community Schools. Additionally, the Coalition for Community Schools garnered the support of more than 150 national, state, and local organizations representing a diverse spectrum of educators, advocacy groups, and SBHCs for their *Community Agenda for America's Public Schools*.[29] Adding community schools and their attendant supportive organizations to the SBHC movement adds breadth to the litany of organizations that can advocate for health, as well as educational policies.

There appears to be no better time to create community schools, firstly because traditionally organized schools serving students with the most need are failing to meet established accountability standards and more generally the comprehensive needs of this population.[20] Secondly, community schools as a politically supported intervention have received significant attention in research centers and federal agencies and present an approach SBHCs should have less trouble inserting themselves into as partners than they would with traditional public schools.[3,5,30]

It would be difficult to find a more natural pairing of institutions committed to holistically intervening on behalf of children and youth than SBHCs and community schools. The data are clear: when children are engaged, healthy, and feel connected with their schools, their interest is sustained and naturally spills over into measurable academic outcomes.[1,22,31–35] It seems equally clear that effectiveness in engaging and maximizing the potential of our children will be enhanced as the SBHC movement takes its rightful place as a partner with FSCS.

REFERENCES

1. Richardson JW. *The Full-Service Community School Movement: Lessons From the James Adams Community School*. New York, NY: Palgrave Macmillan; 2009.

2. Bireda S. Healthy students are better students: health reform bill gives a boost to school-based health centers. Center for American Progress. 2010. Available at: http://www.americanprogress.org/issues/2010/05/healthy_students.html. Accessed April 18, 2011.

3. Center for Mental Health in Schools. Turning around, transforming, and continuously improving schools: federal proposals are still based on a two—rather than a three—component blueprint. 2010. Available at: http://smhp.psych.ucla.edu/pdfdocs/turning.pdf. Accessed April 18, 2011.

4. Cruz A. Bringing health care to children where they are and when they need it. 2010. Available at: http://www.childrensaidsociety.org/community-schools/partnership-press/fall-2010/school-based-health-centers. Accessed April 18, 2011.

5. Harvard Family Research Project. Partnerships for learning: promising practices in integrating school and out-of-school time program supports. 2010. Available at: http://www.hfrp.org/publications-resources/browse-our-publications/partnerships-for-learning-promising-practices-in-integrating-school-and-out-of-school-time-program-supports. Accessed April 18, 2011.

6. Walker SC, Kerns SE, Lyon AR, Bruns EJ, Cosgrove TJ. Impact of school-based health center use on academic outcomes. *J Adolesc Health*. 2010;46(3):251–257.

7. Dryfoos JG. *Full-Service Schools: A Revolution in Health and Social Services for Children, Youth, and Families*. New York, NY: Jossey-Bass; 1994.

8. Dryfoos JG. Full-service community schools: creating new institutions. *Phi Delta Kappan*. 2002;83(5):393–400.

9. Dryfoos JG. A community school in action. *Reclaiming Children and Youth*. 2003;11(4): 203–206.

10. Dryfoos JG, Maguire S. *Inside: Full-Service Community Schools*. Thousand Oaks, CA: Corwin Press; 2002.

11. Dryfoos JG, Quinn J, Barkin C. *Community Schools in Action: Lessons From a Decade of Practice*. Oxford, UK: Oxford University Press; 2005.

12. The Children's Aid Society. Community schools. 2007. Available at: http://www.childrensaidsociety.org/communityschools. Accessed October 25, 2007.

13. Blank MJ, Berg A. *All Together Now: Sharing Responsibility for the Whole Child.* Washington, DC: Association for Supervision and Curriculum Development; 2006.

14. Richardson JW. From risk to resilience: promoting school-health partnerships for children. *Int J Educ Reform.* 2008;17(1):19–36.

15. Coalition for Community Schools. Community schools—results that turn around failing schools. 2010. Available at: http://www.communityschools.org/assets/1/AssetManager/Turning_Around_Schools_CS_Results2.pdf. Accessed April 30, 2011.

16. Bridgeland JM, Dilulio JJ Jr, Morison KB. *The Silent Epidemic: Perspectives of High School Dropouts.* Washington, DC: Civic Enterprises in association with Peter D. Hart Research Associates; 2006.

17. Freudenberg N, Ruglis J. Reframing school dropout as a public health issue. *Prev Chronic Dis.* 2007;4(4):A107.

18. Swanson CB. *Cities in Crisis: A Special Analytic Report on High School Graduation.* Bethesda, MD: America's Promise Alliance and the Bill & Melinda Gates Foundation; 2008.

19. Toldson IA. *Breaking Barriers: Plotting the Path to Academic Success for School-Age African-American Males.* Washington, DC: Congressional Black Caucus Foundation; 2008.

20. US Department of Education, National Center for Education Statistics. *The Condition of Education 2010.* Vol. NCES 2010-028. Washington, DC: US Government Printing Office; 2010.

21. Harris MM, Hoover JH. Overcoming adversity through community schools. *Reclaiming Child Youth.* 2003;11(4):206–211.

22. Basch CE. *Healthier Students Are Better Learners: A Missing Link in School Reforms to Close the Achievement Gap.* New York, NY: The Campaign for Educational Equity, Teachers College Columbia University; 2010.

23. Carey K. State poverty-based education funding: a survey of current programs and options for improvement. 2002. Available at: http://www.cbpp.org/11-7-02sfp.htm. Accessed October 10, 2005.

24. Geierstanger SP, Amaral G, Mansour M, Walters SR. School-based health centers and academic performance: research, challenges, and recommendations. *J Sch Health.* 2004;74(9):347–352.

25. Fiscella K, Kitzman H. Disparities in academic acheivement and health: the intersection of child education and health policy. *Pediatrics.* 2009;123(3):1073–1080.

26. Fletcher JS. Children's lack of access to health care as a barrier to academic performance: a brief summary of issues. *Am J Health Educ.* 2004;35(4):234–237.

27. Hamm EM. Managing asthma in the classroom. *Child Educ.* 2004;81(1):16–20.

28. Hanson TL, Austin G, Lee-Bayha J. *How Are Student Health Risks and Resilience Related to the Academic Progress of Schools?* San Francisco, CA: WestEd; 2004.

29. Coalition for Community Schools. The community agenda for America's public schools. 2010. Available at: http://www.thecommunityagenda.org. Accessed April 10, 2011.

30. US Department of Education, Office of Planning, Evaluation, and Policy Development. *A Blueprint for Reform: The Reauthorization of the Elementary and Secondary Education Act.* Washington, DC: US Department of Education; 2010. Available at: http://www2.ed.gov/policy/elsec/leg/blueprint/blueprint.pdf. Accessed April 10, 2011.

31. Gilroy M. Community schools seek to improve high school achievement and college readiness. *The Hispanic Outlook in Higher Education.* 2011;21(9):14–17.

32. Blank MJ. How community schools make a difference. *Schools as Learning Communities.* 2004;61(8):62–65.

33. Hilliard A III. No mystery: closing the achievement gap between Africans and excellence. In: Perry T, Steele C, Hilliard A III, eds. *Young, Gifted, and Black: Promoting High Achievement Among African-American Students.* Boston, MA: Beacon Press; 2003:131–166.

34. Jehl J. *Connecting Schools, Families and Communities.* Baltimore, MD: Annie E. Casey Foundation; 2007.

35. Jensen JM, Fraser MW. A risk and resilience framework for child, youth, and family policy. In: Jensen JM, Fraser MW, eds. *Social Policy for Children and Families: A Risk and Resilience Perspective.* Thousand Oaks, CA: Sage Publications; 2006:1–18.

About the Authors

Jeanita W. Richardson, PhD, MEd – is an Associate Professor in the Department of Public Health Sciences at the University of Virginia School of Medicine. Her scholarship highlights the inextricable links between health and learning readiness, particularly for disenfranchised children and youth. Her work has been published and presented in numerous national and international journals and conferences. Her consulting energies (Turpeau Consulting Group, LLC) are devoted to supporting healthy children who are ready to learn through the creation of health and educational policy bridges and include five years as a consultant to the W. K. Kellogg Foundation's School-Based Health Care Policy Program. For more information, email TConsultingG@aol.com.

Amanda J. Richardson, MPH – earned her Master's from Tufts University and is currently a Public Health Prevention Service Fellow at the Centers for Disease Control and Prevention (CDC). Her interest in school-based health centers is representative of a larger interest in reducing health disparities through prevention, which also includes work in the areas of food security, youth violence, public–private partnerships, and implementation of the Patient Protection and Affordable Care Act. This chapter was co-authored in her private capacity. No official support or endorsement by the CDC, Department of Health and Human Services is intended, nor should be inferred.

Partnering Around High School Dropout Prevention and Recovery in Massachusetts

Nancy W. Carpenter, Antonia M. Blinn,
and Jeanita W. Richardson

Advocacy has long been used to target improvements in health disparities in diverse population groups. Recently, the Massachusetts Coalition for School-Based Health (hereafter referred to as the Coalition) identified high school dropouts as an issue in need of broad-based advocacy targeting diverse disciplinary and systemic interventions. From a public health perspective, it may not be immediately apparent that many of the factors associated with school withdrawal decisions also are linked to health over the life span.[1,2] Nevertheless, distal factors (e.g., legislative policies and interagency partnerships), as well as proximal agents (family resources, perceptions of the value of a high school diploma, personal income and health) influence this significant decision.[2-9] By identifying the scope and multidisciplinary significance of dropping out of school, the Coalition sought to capitalize on some of its established and emerging relationships with the health, educational, community advocacy, and legislative communities to create a more collaborative advocacy network poised to incite political and practical interventions on behalf of youth. This chapter will describe two meetings organized by the Coalition to accomplish this goal, as well as the outcomes and lessons learned from each.

The number of students dropping out of school has reached epidemic proportions in Massachusetts and across the country, particularly in urban areas and among racial and ethnic minority populations. The estimated scope of the dropout problem and its economic implications are revealed in evaluations of national data sets. During the 2004–2005 school year nationally, only three fourths of high school students graduated on time (e.g., in four years).[10] Native American, African American, and Hispanic/Latino American students are more apt to drop out of school than are Whites or Asians, and in the 50 largest cities in the United States, a little over 50% of children of color graduate from high school.[3,11–13]

Many eventual dropouts can be identified as early as the third grade, 40% can be identified by sixth grade, and 75% by ninth grade.[3,12,14] Yet, as dismal as these statistics are, they still mask the far-reaching implications of not completing high school. Per the Bureau of Labor Statistics, the annual income of a high school dropout compared to a high school graduate, individuals with some college, and those with a bachelor's degree differ by approximately $9,000, $14,000, and $32,000, respectively.[6] Per the US Census Bureau, in 2000, 56% of high school dropouts were unemployed. More recent studies assert dropouts represent 52% of the welfare population, 82% of the prison population, and 85% of the juvenile justice cases.[5] Those without diplomas are more apt, if they are employed, to work in low-skilled, low-paying jobs that do not provide health insurance. They are less likely to participate in the political process and pay taxes and are more apt to experience poor health, need social services, and be victims or perpetrators of crime.[5,11,12,15]

According to the Massachusetts Department of Education, one in five students do not graduate, and dropouts miss an average of 31 days of school before they drop out.[3,11,13] Males drop out at higher rates than do females, and dropouts are highest and increasing among racial/ethnic groups. Relative to Boston, there is great disparity between city graduation rates (57%) and the surrounding suburbs (83%).[11,13,16] Students in Boston who attended less than 90% of the time functioned at a critical dropout threshold. Annually, a Massachusetts dropout collects $5,300 more in cash and in-kind government services than they paid into the Commonwealth's systems, whereas high school graduates and those with a bachelor's degree pay more into the system than they require ($2,124 and $13,620, respectively).[6]

Literature asserts dropping out of school as implied earlier is not an impulsive isolated action impacting youth alone. Instead, dropping out is a culmination of long-term disengagement that profoundly affects families, communities, and the nation.[5] Additionally, singular focus by the educational community is not narrowing the high school dropout trends, and data suggest that allowing students to drop out in the 21st century is the equivalent of passively encouraging economic suicide.[17]

Education has been called the best elixir for health because it manifests its power through three health pathways: health knowledge and behaviors, employment and income (defining housing, insurance, and nutrition options), and social control (e.g., stress and available social and economic resources).[1,9,18,19] As further evidence, male and female college graduates tend on average to live five years longer than those who did not complete high school. Dropouts consistently rate their health as less than very good across race and ethnicity.[9]

School-based health care centers (SBHCs), by virtue of their mission and location in and near schools, are a largely untapped resource in reversing the alarming dropout rates and health disparity trends. Though largely an underutilized support system with respect to dropouts, they have the ability to play a pivotal role in early identification and interventions on behalf of students entering a dropout danger zone. In partnership with schools, SBHCs across the country are beginning to demonstrate their profound effect on learning readiness, which include but are not limited to poor concentration in school, attendance, management of chronic illnesses, and disturbances of normal sequential cognitive development—all precursors to school separation and all of which have been identified as dropout risk factors.[20,21]

Given the recent release of dropout reports and the accountability benchmarks articulated in legislation, many state and local policymakers have become more concerned about the issue. Though clearly an issue that crosses numerous sectors, a barrier to mitigating early school departure trends has been identifying the space and the time for public health, education professionals, policymakers, and grassroots organizations to meet face-to-face to grasp the benefits of collaborating around this issue of common concern.

The sweeping implications and the complex interactions that frame leaving before graduation prompted the Coalition to convene two forums to explore potential collaborations across disciplines that might prove protective of youth and support educational and health resilience. Meetings were designed to bring attention to (1) the role that the health sector can play (especially SBHCs) in reducing school dropout prevalence and (2) potential interagency and multidisciplinary interventions for youth. In May 2008 and again in February 2009, the Coalition invited policymakers and leaders from diverse sectors including health, education, business, philanthropy, and advocacy to explore school dropout as a public health concern. The remainder of this discussion expounds upon each event and the lessons learned.

HOSTING THE DROPOUT FORUMS

Advocacy opportunities come in many forms. In this case, there was a convergence of thought that prompted the Coalition to assume the role of a leader on this topic. Figure 21.1 outlines the order in which events and findings evolved that led to recommendations for other organizations considering similar ventures.

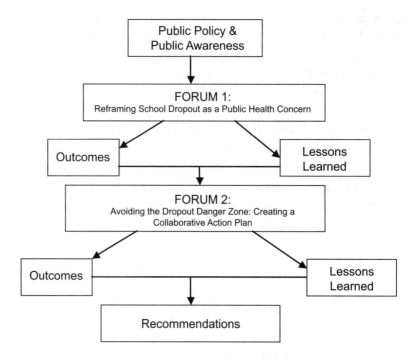

Figure 21.1 — Partnering around dropout prevention and recovery.

Forum 1: Reframing School Dropout as a Public Health Concern

Prior to the first forum, the readiness of health and educational policymakers to consider innovative high school retention strategies in the nation, Massachusetts, and Boston was well documented.[4-7,13,22-24] Shortly after his inauguration, Governor Deval Patrick supported the creation of the Readiness Project Leadership Council and the Child and Youth Readiness Cabinet and commissioned the "Ready for the 21st Century Success" report.[25] In 2004, the Boston Private Industry Council (PIC), whose focus is workforce development, had recognized dropping out as a serious threat and convened The Youth Transitions Task Force, resulting in development of a program to recover students who had dropped out of high school.[26] As a function of their work, they created a DVD entitled "Think Again" and sought venues to promote their program and findings.[27] Reports issued by the Bill and Melinda Gates Foundation, the Business Roundtable, and America's Promise Alliance revealed national dropout trends,[4,7,13] and those issued by the Massachusetts Department of Education mirrored national findings.[11,16] However, press columns, the aforementioned reports, and most research journal articles lacked any acknowledgment that the public health community had a role to play in this presumably education-specific dialogue.[5,15,22,28,29]

However, when the Coalition, through their principal funder W. K. Kellogg Foundation, attained an article by Nicholas Freudenberg and Jessica Ruglis,[1] the relationships between student health and decisions to remain in school became a call to action, particularly given the nature of student contact associated with SBHCs. The article demonstrated how good health is linked to educational attainment, specifically high school graduation. Authors also suggested health professionals could play an important role in reducing dismal high school dropout rates.

The Coalition and its membership were prepared to promote health–education partnerships by virtue of the educational policy monographs,[30,31] and journal articles[18,32] distributed to W. K. Kellogg Foundation School-Based Health Care Policy Program grantees. The Coalition also hosted SBHC practitioners for purposes of building a familiarity with the educational community, and health and learning readiness had been a theme of engagement with schools.

Coalition leadership presented the Freudenberg and Ruglis article to their board and found overwhelming support for pursuing strategies to interject SBHCs in general and student health in particular into the state dropout discourse. Planning meetings ensued, and the first forum was the result.

On May 8, 2008, the first forum was convened. Several speakers discussed the rationale for education–health collaborations around curbing dropout decisions and debuted the DVD "Think Again." Following the speakers, a respondent panel and participant discussion was held. Approximately 50 individuals from various legislative, agency, and foundation offices attended; the audience was intentionally small given the planning committee's intent to engage high-ranking decision-makers. Unfortunately, despite repeated invitations to the educational community, most persons in attendance were associated with the public health sector. Meeting packets included information about the Coalition and its membership, relevant articles, a seating chart, biographical sketches of everyone in attendance, and a participant commitment form that provided various options for post-meeting involvement.

Outcomes and Lessons Learned

Numerous lessons were associated with the first convened forum that informed the planning and execution of the second forum. Staging, location, composition of participants, length of meeting, and whether there will be speakers, discussion groups, or a combination of both matter and influence how the meeting will be perceived. Whether persons are vested in the discourse and whether participants retain an interest post-meeting is a relevant concern. As a result, one of the first things to consider is clearly articulating the goal of the forum and the desired outcomes. That said, host organizations should remain open to additional or alternative outcomes that emerge from participant interactions.

Meeting objectives and the desired post-meeting engagement helps identify who should attend. For example, if state agency change is the long-term goal, participants should be those who can influence that process. Target existing networks to gain access to these individuals and the panelists you believe they will respect. Next, invitations should include those unknown to the host organization's network that fit the profile of empowered political. Organizational actors should model the aspired collaboration. In the Coalition's case, they learned that while high-level policymakers seemed to have difficulty conceptualizing health–education partnerships, participants representing local communities had already begun working on the issue. The forum consisted of expert panel presentations and facilitated discussions with all attendees guided by questions designed to prompt collaboration between educational and health sectors to reduce dropouts.

In retrospect, the Coalition's initial forum goal was a bit ambitious. They wanted to facilitate collaborations between high-ranking health and education policymakers that would ultimately reduce the numbers of youth dropping out of school. Given this meeting objective, it seemed prudent to invite individuals possessing the authority to make commitments and ensure implementation. It became apparent almost immediately that this goal was ambitious because, for most attendees, this appeared to be the first time public health officials were confronted with the symbiotic relationship between dropping out of high school and the potentially protective role of the public health community. In theory the premeeting objective was a valid aspiration; however, disciplinary silos proved more difficult to penetrate than anticipated. Changing views and promoting unconventional approaches requires multiple exposures in varying venues that need to be framed in the priorities of the target audience supported by data.

Relative to logistics several opportunities were missed, which were subsequently addressed at the second forum, described next. First, although evaluation forms were included in packets, there was no system to ensure they would be completed. As a result, there were too few submitted to tabulate. Second, if facilitators of open discussions are not careful, one negative voice can derail dialogue and hinder articulation of innovative solutions. Third, forums are not the place to solicit host organization funding because attempts to do so detract from perceptions of genuine interest in the chosen issue. It might be tempting to use a forum to accomplish multiple objectives, i.e., raise awareness of an issue and seek financial support for the hosting organization. However, fund-raising in this setting can be viewed as self-serving and detract focus from the topic.

Two final lessons from the first forum are significant. Sometimes what is not discussed is as revealing as what is discussed. Coalition staff were taken by the absence of any reference to how student mental health might influence decisions to drop out. Finally, meeting minutes or proceedings are a vital tool to affirm participant contributions and record action items. Some minutes were taken but were not detailed enough to create a formal distributable document. This was a missed opportunity because a document or meeting proceedings can also serve as an advocacy tool.

Several outcomes can be attributed to the first forum. The executive director of the Boston PIC has become an outspoken ally and invited the Coalition's executive director to join the organization's Youth Transitions Task Force. He was also instrumental in having pending legislation amended—the Dropout Prevention and Recovery Commission composition was changed to include the Commissioner of Public Health as a member. The Coalition leadership using the forum's outcomes as an entree met with the newly appointed Secretary of Education to introduce him to the Coalition and the SBHCs and to discuss the health sector's vested interest in reducing the achievement gap in general and dropout rates in particular. Building on a need to understand better why educators might not have found the forum worth attending, Coalition leadership contacted individuals hosting the annual Massachusetts School Committee (similar to local school boards) and Superintendent's conference for permission to attend. Not only was the Coalition welcome, they were encouraged to set up an information booth, which provided valuable contacts, information, and education community exposure for the Coalition.

Forum 2: Avoiding the Dropout Danger Zone: Creating a Collaborative Action Plan

It was clear from the first forum and subsequent investigations that the energy to reduce dropouts and craft innovative collaborations had taken root at the community or grassroots level as opposed to state agencies. Several other events and relationships influenced the planning and implementation of the second forum. The Governor's cabinet and commissions had been convened and were charged with reducing premature exits from schools. The Rennie Center released another report on the issue as did the Governor's administration.[25,33] Essentially, the Rennie Center report confirmed findings of the national studies cited earlier about the dropouts with a particular focus on Massachussetts. The Coalition staff had gained entry into educational decision-maker circles after attending the previously mentioned Massachusetts Association of School Committees and Superintendents annual meeting.

The goal of the second forum was imbedded in its name, leveraging knowledge and commitment to begin creating a network and action plan for students at risk of dropping out. Speakers represented diverse perspectives on the issue and were engaged more strategically in forum planning through one-on-one conversations outlining anticipated contributions, and the expectation comments would be submitted for inclusion in conference proceedings. Rather than a whole group discussion after the informational panels, each roundtable was staffed with a facilitator and student note taker to capture dialogue. Facilitators were provided a guide for engagement and specific table discussion questions crafted by the Coalition. There was also a skilled note taker for the panel discussions as well as video to ensure events were accurately recounted in proceedings. Packets included the agenda, biographical sketches of speakers, supporting articles, relevant legislation descriptions, fact sheets on SBHCs' impact on student mental, behavioral, and physical health; evaluation and information forms; and a Coalition-sponsored article articulating an innovative SBHC program in a local elementary school. Serendipity also lent a hand when the night before the forum President Obama, in a speech to a joint session of Congress, specifically addressed the high cost of allowing students to drop out of high school.

Outcomes and Lessons Learned

Greater diversity was achieved at this forum, as evidenced by 31% attendees self-identifying as associated with education, 29% health, 15% government, 15% multiple affiliations, and 11% other, which included advocacy organizations, a parent, and a youth developmental agency, for example. Participant information and evaluation forms were judiciously collected and analyzed, and as a result, the findings are drawn from participant perspectives.

It was discovered that most of the forum participants were already engaged in working to reduce the numbers of dropouts (83%). A sample of reported interventions included using in-school and out-of-school programming, mentoring, peer mentoring, casework, and prevention strategies to identify and support students at risk; targeting specific student populations for support (e.g., overage, truant, low income, pregnant, homeless); forging partnerships between schools and community-based organizations; providing health care to students in schools and identifying health needs; and providing academic support and encouragement.[34]

In order to help students stay in school, participants felt that it would be beneficial to have a better understanding of the myriad agencies that support youth and promote greater communication and coordination between and among these agencies (29%). Targeted interventions best suited for this issue were believed to be more youth programming and resources and a better understanding of how to facilitate youth resilience, particularly in light of the prevailing belief that a chief contributor to dropping out was a lack of connectedness (43%). Respondents thought that families stressed by economic disadvantage exhibited diverse needs which, if not addressed, trickle into a student's decision-making process (29%). Another underlying cause of dropping out was believed to be early academic and health difficulties and a subsequent absence of support complicated by school climates not conducive to nurturing student–adult relationships (51%). A key element of reversing current trends was considered to be rooted in ensuring students were connected with a caring adult (35%).

Participants recommended additional forums and opportunities to network and collaborate (48%). There was some consensus that federal, state, and local policies would have to be adjusted to ensure this issue is addressed (25%). Prevention programming and early identification strategies should be more widely available to equip the community (educators, SBHCs, advocates, and so on) to intervene at a time most apt to yield positive results (27%). Finally, recommendations to the Dropout Commission and the Child and Youth Readiness Cabinet included framing the dropout issue more holistically (e.g., acknowledge the roles of race, ethnicity, class, health, and gender), consider engaging multiple stakeholders with the goal of creating year-round programming and support for students, include the student voice when crafting interventions and programs, and include provisions for professional development and training for those most apt to work with students in the dropout danger zone.[34]

As evidence of inroads into the educational decision-making circles, the Coalition organized a series of sessions to address formally the value of health–education partnerships for district school committee members and superintendents at a subsequent statewide conference. The data provided in the proceedings have served as a useful advocacy tool across education and health disciplines for initiating dialogue in some cases and deepening understanding in others. Perhaps most significantly, the Coalition placed school dropouts into a public health lexicon calling attention to multiple social determinants influencing youth leaving high school before graduation.

RECOMMENDATIONS

Relative to replicated use of an issue as a focus for advocacy coalition building, the Coalition offers the following recommendations:

- Ensure selected issues are highly relevant across disciplines and congruent with the partner organization's existing priorities;
- Ground the issue in the host organization's mission, and articulate meeting goals and outcomes prior to developing an invitation list;
- Think strategically about the meeting logistics, location, venue for information sharing, and level of decision-making required to implement suggestions evolving from the meeting;

- Allow time for a learning curve, particularly if collaboration around the target dilemma is a novel approach;
- Protect time for meaningful dialogue and networking for participants and remain open to nontraditional approaches to the problem;
- Listen carefully to what is not said and not being done to mitigate the detrimental aspects of the issue;
- Capture proceedings in writing or on video—data are vital to ongoing dialogue. As a result, make sure evaluation forms are well crafted, collected, and included in proceeding documents;
- Do not assume that all facilitators are equally equipped for the task at hand—provide briefs and trainings as necessary before the event; and
- Determine the most utilitarian post-meeting products and develop follow-up strategies to capitalize on progress toward your ultimate objectives.

There continues to be residual enthusiasm about partnering to rescue students from the "dropout danger zone." Participants expressed the value of the meetings as a networking opportunity because many felt as though they had been working on this issue in isolation. By stepping out of their comfort zone, the Coalition charted an unconventional pathway to advocacy coalition building that resonated with multiple state and local legislative bodies and health and educational agencies. By hosting the forums, the Coalition is now seen as an organization with multidisciplinary interests, as opposed to one that supports traditional conceptions of SBHCs alone.

REFERENCES

1. Freudenberg N, Ruglis J. Reframing school dropout as a public health issue. *Prev Chronic Dis*. 2007;4(4):A107.

2. Commission to Build a Healthier America. *Beyond Health Care: New Directions to a Healthier America*. Princeton, NJ: Robert Wood Johnson Foundation; 2009.

3. Balfanz R, Allensworth E, Jerald C. *Improving the Transition From Middle Grades to High Schools: The Role of Early Warning Indicators*. Forum Brief. Washington, DC: American Youth Policy Forum; 2008.

4. Bridgeland JM, Dillulio JJ Jr, Morison KB. *The Silent Epidemic: Perspectives of High School Dropouts*. Washington, DC: Civic Enterprises in association with Peter D. Hart Research Associates; 2006.

5. Christle CA, Jolivette K, Nelson CM. School characteristics related to high school dropout rates. *Rem Spec Ed*. 2007;28(6):325–339.

6. McLaughlin J, Sum A, Khatiwada I, Palma S. *State and Local Fiscal Consequences of High School Dropout Problems in Massachusetts*. Boston, MA: Boston Youth Transition Funders Group; 2007.

7. Sum A, Harrington P. *The Hidden Crisis in the High School Dropout Problems of Young Adults in the U.S.: Recent Trends in Overall School Dropout Rates and Gender Differences in Dropout Behavior*. Boston, MA: The Business Rountable and the Center for Labor Market Studies at Northeastern University; 2003.

8. Toldson IA. *Breaking Barriers: Plotting the Path to Academic Success for School-Age African-American Males*. Washington, DC: Congressional Black Caucus Foundation; 2008.

9. Egerter S, Braveman P, Sadegh-Nobari T, Grossman-Kahn R, Dekker M. *Education Matters for Health*. Issue Brief. Princeton, NJ: Robert Wood Johnson Foundation; 2009.

10. Planty M, Hussar W, Snyder T. *The Condition of Education 2008*. Washington, DC: National Center for Education Statistics, Institute of Education Sciences, US Department of Education; 2008. NCES 2008-031.

11. Massachusetts Department of Education. *Dropouts in Massachusetts Public Schools: 2003-04*. Malden: Massachusetts Department of Education; 2005.

12. Van Dorn RA, Bowen GL, Blau JR. The impact of community diversity and consolidated inequality on dropping out of high school. *Family Relat*. 2006;55(1):105–118.

13. Swanson CB. *Cities in Crisis: A Special Analytic Report on High School Graduation*. Bethesda, MD: America's Promise Alliance and the Bill & Melinda Gates Foundation; 2008.

14. Matthews MS. Gifted students dropping out: recent findings from a southeastern state. *Roeper Rev*. 2006;28(4):216–223.

15. Patterson JA, Hale D, Stessman M. Cultural contradictions and school leaving: a case study of an urban high school. *High Sch J*. 2007–2008;91(2):1–15.

16. Massachusetts Department of Education. *Dropouts in Massachusetts Public Schools: District Survey Results*. Malden: Massachusetts Department of Education; 2006.

17. Rennie Center for Education Research & Policy, Boston Private Industry Council, Massachusetts Department of Elementary and Secondary Education. *Signs That Matter: Using Early Indicators to Lower the Dropout Rate*. Boston, MA: Rennie Center for Education Research & Policy; 2008.

18. Richardson JW. Building bridges between school-based health clinics and schools. *J Sch Health*. 2007;77(7):337–343.

19. Richardson JW. From risk to resilience: promoting school–health partnerships for children. *Int J Educ Reform*. 2008;17(1):19–36.

20. Lear JG. Children's health and children's schools: a collaborative approach to strengthening children's well-being. In: Lear JG, Isaacs SL, Knickman JR, eds. *School Health Services and Programs*. San Francisco, CA: Jossey-Bass; 2006:3–38.

21. Lear JG. Health at school: a hidden health care system emerges from the shadows. *Health Aff (Milwood)*. 2007;26(2):409–419.

22. Cassidy W, Bates A. "Drop-outs" and "push-outs": finding hope at a school that actualizes the ethic of care. *Am J Educ.* 2005;112(1):66.

23. Hanson TL, Austin G, Lee-Bayha J. *How Are Student Health Risks and Resilience Related to the Academic Progress of Schools?* San Francisco, CA: WestEd; 2004.

24. Suh S, Suh J. Educational engagement and degree attainment among high school dropouts. *Educ Res Q.* 2006;29(3):11–20.

25. The Patrick Administration Education Action Agenda. *Ready for 21st Century Success: The New Promise of Public Education.* Boston, MA: The Patrick Administration Education Action Agenda; 2008.

26. Boston Youth Transitions Task Force. *Too Big to Be Seen: The Invisible Dropout Crisis in Boston and America.* Boston, MA: Boston Private Industry Council; 2006.

27. Boston Private Industry Council. *Think Again.* Boston, MA: Commonwealth Corp; 2008.

28. Byrd RS, Weitzman ML. Predictors of early grade retention among children in the United States. *Pediatrics.* 1994;93(3):481–487.

29. Peltzman A, Jerald C. *High Standards and High Graduation Rates.* Washington, DC: National Association of State Boards of Education; 2006.

30. Richardson JW. *SBHC Policy Program: Public K–12 Grantee State Educational Policy.* Battle Creek, MI: The W. K. Kellogg Foundation; 2006.

31. Richardson JW. *Public K–12 Federal Educational Policy.* Battle Creek, MI: The W. K. Kellogg Foundation; 2006.

32. Geierstanger SP, Amaral G, Mansour M, Walters SR. School-based health centers and academic performance: research, challenges, and recommendations. *J Sch Health.* 2004;74(9):347–352.

33. Rennie Center for Education Research & Policy. *Meeting the Challenge: Promising Practices for Reducing Dropout Rate in Massachusetts Schools and Districts.* Boston, MA: Rennie Center for Education Research & Policy; 2009.

34. Massachusetts Coalition of School-Based Health Centers. School dropout as a public health concern. In: Carpenter NW, Blinn AM, eds. *Avoiding the Dropout Danger Zone: Creating a Collaborative Action Zone.* Boston: Massachusetts Coalition of School-Based Health Centers; 2009.

About the Authors

Nancy W. Carpenter – is Executive Director of the Massachusetts Association for School-Based Health Care. Carpenter has a background in public health policy, planning, and program development. During her 12-year tenure at the Massachusetts Department of Public Health, Carpenter was appointed as the first director of the Health Resource Office, responsible for developing the state's policy, education, research, and service response during the initial years of the AIDS epidemic. Previously, Carpenter worked independently as a health care consultant on topics concerning the health care safety net, access for uninsured and vulnerable populations, and Medicaid managed care. She received her Master's degrees in Public Health and Urban Affairs from Boston University.

Antonia M. Blinn – is the Program Director for the Massachusetts Association for School-Based Health Care. Her career has focused on social justice and improving health services access for children and families who rely on publicly funded programs. Blinn utilizes policy, advocacy, outreach, and community engagement to expand collaborations and increase funding for school-based health services. Ms. Blinn has a Bachelor of Science in Community Health Education from the University of North Carolina at Greensboro and is a Certified Health Education Specialist (CHES). Blinn is an alumnus of the Blue Cross Blue Shield of Massachusetts Foundation, Massachusetts Institute for Community Health Leadership.

Jeanita W. Richardson, PhD, MEd – is an Associate Professor in the Department of Public Health Sciences at the University of Virginia School of Medicine. Her scholarship highlights the inextricable links between health and learning readiness, particularly for disenfranchised children and youth. Her work has been published and presented in numerous national and international journals and conferences. Her consulting energies (Turpeau Consulting Group, LLC) are devoted to supporting healthy children who are ready to learn through the creation of health and educational policy bridges and include five years as a consultant to the W. K. Kellogg Foundation's School-Based Health Care Policy Program. For more information, email TConsultingG@aol.com.

Post-Disaster Roles and Challenges of School-Based Health Centers in the Aftermath of Hurricane Katrina

Marsha Broussard

WHAT IS CHAOS?

Today, and no doubt for years to follow, Southeast Louisianans will reference time and significant events as occurring pre- or post-Hurricanes Katrina (August 30, 2005) and Rita (September 8, 2005). Hurricane Rita made landfall in Southwest Louisiana almost a month following Katrina. Though not as devastating as Hurricane Katrina, Rita did significant damage to communities in coastal Louisiana and Texas with a 15-foot storm surge, closing two schools and destroying the majority of homes and businesses in the small town of Cameron, Louisiana. As everyone who was there witnessed, the immediate post-Katrina/post-Rita environmental context was that of complete disorder and confusion. It was chaos, aptly characterized as a complete breakdown of all of segments that undergird our understanding of "community." Katrina had an impact on all basic service and business sectors affecting the residents of New Orleans and a substantial portion of the surrounding parishes (counties), including housing, primary to higher education, primary and tertiary health care institutions, local religious institutions, human service organizations, local government, personal and public transportation, and employment.

One useful approach to describing the aftermath of these storms, particularly for the hardest hit areas, is to examine their devastating impact through specific lens. As it relates to this chapter, the lens of interest is school-based health centers (SBHCs). Since SBHCs are bound to the schools in which they operate, this discussion cannot be completely separated from the impact of Katrina and Rita on schools and student enrollment. An April 2007 report, published by the Public Affairs Research Council of Louisiana, stated that from the 2004–2005 school year to the 2006–2007 school year, the percentages of operating schools were 44.5% in Orleans Parish and 20.0% in St. Bernard Parish.[1] Although Jefferson Parish avoided much of the flooding that devastated St. Bernard, Plaquemines, and Orleans Parishes, 70 out of 85 schools sustained significant wind damage.[1] Schools across the state experienced surges in enrollment due to an estimated 186,000 students who were dispersed across the state and country.[2] More than 6,000 new students enrolled in the East Baton Rouge Parish system, precipitating large evacuee communities such as those in Baton Rouge, Houston, and Atlanta, and smaller communities throughout the entire country.[1]

SCHOOL-BASED HEALTH CENTERS SERVING STUDENTS

In the months and years that followed, short-term and long-term recovery activities were a preoccupation across public service sectors in Orleans and other severely affected Parishes, and public education was always at the forefront of these activities. Orleans public schools experienced damage or complete destruction at 90% of its public school facilities. At the same time, the Louisiana Legislature hotly debated the best fate for Orleans schools and placed 107 under state control through the Recovery School District (RSD).[1] RSD leadership soon began a massive restructuring of Orleans schools into Charter organizations aimed at improving school performance, but inadvertently created disaggregated administrative bodies that were complex to navigate in an environment already taxed by recovery challenges in all other sectors.

Although a smaller school district, 100% of St. Bernard Parish school facilities were damaged or destroyed. All schools in Plaquemines Parish were damaged or destroyed except those located in Belle Chase, a community that is located more inland and not on the peninsula which is surrounded by water. Although the damage to school facilities in neighboring Jefferson Parish were limited, Jefferson Parish schools were inundated with students from the other three parishes.

Three of the five Orleans SBHCs operating pre-Katrina were totally destroyed, and two ceased to operate due to the inability of the school or the SBHC provider to resume the service. When the first schools began reopening, Orleans SBHC providers, anxious to address the needs of students, began negotiating to reopen SBHCs in new locations as schools reopened and began accepting students. The SBHC at George Washington Carver High School, the first SBHC in the state of Louisiana, was located in the completely destroyed Desire community of New Orleans. By early 2006, Clint Ball and Joan Thomas, the SBHC Coordinators for the SBHCs sponsored by the City of New Orleans who operated the Booker T. Washington

High and G. W. Carver SBHCs, had negotiated relocations. The Booker T. Washington High clinic was moved to the O. Perry Walker High School in Algiers, a community on the West Bank of New Orleans that did not flood, and G.W. Carver's clinic was relocated to McDonogh 35 High School in the Tremé community.

Within the first year following Katrina and despite their personal struggles, leaders from four of five SBHCs in Orleans had reopened their SBHCs in new school locations, demonstrating phenomenal resilience and commitment to the health needs of students. Dr. Ryan Pasternak and Colleen Bodet, ANP, SBHC leaders from Louisiana State University Health Sciences Center, Department of Pediatrics, Adolescent Medicine, relocated the SBHC at John McDonogh High to New Orleans Charter Science and Math High School, and Methodist Foundation relocated the SBHC at Abramson High School to Sarah T. Reed High in the East. Only the Lawless High SBHC did not reopen in a new location, and Lawless High School will not be rebuilt. Amazingly, three of these five arrangements have survived, despite the tumultuous landscape for public schools in Orleans, which were being simultaneously launched into the most aggressive and transformative chartering process in the entire country. In this uncertain school administrative environment, the Louisiana State University Health Sciences Center team also managed to open a new SBHC site at McMain High School in the second year after Katrina.

The W. K. Kellogg Foundation (WKKF) was a strategic catalyst in the recovery of SBHC services and the rebuilding of Louisiana's SBHC infrastructure in the aftermath of Katrina. SBHC leaders, with assistance from the Louisiana Assembly of School Based Health Centers and the Louisiana Public Health Institute (LPHI), engaged the assistance of Terri D. Wright from WKKF, who led the Kellogg response. Their strategic and well-funded response included major funding that supported SBHC short-term operations and recovery and expanded SBHC services in Orleans, Jefferson, St. Bernard, and E. Baton Rouge Parishes. The response also resulted in leveraged state, local, and other private funding.

Orleans Parish's WKKF funding supported the operations of the newly relocated sites, financed capital developments for five new or renovated facilities, funded enhanced mental health services in SBHCs through adding psychiatry, and offered mental health services to high-need public elementary schools without SBHCs. This work was guided by the Orleans SBHC stakeholders, who worked with LPHI to form the School Health Connection (SHC) program and use WKKF funds for local SHC program staff to implement the projects and plans. The State of Louisiana also funded two capital projects resulting in eight SBHCs now available in Orleans Parish.

St. Bernard Parish School District was reduced to one public school operating from a modular campus. When SHC offered WKKF support to open an SBHC at Chalmette High School, Doris Voitier, the school superintendent, reluctantly accepted assistance. With strong support from Cameron Barr of the Methodist Foundation, a temporary SBHC in one of the modular classroom structures was opened within a year post-Katrina. It immediately began seeing more that 60 students a day, providing primary care and mental health services. In this small community reduced to 4,000 residents, this SBHC offered the only pediatric care available for students. Several years later, a first class, permanent SBHC facility opened in Chalmette High School, spearheaded with WKKF funding and attracting other private funds.

Jefferson Parish, which had only one SBHC pre-Katrina, was also inundated with displaced Orleans students. Jefferson Parish School Board experienced an intensified need to address health services for these new students, as well as to serve regular students and families who were experiencing extraordinary stressors. Angie Ruiz, the SBHC leader from Jefferson Parish School District, worked with SHC and led the development of three new WKKF-supported SBHC facilities. Jefferson Parish also secured a state grant and local district support to develop a fourth new SBHC in the Jefferson Parish School District three years post-Katrina.

Immediately post-Katrina, Scotlandville, Louisiana, became home to Renaissance Village, the largest and most-concentrated settlement of Katrina evacuees in the country. Renaissance Village was a FEMA[a] trailer park, remotely located, and housing over 3,000 evacuees from 2006 to late 2008. Only the neediest residents were forced to such accommodations, and access to health care, transportation, and other essential services was limited. As a result of the influx of new students from Renaissance Village, the East Baton Rouge School District opened a new middle school in Scotlandville and even staffed it with evacuees. With support from WKKF, Sue Catchings from Health Care Centers in Schools, Inc,[b] opened an SBHC at Scotlandville Middle School to serve students from Renaissance Village, and also hired 10 new social workers for several months to float through the school district to address mental health needs of evacuee students.

As mentioned, the mental health needs of students were exacerbated post-Katrina, although under-recognized compared to other acute needs such as food or housing. Disaster trauma studies show that children are more likely than adults to suffer post-traumatic stress disorder, and they often express their trauma in ways that adults misinterpret, e.g., sleep problems, separation anxiety, avoiding situations that remind them of the trauma, depression, social alienation, and aggres-

---

[a] FEMA, the Federal Emergency Management Agency, manages the placement of evacuees and the recovery and rebuilding of individuals and communities affected by national disasters.
[b] Health Care Centers in Schools is a nonprofit organization that provides health services to public schools in East Baton Rouge Parish, Louisiana.

sion.[3] WKKF and many agencies including FEMA, the Children's Trust Fund, Save the Children, and others from across the country responded to the acute mental health needs of students in the aftermath of Katrina.

SBHCs offered a significant access point for primary mental health care in the schools in Jefferson, Orleans, St. Bernard, and East Baton Rouge Parishes, and 53% of SBHCs statewide reported an increase in patient volumes, with 18% related to behavioral issues such as physical fights, truancy, sexual promiscuity, and parental conflicts.[4] The SBHC care model effectively integrates mental health and primary care services, detecting many underlying mental health problems. Emotional and behavioral concerns are often the first or second most-common presenting complaint for SBHC visits. Through WKKF funding, Orleans and St. Bernard SBHCs were able to integrate the services of a psychiatrist who rotated through the clinics. The impact of seamlessly integrating this higher level of mental health care in the SBHC model was an inspired strategy for meeting post-disaster needs of youth. Although the savings realized from these early interventions may never be quantified, these investments made a profound impact on the recovery of youth and families.

LESSONS LEARNED

In January 2010, SHC-LPHI conducted a quasi-experimental study to evaluate the impact of SBHCs in Orleans. In spring 2009, 1,924 students from six public high schools, three with and three without SBHCs, were surveyed to assess students' perceptions regarding their health, health care seeking behaviors, and other aspects of their lives, including their mental and physical well-being. The results offered a very favorable snapshot of the impact of the SBHCs, indicating that SBHCs filled a gap for students who might have otherwise had inadequate access to quality, age-appropriate health services at a critical time.[5] It also indicated that SBHCs reduced emergency room and hospital utilization and had a positive impact on youth risk behaviors and their mental health status.

There were lessons learned through this process of recovery and rebuilding. Although there was a sense of urgency to replace SBHC infrastructure in Orleans, the construction of the new SBHCs outpaced the school districts plans to rebuild the massive public school infrastructure, which took several years to plan. As a consequence, two of the early SBHC facilities in Orleans Parish are in schools that, seven years later, are being moved or renovated. Because of the impact that SBHCs made over a short period, the Orleans Recovery School District and the Orleans Parish School Board has assured SHC that the school districts are committed to incorporating SBHC facilities in the plans for renovations and replacement schools.

Although this strategy of quickly expending funds on more permanent SBHCs can be viewed as a success, it still calls into question the higher cost–benefit compared to its alternative: utilizing mobile or more temporary facilities immediately following a major disaster. This latter approach might save some funds in the short term, allowing more time for synchronization with the overall community rebuilding process before investing in building more permanent SBHC structures. The chosen alternative of permanent SBHCs realized savings from the provision of preventive physical and mental health services and, comparatively speaking, SBHC facilities are less costly to construct than are other health facilities.

Utilizing local coordinating agencies to convene stakeholders and provide on-the-ground project management was also a sound strategy. Large sums of money are entrusted to causes in post-disaster communities. Having a local, fiscally sound agency, such as the LPHI, to coordinate the SBHC rebuilding project yielded a more cohesive result, the building of long-term relationships with local school officials, and the opportunity to leverage many more dollars from other projects occurring within and associated with the LPHI organization. One example is that LPHI was concurrently administering a $100 million dollar federal appropriation to rebuild and expand primary infrastructure in the greater New Orleans area, and SBHCs directly benefited from being able to access these additional funds.

Also, because of its influence with other foundations, LPHI was able to attract nearly $1 million in funding from the Robert Wood Johnson Foundation to work on an electronic health record (EHR) project for the new system of SBHCs. EHRs are part of the vision for more efficiently operated community health systems and have been shown to be particularly vital in disaster-prone areas to ensure continuity of care for displaced evacuees.

In conclusion, although surviving students and families were badly bruised by Katrina and Rita, there were many pots of gold left as residual benefits. Today, an expanded system of quality community-based health care is available for children and families, which includes SBHCs as an access point. New school facilities and educational approaches are available to students in Orleans and the surrounding areas, and improved housing and better transportation options are now available. Indeed, there is a great deal about which to be optimistic.

Louisiana SBHCs are facing a new challenge, which is to define their role in the emerging Medicaid managed care system that will be launched in July 2011. In spite of their proven relevancy to the health needs of vulnerable youth, SBHCs have not been ensured a place in the Community Care Networks that are the hallmarks of the new Medicaid managed care system. Although the challenges are never ending, SBHCs remain a highly adaptable model of care that is dedicated to the principle that children are well served by easily accessible services delivered in their schools that are seamlessly connected to the broader system of community health care providers.

REFERENCES

1. Rowley K. An examination of the impact of Hurricanes Katrina and Rita on public school districts in 15 communities. *GulfGovReports: Education.* 2007. Available at: http://www.rockinst.org/gulfgov. Accessed February 1, 2011.

2. Lafronza V, Burke NS. *Life After Katrina: Where Do We Go From Here?* Washington, DC: CommonHealth ACTION; 2005.

3. Dean KL, Langley AK, Kataoka SH, Jaycox LH, Wong M, Stein BD. School-based disaster mental health services: clinical, policy, and community challenges. *Professional Psychology: Research and Practice.* 2008;39(1):52–57.

4. Madrid PA, Garfield R, Jaberi P, Daly M, Richard G, Grant R. Mental health services in Louisiana school-based health centers post-hurricanes Katrina and Rita. *Prof Psychol Res Pr.* 2008;39(1):45–51.

5. School Health Connection Program. *School-Based Health Centers Are Making a Difference: An Evaluation Study of School-Based Health Centers in Orleans Parish Schools.* New Orleans: Louisiana Public Health Institute; 2010. Available at: http://itg.lphi.org/ home2/section/3-30-32-90-326/evaluation-study%3A--sbhc%27s-making-a- difference. Accessed February 1, 2011.

About the Author

Marsha Broussard, DrPh, MPH – is a public health leader who serves as the Program Director and Principal Investigator for the School Health Connection program and the Orleans Teen Pregnancy Prevention Program at the Louisiana Public Health Institute (LPHI). LPHI, an independent, nonprofit public health organization, strives to improve health and quality of life in Louisiana. Under Dr. Broussard's leadership, LPHI has become a key stakeholder in school health services, including school-based health centers, health and wellness programs, and risk reduction programs, all targeting adolescents. Success has required coalition building across state and local governmental agencies, universities, foundations, and local partners.

A Funder's Perspective— Supporting Local Policy Change to Sustain Investments

Edgar G. Villanueva

"Students who are hungry, sick, troubled or depressed cannot function well in the classroom, no matter how good the school."

—*Carnegie Council on Adolescent Development*

INTRODUCTION

Children and adolescents are among the most underserved populations in America's health care system and are often overlooked in the larger health care reform debate.[1] As a result, many children and young adults face difficulty in accessing primary health care because of a lack of medical providers in the community, socioeconomic status, medical insurance coverage, and other factors.

The issue of access to quality medical care is one that affects not only our youth, but their parents, their lifestyles, and their overall well-being. One way to address this issue is to consider school-based health centers (SBHCs) as an access point to comprehensive health care for younger populations. SBHCs are partnerships created by school and community health organizations to provide the medical services that promote the health, wellness, and emotional success of school-age youth. Through SBHCs, students are able to access a wide array of health care services such as primary, dental, and mental and behavioral health care, and receive referrals for other health services.[2] Because parental consent is required for any student treatment, and SBHCs vary by location, services are determined at the local level through parental and community input. The SBHC model is a unique and successful approach to providing quality comprehensive medical care to vulnerable populations. For many individuals SBHCs are a medical home, yet SBHCs have struggled to be identified with traditional safety net providers and to benefit from legislation impacting those providers.

Recognizing the important benefit of SBHC services and the national movement around SBHC policy, the Kate B. Reynolds Charitable Trust ("the Trust"), a private, statewide foundation based in Winston-Salem, North Carolina, engaged in efforts to create additional access to health services and to advance favorable policy for school-based health care in the state of North Carolina. The hope was to create sustainable access to medical homes for some of the state's most at-risk residents. The Trust was established in 1947 to improve the quality of life and health for the financially needy of North Carolina. Since then, the Trust's assets have grown to over $600 million, making it one of the largest health foundations in the state. Over the past 60 years, the Trust has invested more than $450 million dollars toward improving life and health for disadvantaged North Carolinians. In order to be a strategic catalyst for community change, the Trust is dedicated to impact, that is, to fund innovative solutions that tackle challenges to health, to use the Trust's influence to leverage and support organizations, and to be a voice for the vulnerable, the underserved, and the economically disadvantaged.

Through strategic grantmaking, the Trust has been able to influence and support significant SBHC policy efforts and operations, resulting in additional access to health services for vulnerable youth. In addition to the Trust's grantmaking program, the Trust seeks to reverse negative health outcomes through multiple avenues such as engaging in partnerships and collaborations, convening key stakeholder groups, supporting public policy change, providing capacity-building opportunities, and offering leadership development opportunities. This chapter will highlight the impact of the Trust's approach to and perspective of systemic change through support of the SBHC movement in North Carolina.

The Trust's interest in supporting school-based health care services in North Carolina over the years has been an obvious choice that was justified due to the scope of the services being aligned with the Health Care Division's funding priorities. Over the past 13 years, the Trust has made a total of 30 grants to organizations based in 21of the 100 counties in North Carolina. The bulk of these grants have supported direct operating costs such as start-up and expansion of services (i.e., staff salaries, technology, capital). As the Trust became increasingly more focused on the provision of a medical home through its Access to Primary Medical Care Program Area, the interest in expanding SBHCs grew. In North Carolina, SBHCs serve as a medical home for many, specifically because they provide core services such as preventative care, mental health services, and integrated community-based primary medical care. After years of investing in direct services, the conversation about sustaining these services through favorable policy advancement began.

HISTORY OF THE SCHOOL-BASED HEALTH CENTER MOVEMENT IN NORTH CAROLINA

In 1991, the North Carolina Department of Public Health and its partners conducted a statewide survey, which revealed that there was limited access to health care providers for adolescents. At that time, there were fewer than six SBHCs in the state. The following year, the North Carolina General Assembly appropriated funds to establish four Comprehensive Adolescent Health Care Projects in the form of school-based and school-linked centers, and funded an additional ten centers in 1993. In 1995, the North Carolina Division of Women's and Children's Health received a Robert Wood Johnson Foundation (RWJF) Making the Grade infrastructure grant to develop and implement policies and programs to support the development of SBHCs. Over the next few years, dollars were spent to plan and develop additional sites through funding from The Duke Endowment and the State of North Carolina appropriations. The most important milestone around SBHC policy occurred in 1998, when the state's Division of Public Health, Women's and Children's Health Section, in partnership with the North Carolina Division of Medical Assistance, agreed to include credentialed SBHCs in the North Carolina Medicaid provider reimbursement network. Currently, centers in North Carolina are credentialed by the Department of Health and Human Services to assure quality comprehensive services for youth. Credentialed standards include rigid guidelines that require centers to use nationally accepted pediatric and adolescent health care standards in all services provided. Today, the state provides partial funding support for 28 SBHCs in 15 counties, with 25 being credentialed. State funding for SBHC efforts has remained fairly flat since 2001.[3]

TRUST PARTNERSHIP WITH THE ALLIANCE

The North Carolina School Community Health Alliance ("Alliance") was incorporated in 1998 as a voluntary network to build statewide support for school-based and school-linked health centers, to ensure financial stability for the centers and the association, and to foster linkages and benefit centers. The mission of the Alliance includes a commitment to affordable quality health care and health education that will improve the lives of underserved young people and their families. The original network was originally funded through a RWJF state program office grant under their SBHC initiative.

In 2000, the Trust made a grant to the Alliance in the amount of $48,181 in an effort to support a centralized, staffed office; to provide technical assistance to centers; and to lead the effort to advocate and raise awareness about the importance of SBHCs in North Carolina, particularly in rural areas. In North Carolina, school health centers are predominantly located in communities where access to care is limited for a significant number of children, either because of low wealth, lack of health insurance, lack of primary care providers, or geographic isolation. The success of the SBHC policy movement in North Carolina began with the formation of this association. This first investment in 2000 was a one-year grant to support a part-time Executive Director and infrastructure to get the organization started. As a result, the Alliance was able to secure several small grants, but sustainability remained a challenge. The organization was not able to sustain the Executive Director position, yet the movement continued through a group of dedicated volunteers.

After many years of investing millions of dollars into direct service in SBHCs, the Trust desired to have a broader, deeper impact that would sustain these services for low-income youth. The Trust, in partnership with the Alliance, began planning to make the state association more robust in order to have the capacity to advocate on behalf of and raise the awareness of the work of SBHCs. The Trust recognized the Alliance's success across the state in spite of not having a steady paid staff or formal infrastructure. However, a strengthened state association would provide a network for individuals and communities to establish and expand SBHCs, jointly advocate for additional funding, and work in conjunction with the North Carolina Department of Health and Human Services School Health Center Program to assist in data collection and technical assistance to centers. In 2007, the Trust made a three-year operating support grant to the Alliance in the amount of $310,759. This grant was to support a full-time Executive Director and for clerical support for the association. The role of the more robust association was to continue to build the capacity of the association, promote center expansion, and to take a stronger lead in education and advocacy at the local, state, and national policy levels. The grant was an effort to maintain and expand the momentum of the Alliance's work due to school-based health being closely aligned with the funding goals of the Trust. The Trust understood that without support, sustainability for existing SBHCs would be even more challenging.

With the successful establishment of the Alliance, the Trust considered another critical factor influential in sustaining the investments in the SBHC movement—

advancing favorable policy. The Trust began to build a relationship with the W. K. Kellogg Foundation (WKKF). As an inexperienced public policy funder, the Trust sought to leverage WKKF investments in the Alliance by seeking to have North Carolina included in WKKF's national school-based health initiative. Not only would this partnership between national and state funders bring additional financial resources to North Carolina, but the Trust and the Alliance would have the unique opportunity to benefit from WKKF's wealth of technical assistance in advancing favorable policy. As a result of the Trust's intervention and partnership with WKKF and the Alliance, public policy has been impacted and the SBHC movement momentum continues.

NORTH CAROLINA SNAPSHOT AND KEY ACCOMPLISHMENTS

The Alliance has been the leader in advancing favorable school-based health care policy in North Carolina and has been critical in opening new centers, supporting existing centers, impacting community perceptions, and serving as an advocate for disadvantaged youth. Currently, there are 56 school health centers in 23 North Carolina counties: 50 are school-based fixed sites, 4 are school-linked community sites, and 2 are mobile units that serve multiple schools. Twenty-two SBHCs are located in high schools, 17 in middle schools, 5 in elementary schools, and 6 are combination centers. In addition to the Trust's financial support, the North Carolina Department of Health and Human Services currently funds 28 of the 56 SBHCs in the state, with four new high school centers opening in 2011. Presently, centers who are members of the Alliance are reaching approximately 34,000 young people in the 5- to 18-year age group with 48% to 65% of enrollees having Medicaid or CHIP and an additional 10% to 22% being uninsured.[2] The Alliance has been essential in informing legislators in the state, which led to the development of champions for school health centers and significant policy changes that were implemented in 2008, including identifying school health centers as part of the safety net of health providers in recurring and nonrecurring public grant funds.

Leadership has played a strong role in the success of the SBHC movement in North Carolina. A more robust state alliance can take a stronger stance in public policy advocacy at all levels and in engaging key stakeholders in the value of the movement. North Carolina's Alliance has several key accomplishments that have been critical to the sustainability of SBHCs in the state. Major achievements include:

1. Establishment of statewide partnerships led by the Alliance and its centers to raise the awareness of the value of school health centers to both schools and the health care professions. Empowered youth have been critical to this movement.

2. Secured public grant funding to provide $25,000 mini-grants to 10 school health centers to prevent youth suicide.

3. The Alliance's participation in the North Carolina Institute of Medicine Adolescent Health Taskforce resulted in SBHCs, along with school health education curriculum and key contributors to ongoing policy, making recommendations to the North Carolina Legislature.

4. Cosponsored the Training of Trainers grant award from the National Assembly on School-Based Health Care to the North Carolina Department of Public Health to provide technical assistance funding for cooperative educational opportunities to seven center professionals, as well as trainers from three others states.

5. Secured additional funding in the amount of $150,000 from the WKKF to advance favorable policy for SBHCs in North Carolina. The Alliance plans to enhance youth involvement and data collection at the state level, as well as to expand technical capabilities to serve the centers, which models itself after the WKKF School-Based Health Care Policy Program.

6. Through partnership with the National Assembly on School-Based Health Care, the Alliance has been actively involved in introducing and supporting a federal authorization bill that if passed will establish a separate funding stream for centers across the country. Alliance staff and representatives also participated in an outreach campaign and have an extensive working relationship with North Carolina congressional offices.

7. The education of state legislators about the role and benefits of SBHCs developed champions for centers that helped to designate SBHCs as a part of the safety net of health care providers, making them eligible for grants from a $5 million appropriation and carving out a $375,000 appropriation that was used as a cost of operations increase. This also increased state program funding for the centers on a recurring basis, because safety net providers are exempt from state-mandated Medicaid reimbursement freezes.

As a result of the ongoing partnership with the Alliance and other key partners, the Trust has had a unique opportunity to influence SBHC policy efforts.

LESSONS LEARNED

Historically, the Trust has been a funder of direct health care services throughout the state of North Carolina. Prior to the Trust's investment in the SBHC movement in the state, the Trust had little experience in supporting community advocacy efforts. Acknowledging that the Trust had limited experience as an advocacy funder, support was sought from a national colleague to share expertise in that area. Through partnership with a national foundation like the WKKF, the Trust was better positioned to support SBHC policy and advocacy work within North Carolina and nationally. As a result, the Trust has embraced the high impact value of funding public policy advocacy in addition to direct services in order to achieve systemic change around health issues in North Carolina. There are several key learning lessons that can be illustrated by the Trust's approach including the importance of partnerships and collaborations, leveraging resources, and making timely, calculated risks.

Being known across the state as a funder of direct medical and health care services to disadvantaged and vulnerable individuals did not limit the action of the Trust in making an investment in the Alliance to sustain investments in direct services. The resulting benefits have no doubt in improved quality of care for youth by providing early intervention and prevention services, addressed health disparities and service gaps in minority communities, supported and expanded the safety net structure to increase access, increased access to mental health and behavioral services, and supported working parents through health care delivery in a convenient location. Not only have direct services improved and expanded, there are potentially positive gains associated with the youth empowerment work grounded in their direct advocacy for their own school-based health care sites.

It is imperative to understand the power of true partnership and collaboration from a funder's perspective. True partnership extends beyond writing grant checks or letters of support. True partnership requires hours of engagement, planning, and hard work as exhibited by the benefits that accrued to the Trust from the WKKF and to the Alliance from the Trust. This approach was successful due to the engagement of the Trust staff with the WKKF, resulting in the brokering of additional resources to allow the Alliance to maximize marketing/communication efforts, youth empowerment and engagement, and evaluation of the initiative, all designed to influence decision-makers around the state. Due to the unique partnership between the Trust and WKKF, the Alliance was able to not only secure funding under WKKF's national school-based health initiative but also access the valuable technical assistance offered to WKKF's SBHC state association grantees to build their capacity to influence policy. Further, the two foundations have utilized their relationship with Grantmakers in Health to create a platform for the mutual work of funders with school health centers. This platform has allowed for cross-foundation learning and sharing. Finally, it is also important to recognize the impact of the Trust's and the Alliance's partnership with the North Carolina Department of Health and Human Services. Through the Trust's funding support of SBHCs and of the Alliance, the Trust has been positioned to influence decision-makers in state government. The Trust is now seen as a critical partner by all in the SBHC movement in North Carolina.

In conclusion, one of the greatest gains from the Trust's support of SBHC services and public policy work is the return on investment realized from the support of advocacy efforts. Advocacy is one of the most effective strategies for implementing a systems approach to achieving significant community change.[4] The Trust's support of the SBHC efforts began because the work was directly aligned with the mission of the foundation. However, as understanding grew about the complex challenges impacting SBHC sustainability, going the extra mile to create partnerships, opportunities, and leverage additional expertise and dollars for the state necessitated expanding beyond the traditional funding scope. The investment has yielded much greater opportunities for North Carolina SBHCs and the Alliance to sustain their work through favorable policy change. Funding direct services often meets immediate needs; however, when direct service providers are also empowered and equipped to advocate for their programs, long-term impact can be accomplished. Further, by funding the SBHC effort in North Carolina, the Trust was able to provide a timely voice to an issue that may have never been heard otherwise. Finally, the support of the Trust demonstrates an investment in systemic reform can result in tremendous outcomes for school-based health care services and in public policy in the state of North Carolina.

REFERENCES

1. Okrent D. Public health. In: [no editors]. *Covering Health Issues, 5th Edition.* Washington, DC: Alliance for Health; 2010. Available at: http://www.allhealth.org/sourcebook-content.asp?CHID=75. Accessed November 2, 2010.

2. Health Foundation of Greater Cincinnati. *A Prescription for Success: How School-Based Health Centers Affect Health Status and Health Care Use and Costs.* Cincinnati, OH: Health Foundation of Greater Cincinnati; 2005.

3. North Carolina Department of Health and Human Services. *North Carolina Annual School Health Services Report for Public Schools: Summary Report of School Nursing Services School Year 2006–2007.* Raleigh: North Carolina Department of Health and Human Services; 2007:2. Available at: http://www.ncdhhs.gov/dph/wch/doc/stats/School_%20Health_Services_2006-07_eoy.pdf. Accessed August 3, 2011.

4. Jagpal N, Dorfman A, Powell JA, Craig J, Ranghelli L. *Criteria for Philanthropy at Its Best.* Washington, DC: National Committee for Responsive Philanthropy; 2009.

About the Author

Edgar G. Villanueva, MHA, BSPH – is a philanthropic and nonprofit consultant who served as a Senior Program Officer at the Kate B. Reynolds Charitable Trust in North Carolina from 2005 to 2011. He has worked with public and private organizations throughout North Carolina and the United States on a variety of programs that address health care for the underserved. He holds a bachelor's in Theology, a BSPH in health policy and administration, and a Master of Health Care Administration (MHA) from the University of North Carolina at Chapel Hill. Mr. Villanueva is a Fellow with Grantmakers in Health (2011) and the American College of Health Care Executives (2009) and is a Hull Fellow with the Southeastern Council of Foundations (2006).

SECTION IV

School-Based Health Care: Looking to the Future

OVERVIEW

This final section builds on the historical and most current advances of school-based health care by taking what is known and applying it in the service of school-age youth in the 21st century and beyond. It wrestles with the knowledge that the challenges faced by today's youth are multifaceted, complex, and daunting. Consider this: almost 25% of young people under 18 are living in poverty[1]; 23% now live in food insecure households[2]; 7,000 students drop out of high school every school day, 1.2 million each year[3]; one third of all high school students say that violence is a big problem at their school, and one in four say they do not feel safe at school.[4] And finally, approximately 12.8 million days of school are missed each year due to asthma, making it the leading cause of absenteeism for school-age youth.[5]

The preceding chapters in this volume provide the theoretical, practice-, and evidence-based pathways for school-based health centers (SBHCs) of the future to be well positioned to expand their impact into strategies and guidance for supportive school environments. The following chapters offer the rationales for consideration.

The section begins with a reprint authored by Richardson (Chapter 24) that illuminates the multiple dimensions of risks associated with poverty and experienced by school-age youth. The chapter provides a grounded rationale for educators and health practitioners to collaborate and redirect their energies toward the promotion of resilience as opposed to the amelioration of risk, particularly when many of the root causes of risk are beyond their purview of influence.

In Chapter 25, Horton and Lima-Negron share the experience of one state school-based health association to encourage and support the collaborative efforts of sponsoring health agencies of SBHCs with prospective school districts in high-need communities. Insights and lessons learned from the process are shared.

Over 27% of the nation's SBHCs are in rural communities,[6] mitigating the access issues related to geography and topography in states such as New Mexico and upstate New York. This has been an area of growth and a departure from the historical beginnings of SBHCs.[7] In Chapter 26, North and Kjolhede share the unique opportunities and challenges of SBHCs providing a medical home to otherwise isolated students.

Almost 57% of SBHCs serve urban environments[6] where the students are challenged by complex circumstances as articulated in the opening chapter of this section. Ruglis and Freudenberg, in Chapter 27, take a special look at high schools and call for a social movement that would improve school achievement and graduation rates. This approach proposes to integrate public health and educational reform by creating a school environment that engages youth in promoting lifelong health and preventing not only chronic diseases but also violence.

In Chapter 28, Wright follows with a discussion on school violence such as bullying and its devastating impact on young people, with chronic absenteeism and suicide being the most visible outcome. SBHCs can and should play a vital role by incorporating a public health approach to creating a safe and violence-free school community. The examples of five students compel the reader to carefully examine how SBHCs can be the catalyst for change. Resources for learning more are provided at the end of the chapter.

Critical to the expansion and future of school-based health care is the engagement of multiple sectors. The focus shifts to how much money can be saved with the provision of health care in schools. Thus far, the research and evaluations have demonstrated that SBHCs contribute to reductions in the inappropriate use of emergency rooms,[8] fewer hospitalizations,[9] and a reduction in Medicaid expenditures.[10] The next two chapters provide further examination of SBHCs from the business perspective. Chapter 29, by Guo and colleagues, shares the empirical findings of a cost–benefit analysis across four school districts that revealed substantial net savings over a three year period. Estimates of savings to the Medicaid program are provided.

Next, Brimfield and colleagues (Chapter 30) provide a compelling presentation of the numerous reasons for the business community to embrace, support, and advocate for SBHCs. As stated earlier and throughout this volume, the evidence supporting the virtues of school-based health care has grown substantially in the last 10 years. Collectively, an effective case is made for the business community to invest in school-based health care predicated on the savings in medical care costs and the potential contributions to the workforce.

As we look to the future, it is important to acknowledge that SBHCs (as well as other health care delivery models) function on the precipice of unprecedented changes in the nation's health care system. The United States witnessed the historical signing of health care reform in the Patient Protection Affordability Care Act 2010 (aka, the Affordable Care Act). Several provisions of the Affordable Care Act pose unprecedented opportunities for SBHCs while others invite concern. Holmes, in Chapter 31, provides a comprehensive analysis of the impact of this law on SBHCs and includes the definitions of key terms and concepts. More importantly, she outlines how SBHCs can now chart their own course as health care providers and potentially move into the mainstream. Indeed their future in a "reformed" environment depends on their tenacious and persistent leadership.

And finally, Wright, in Chapter 32, closes this volume by drawing on the years of practice and empirical evidence to substantiate a strategic proactive direction for school-based health care and SBHCs. Specifically, they must expand their footprint beyond the clinic walls and into the school population as a community of focus for public health. They have the opportunity to leverage the trust they have earned and the reputation they have established to be a catalyst and a leader for the health and educational equity for our nation's most vulnerable children and adolescents. The chapter provides a description of the Center for School, Health, and Education that is positioned within the American Public Health Association to champion this new and expanded direction for school-based health care.

REFERENCES

1. CBS. Hard times generation. *60 Minutes*. First aired on March 6, 2011.

2. Food Research and Action Center. Hunger data. 2010. Available at: http://frac.org/reports-andresources/hunger-data. Accessed March 18, 2011.

3. Alliance for Excellent Education. The high cost of high school dropouts: what the nation pays for inadequate high schools: Issue brief. 2007. Available at: http://www.all4ed.org/files/archive/pubications/HighCost.pdf. Accessed September 22, 2008.

4. Josephson Institute Center for Youth Ethics. Ethics of American Youth Survey. 2010. Available at: http://www.charactercounts.org/programs/reportcard/2010/index.html. Accessed March 18, 2011.

5. Centers for Disease Control and Prevention. Families, clinicians, and schools: working together to improve asthma management. 2010. Available at: http://www.cdc.gov/Features/ManageAsthma. Accessed January 14, 2011.

6. Strozer J, Juszczak L, Ammerman A. *2007–2008 National School-Based Health Care Census*. Washington, DC: National Assembly on School-Based Health Care; 2010.

7. Brindis CD, Klein J, Schlitt J, Santelli J, Juszczak L, Nystrom RJ. School-based health centers: accessibility and accountability. *J Adolesc Health*. 2003;32(Suppl 6):98–107.

8. Key JD, Washington EC, Hulsey TC. Reduced emergency department utilization associated with school-based health center enrollment. *J Adolesc Health*. 2002;30(4):273–278.

9. Santelli J, Kouzis A, Newcomer S. School-based health centers and adolescent use of primary care and hospital care. *J Adolesc Health*. 1996;19(4):267–275.

10. Adams EK, Johnson V. An elementary school-based health center: can it reduce Medicaid costs? *Pediatrics*. 2000;105(3):780–788.

From Risk to Resilience: Promoting School–Health Partnerships for Children[*]

Jeanita W. Richardson

Across the globe, educational and health practitioners wrestle daily with the paradoxes of risk and resilience. Though the causes of risk are generally outside the control of professionals, manifestations of disadvantage directly affect service delivery and the realizing of accountability benchmarks. This article proposes a shift in attention from risk to resilience as being empowering and proactive for students and those vested in maximizing their potential. Given that resilience has been deemed an ecological phenomenon, the ecology of human development framework posited by Uri Bronfenbrenner (1979) was applied to advance the rationale for resiliency partnerships between schools and school-based health clinics.

Poverty can create risk in every dimension of a child's life. Impoverished youngsters around the world are more apt to be born underweight and to be malnourished, as well as susceptible to disease and environmental toxins. Furthermore, implications of these poverty markers do not disappear after birth or early childhood but rather persist into adulthood (Borman & Overman, 2004; Guo & Harris, 2000; Jenson, 2007; Richardson, 2006). Lest the focus on child poverty and the risk it creates target emerging nations alone, it is important to remember that citizen status in wealthy nations such as the United States does little to protect youngsters from economic disadvantage, particularly if they belong to racial and ethnic minorities. Whether residing in developed or emerging nations, babies

[*] This research was conducted with the generous support of the W. K. Kellogg Foundation's School-Based Health Care Policy Program. Reprinted with permission. Richardson JW. From risk to resilience: promoting school health partnerships for children. *Int J Educ Reform*. 2008;17(1):19–36.

and youth are subjected to a toxic risk cocktail if they are poor, by their nation's definition. In and of itself, the term poor is relative and contextual. For purposes of this article, the word refers to family resources that are insufficient to ensure adequate housing, health, and educational opportunities undergirding optimal child development.

Volumes have been written about economic deprivation and risk. Far fewer have concentrated on resilience as a framework for child health and educational interventions; however, this focus is changing. As an example of paradigmatic shifts UNICEF (United Nation's Children's Fund) deems child survival as being dependent on integrated approaches to ensure child well-being. Especially in impoverished communities, it is imperative that essential services be packaged as a matter of efficiency, cost-saving, and effectiveness. Furthermore, partnerships need to reflect community priorities and so create a strategic continuum of care for youngsters (UNICEF, 2005).

A model espoused by UNICEF, UNESCO (United Nations Educational, Scientific, and Cultural Organization), and other organizations to mitigate risk and promote resilience involves the use of schools as the site for health care delivery. In a U.S. context, a collaboration that holds great potential in the quest to optimize childhood intellect and wellness involves schools and school-based health centers (SBHCs) or school-linked health facilities. This article considers the efficacy of programmatic and policy collaborations between education and health professionals that are designed to facilitate resilience in youngsters, as opposed to focusing singularly on risk, primarily in the United States. That said, the rationale for such partnerships has merit because many nations seek to provide for impoverished children.

At the heart of the childhood risk and resilience puzzle is the inability to come to consensus about comprehensive definitions of both terms; formulae that could be applied to predict successful interventions designed to mitigate risk and facilitate resilience; and the role of institutional partnerships in the quest to protect and enhance childhood potential. In addition, strategic partnerships and program collaboration are sorely lacking given that programs often function in disciplinary silos (Jenson, 2007; Jenson & Fraser, 2006).

Uncontested is the impact that stressors associated with child poverty create for health and learning, which can persist into adulthood and hinder educational attainment, thereby presenting another benefit for school-health alliances (Freudenberg & Ruglis, 2007; Halterman et al., 2001; Richardson, 2006). Because economically challenged families do not command the resources to completely mitigate problems linked to childhood poverty, they are in the greatest need of targeted government and nongovernmental organization interventions.

The shear numbers of poor and near-poor children in the United States provides sufficient impetus to consider their plight across developed and emerging nations. Specifically, 63% of American Indian children, 61% of Latino children, 60% of Black children, 27% of Asian children, and 26% of White children are supported by poor and near-poor families. Low-income children in the wealthiest nation in the world are disproportionately both victims and perpetrators of crime and in jeopardy relative to health and academic attainment. Families of these youth subsist as a function of their economic status, which creates a cycle of stress that affect the physical and emotional development of children (Annie E. Casey Foundation, 2007; Children's Defense Fund, 2004, 2006a, 2006b; Federal Interagency Forum on Child and Family Statistics, 2007).

To ascertain why it is reasonable for schools and health providers to function as collaborators against the consequences of economically driven childhood factors, this discussion begins by considering how risk and resilience manifest themselves in health and learning outcomes.

RATIONALE

In nations across the globe, educational and health practitioners wrestle with the paradoxes of risk and resilience, particularly in the case of poor youth. Given the time that children spend in school, educators and health staff are well aware of risk manifestations. Unfortunately, the causes of risk are most often outside their control. Thus, although it is useful to be knowledgeable about poverty-based risk factors, a more efficient expenditure of energy would be to apply an understanding of risk to organizational alliances that could promote resilience.

Risk tends to refer to any factor or combination of factors that interfere with optimal development. Risk is not relegated solely to children of low status; presumably, it is universally experienced by children, irrespective of race, ethnicity, gender, religion, socioeconomic status, and sexual preference. When wealthy parents fail to provide a loving, nurturing, and affirming environment, their children are at developmental risk (Brendtro & Longhurst, 2005). Intellectually gifted youngsters are at risk when stifled by unstimulating curricula (Reiss, Colbert, & Hebert, 2005). However, when reflecting on those in greatest jeopardy, one commonly assumes that poor children are exposed to sustained multiple risk factors that forecast academic and health difficulties with higher probability than that of their upper-income counterparts.

Most poor children in the United States, for example, are supported by at least one working caretaker who tends not to possess the full complement of health insurance, access to transportation, and paid leave to ensure youngster's health.

As well, health markers of asthma, lead poisoning, and minimal access to care are emblematic of the types of housing that families can afford. In turn, housing location largely determines the type of schools that children attend, and as noted by several sources, poor children are most apt to attend underresourced public schools. Academic outcomes of youth in high-poverty neighborhoods (some of which are manifestations of health issues) also diminish the likelihood that the cycle of poverty will be broken (Annie E. Casey Foundation, 2007; Children's Defense Fund, 2006a, 2006b; Dorn, 2007; Douglas-Hall & Koball, 2006; Fass & Cauthen, 2005; Federal Interagency Forum on Child and Family Statistics, 2007; National Center for Children in Poverty, 2007a, 2007b; National Center for Education Statistics, 2006). Risk is pervasive, and no dimension of a child's life is immune; thus, researchers have called for a holistic approach to its reduction. Furthermore, if children are subjected to one deterrent to development, it is highly likely that they will experience other risk factors concomitantly (Reiss et al., 2005).

Whereas some poor families are fragile entities, others are not. As such, families of similar economic status should not be viewed monoliths, because despite the challenges of low income, there are those who possess the tenacity to protect youngsters from the consequences of poverty and so promote resilience. For example, some families have demonstrated their ability to "beat the odds" by creating support networks that create a safety net of services for children (Orthner, Jones-Sanpei, & Williamson, 2004). Thus, there is a need to not only acknowledge the inherent strengths that many low-income families demonstrate but also examine the social systems best positioned to promote similar outcomes (i.e., resilience) in children and youth (Orthner et al., 2004).

Each author contributes a piece to the puzzle of resilience predictability by building on a few basic tenets. Common across the generic definitions of resilience is thus: the ability to defy negative predictions as a function of meaningful protective factors or interventions (Jenson & Fraser, 2006). Stated another way, resilience is the ability to (a) overcome adversarial factors that would typically predict failure and (b) survive and recover from trauma (Brooks, 2006; Edwards, Mumford, Shillingford, & Serra-Roldan, 2007; Jenson, 2007; Kitano & Lewis, 2005).

Childhood resilience manifests itself as personal flexibility, adaptability, motivation, social responsibility, and creativity. Institutions, as well as individuals, can nurture resilience through responsive atmospheres and well-run organizations (Mandleco & Perry, 2000). Educational resilience has been defined as "the heightened likelihood of success in school and other life accomplishments despite environmental adversities brought about by early traits, conditions, and experiences" (Reiss et al., 2005, p. 111). Considering health, resilience is a function of culturally sensitive, integrated structural and programmatic processes for children (Mykota

TABLE 24.1—FACTORS INFLUENCING RESILIENCE

Protective Factors	Research
Resilience is influenced by internal and familial attributes	Bellin & Kovacs, 2006 Brendtro & Longhurst, 2005 Edwards et al., 2007 Kitano & Lewis, 2005 Mandleco & Perry, 2000 Orthner et al., 2004 Reiss et al., 2005
Resilience is influenced by relationships, systems, institutions, and programs	Bellin & Kovacs, 2006 Brendtro & Longhurst, 2005 Edwards et al., 2007 Mandleco & Perry, 2000 Orthner et al., 2004 Reiss et al., 2005
Protective factors are complex integrative	Arrington & Wilson, 2000 Bellin & Kovacs, 2006 Edwards et al., 2007 Mandleco & Perry, 2000 Orthner et al., 2004 Vinson, 2002
Resilience is sensitive to gender, race, ethnicity, socioeconomic status	Arrington & Wilson, 2000 Bellin & Kovacs, 2006 Borman & Overman, 2004 Orthner et al., 2004 Reimer, 2002 Reiss et al., 2005 Renn, 2003
Resilience is sensitive to health	Mandleco & Perry, 2000 Orthner et al., 2004 Vinson, 2002
Strategic support of resilience should take an ecological approach	Bellin & Kovacs, 2006 Bernard, 2004 Brooks, 2006 Edwards et al., 2007 Reiss et al., 2005

& Muhajarine, 2005). All of these definitions and those noted in Table 24.1 posit at least three ideas in common.

First, a person has to be exposed to a degree of adversity that increases the probability for negative emotional, psychological, social, and/or behavioral outcomes (Bellin & Kovacs, 2006; Brooks, 2006; Kitano & Lewis, 2005; Reiss et al., 2005).

Second, the quality of adaptation, or the ability to mitigate the consequences of adversity, varies. And third, protective or resiliency factors deflect negative outcomes (Bellin & Kovacs, 2006; Reiss et al., 2005). In its most inclusive form, "resilience is an ecological phenomenon. It cannot be developed by sheer willpower within the at-risk person; it is developed through interactions within the environment, families, school, neighborhoods, and the larger community" (Brooks, 2006, p. 70).

As indicated in Table 24.1, resilience has been deemed a dynamic phenomenon rather than a static one (Bellin & Kovacs, 2006; Bernard, 2004; Reiss et al., 2005). Interventions designed to support youth resilience need to take into account that singular interventions and one-size-fits-all programs do not yield the greatest results in children. As youngsters grow and familial needs change, so do the structures needed to nurture resilience.

Race, ethnicity, and socioeconomic status are presumed to impose multiple dimensions of risk (Arrington & Wilson, 2000; Bellin & Kovacs, 2006; Borman & Overman, 2004; Orthner et al., 2004; Reimer, 2002; Reiss et al., 2005; Renn, 2003). Unfortunately, potential harm can be translated into predictable failure, and children can be discounted prematurely (i.e., blaming the victim; Arrington & Wilson, 2000; Edwards et al., 2007). This is one inherent danger of continuing discourse around "at-risk youth" and risk factors. However, attention to protective factors is more positive than exclusive attention to frameworks informed by knowledge of risk.

What becomes clear in a survey of the literature is that possessing the capacity to bounce back from challenges typically predictive of failure requires a combination of personal attributes, positive relationships, and institutional supports. Thus, when used in tandem, internal and external strengths most often aid in overcoming challenges that manifest themselves in dynamic, contextual, and culturally influenced ways. Furthermore, resilience is highly dependent on relationships and programs at the places where children spend the bulk of their time: school and home.

Between studying risk and resilience, researchers have included protective factors as those resources that minimize or mitigate risk. Protective factors can be internal or external to individuals. Individual physiological, emotional, and intellectual characteristics—such as general health, IQ, and coping ability—are considered internal contributors to resilience. Families and other organizations, such as schools and health care agencies, are considered external protective factors (Mandleco & Perry, 2000). Protective factors can also differ on the basis of context. Bearing all these attributes in mind, effective protective factors are the nexus between need and outcome. Different protective factors may insulate youth at one point and be ineffective at other junctures because needs change, children develop, and challenges vary. Table 24.1 and the combinations cited in the literature help make the case for school–health collaborations being important in building capacity to overcome childhood risk.

As noted earlier in the text, families are pivotal in creating buffers against poverty-based risk. Community relationships can also serve as protective factors that are not sensitive to income. Caring, supportive relationships between adults and youth are affirming to youth and, whether generated in schools, communities, or families, serve as protective factors (Brooks, 2006; Edwards et al., 2007; Orthner et al., 2004). However, family and general community influence on resilience are, for the most part, outside the locus of school and SBHC control.

If we combine what is known about poverty-based risk with characteristics of resilience, we can see the inefficiency and ineffectiveness of silo interventions. As it pertains to the relationship between health and learning, low-income children with fair or poor health status were 6 times as likely to have a learning disability and 3 times as likely to have attention-deficit/hyperactivity disorder (Bloom & Dey, 2006). School interventions, caused by learning disabilities, for example, have historically been triggered by student failure, as opposed to preventative measures geared toward resilience. School-based services typically become available after risk factors manifest themselves (such as through noncompliant behavior). As it relates to health, the public health community is committed to preventative services; however, many poverty-related safety-net services and other dimensions of low status perpetuate health risk in children (Edwards et al., 2007; Jenson & Fraser, 2006). For example, it is only after a child has been identified as being lead poisoned that certain health and housing supportive services become available (Richardson, 2005). Attention to resilience and the creation of protective partnerships would represent a paradigm shift to a prevention-based approach, as opposed to waiting until the negative consequences of poverty manifest themselves.

There is ample evidence of the links between health and learning readiness, as well as economic stability and educational attainment, which has fueled calls for multidisciplinary interventions in general and for support of resilience in particular. Noteworthy for purposes of this article are the potential benefits of health and educational partnerships, as exemplified by the following testimony. First, in his article on school health policies and programs, Kolbe (2006) writes, "Today, more than ever, school health programs could become one of the most efficient means available to improve the health Please of our children and their educational achievement" (p. 226). Similarly, in an article concerned with school–community partnerships, Lee-Bayha and Harrison (2002) posit, "The best of teaching cannot always compete successfully with the challenges many students face outside of school" (p. 1). Other authors concur that it is not possible to eliminate health disparities without simultaneously reducing educational attainment disparities (Freudenberg & Ruglis, 2007). Given that economically disenfranchised children are more sensitive than their upper-income counterparts to social systems and their integration, Uri Bronfenbrenner's ecological model of human development and education (1976, 1979) sets forth a theoretical framework that supports the efficaciousness of schools and health professional partnerships.

THEORETICAL FRAMEWORK

Interactive risk factors influence whether the normal versus disturbed developmental processes ensue. As a result, resilience has been identified as an ecological phenomenon because an ability to surmount challenges is not believed to exist solely within a persona. In addition, because risk and resilience factors do not occur in isolation but perpetually interact, there is a call to think about childhood interventions at critical junctures via an approach inclusive of families, social systems, programs, and communities (Bellin & Kovacs, 2006; Brooks, 2006; Mandleco & Perry, 2000).

The ecology of human development (EHD) framework posited by Bronfenbrenner (1979) has been widely used to explain why some children might be more resilient than others. It has not, however, been pervasively applied to validate the merit of school–SBHC partnerships as a way to improve the lives of children. An ecological approach to resilience in this context presumes certain things: It requires that more than a singular vulnerability factor be at work in a student's life, and it assumes that interventions at multiple levels (personal, family, community, institutional, and broader society) take place concurrently (Edwards et al., 2007).

Three fundamental concepts undergird the EHD framework. First, the EHD model asserts persons as dynamic entities upon whom environments exert influence. Second, individuals and their environment reciprocally interact, thereby creating a need to accommodate each other in the developmental process. Third, environments and developmental processes are not one-dimensional but rather extend between settings, emanating from narrow to broad contexts (Bronfenbrenner, 1979). Each of these assumptions aligns with the characteristics of protective factors and resilience already discussed. Concentric circles representing micro-, meso-, exo-, and macrosystems are most often used to represent the perpetual interaction of multiple contexts (see Figure 24.1).

Central to development are child–adult relationships formed as one-on-one exchanges that occur between youth and significant others, such as parents and teachers. Microsystems (i.e., one-on-one exchanges) take place in settings such as homes, day cares, and schools, and they occur where childhood experiences influence development (Bronfenbrenner, 1976, 1979; Mertensmeyer & Fine, 2000).

Interrelations between two or more settings, such as home and school, home and community organizations, are criteria for mesosystemic influence. In schools,

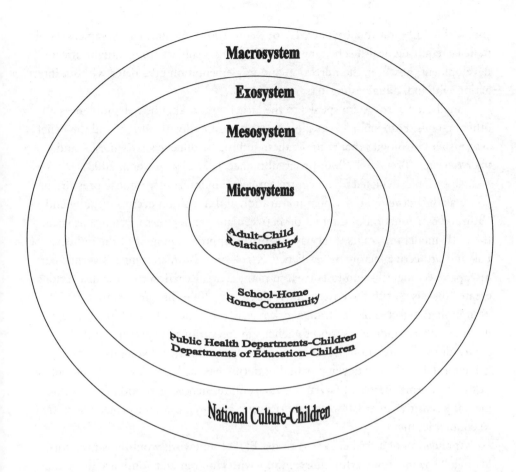

Note. Adapted from Bronfenbrenner (1976 and 1979) and Brendtro (2006).

Figure 24.1 — Ecology of human development.

a developing child is forced into a new setting, requiring an adjustment to new norms, behaviors, and expectations. Mesosystems, like microsystems, are settings where children spend most of their time. By virtue of the hours spent in school, for example, opportunities exist to foster relationships and implement interventions that shape early learning, health, and behavior (Mertensmeyer & Fine, 2000). Another way to conceptualize a mesosystem would be to envision a network of microsystems (Bronfenbrenner, 1979).

Settings that extend their influence to a child but do not directly involve the child are considered exosystems (Bronfenbrenner, 1979). Formal social welfare agencies charged with distributing resources and dictating practices in schools and public health departments at the federal, state, or local level are examples

(Brendtro, 2006; Bronfenbrenner, 1976; Renn, 2003). As another example, school policies requiring health screenings and designating subjects to be taught affect development; however, their creation and implementation take place without interaction with individual youngsters.

Finally, a macrosystem speaks to the larger culture that heavily influences all other systems. For example, the global economy, a national culture, and the belief systems and ideologies that support them indirectly influence exo-, meso-, and microsystems (Brendtro, 2006; Bronfenbrenner, 1976, 1979; Renn, 2003).

All systems, depicted as concentric circles, simultaneously impose pressure on youth as they develop. Individual maturation and transition occur normally and naturally as a function of interaction between and among these systems; as such, the EHD model proves its utility as a heuristic approach in light of the influence of risk and protective factors on resilience. Risk—or in Bronfenbrenner's vernacular, disruptive ecologies—manifests itself in many ways. Reaction to these disruptions create "dis-ease" with the environment (Brendtro, 2006; Bronfenbrenner, 1976). Terminology selected in this framework rejects the notion that children possess deficits; rather, children respond to deficits in the various dimensions of their environment. Transactions occur among children, adults, and systems that create behavioral, health, and developmental patterns that facilitate normal development or thwart normal patterns. Given our focus on resilience, disruptions to developmentally sensitive interactions create risk that creates a need for protective factors to counteract them.

Application of a resiliency lens to the EHD framework would posit the following: "The most powerful interventions with children and youth are those that seek to build a supportive ecology around a child" (Brendtro, 2006, p. 165). As it applies to Bronfenbrenner's work, the problem with risk and resilience is not so much a child-based problem as it is a need to introduce protective factors into high-risk ecologies. Applied to education, Bronfenbrenner (1976) noted,

> Whether and how people learn in educational settings is a function of sets of forces, or systems, at two levels: a. The first comprises the relations between the characteristics of the learners and the surroundings. . . . b. The second encompasses the relations and interconnections that exist between these environments. (p. 5)

That said, schools and the services offered within them are prime locales for protective interventions.

This text begins by making the argument that children of poverty are in great need of systemic interventions that support optimal learning readiness and health because their families do not command as many resources as do their upper-income counterparts. With poor and near-poor children most apt to being uninsured or underinsured, not having access to care, and attending schools that lack requisite resources, partnerships hold the possibility of building shields around childhood potential via micro-, meso-, and exosystems.

SBHCS AND SCHOOLS PROMOTING RESILIENCE TOGETHER

Risk, protective factors, and resilience coexist on the life continuum of a child, exerting pressures on him or her to adapt to circumstances. Mental and physical health, social, emotional, and cognitive development are also influenced by various systems, programs, and institutions (Hair, Halle, Terry-Humen, Lavell, & Calkins, 2006; Jenson & Fraser, 2006). One of the dangers of yet another article about risk is that for the most part, public health and educational professionals have no control over childhood risk factors, such as income, race, family stability, and community resources. They do, however, have the capacity to construct targeted collaborative interventions that bolster resilience by providing holistic services, as would be supported by the EHD framework. A pertinent question to pose at this juncture is why, given the many responsibilities that schools and SBHCs manage, should they consider collaborating formally around resilience?

Rationale for forging collaborative health–education resilience partnerships is rooted in the vulnerability of poor and near-poor children to government supported systems, programs, and services. In addition, researchers concur that educational attainment and health are perhaps the greatest capital sources in breaking the cycle of poverty-induced disadvantage (Freudenberg & Ruglis, 2007). In an international context, poor health has been confirmed to influence low school enrollment, absenteeism, poor classroom performance, and early school dropouts.

Although no singular pathway unequivocally destines economically deprived youth to school failure and poor health, the focus on institutional dimensions of resilience is most appropriate given the mission of schools and the contact hours involved. Academic organizations, health facilities, and community organizations have been identified as being pivotal to resilience, relative to two dimensions: formal programming and adult–child relationships (Edwards et al., 2007). Institutions such as schools are examples of organizations that, by virtue of their mission and location, have high contact with "at-risk" youth and can directly and indirectly serve as a protective factor.

Furthermore, schools tend to be one of the last institutions that all communities have in common and so are a most logical place to provide health services.

Ninety percent of school-aged children in the United States attend publicly funded schools and, as such, are the one place that children dependably convene. Furthermore, the relationship between health and learning readiness is fluid and reciprocal. The Foundation for Child Development indicates that good health, cognitive and literacy skills, and motivation are key predictors of academic achievement and that childhood access to health services is crucial to facilitating transition to productive adulthood (Takanishi, 2004). According to Freudenberg and Ruglis (2007), education is one of the strongest predictors of health and economic stability; conversely, health exerts direct and indirect effects on degree attainment. This may be why some researchers have suggested that schools develop partnerships with families, communities, and other entities to facilitate a resilient environment for youth, based on the premise that schools and school-linked services such as SBHCs can promote early protective interventions in an effective, efficient culturally relevant way (Dryfoos, 2006).

Provision of health services in schools, particularly in low-income communities, is not a new concept. Several programs are in various stages of implementation in numerous countries (e.g., Benin, Mozambique, Sierra Leone) and are tied to international nongovernmental organization initiatives. In the United States, there are over 1,500 SBHC facilities. As a result, the significant cross-section of organizations invests in school-based and school-linked health facilities as part of their commitment to basic education quality (UNESCO, 2002, 2007).

For example, the FRESH programs (Focusing Resources on Effective School Health) are supported by a partnership among UNESCO, UNICEF, the World Health Organization, the World Bank, the World Food Programme, the Partnership for Child Development, Education International, and Save the Children US. The FRESH framework focuses on health-related school policies, safe water, and sanitation; skills-based health and nutrition education; and access to health and nutrition services. Much like U.S.-based SBHCs, services are determined by local communities and are supported by school–community–health partnerships, with schools as the service delivery sites (United Nations System Standing Committee on Nutrition, 2002).

An initial barrier to the proliferation of school–health partnerships in the United States is the educational community's unfamiliarity with SBHCs. As such, SBHCs are created as collaboratives among schools, a health organization, and community. They do not take the place of a school nurse; rather, they expand the health services that are available to children, going beyond the authorized scope of school nurse duties. Models of care and the personnel on site who deliver services are dictated by the needs and priorities of idiosyncratic communities, the school site, and the health organization that is supporting the enterprise. Services are age appropriate and can include, but are not limited to, primary care for acute and chronic conditions (such as asthma, diabetes, and on-site injuries), nutrition education, health education, mental and dental health services, and substance abuse services (Juszczak, Schlitt, Odum, Barangan, & Washington, 2006; National Assembly on School-Based Health Care, 2002).

Given the sensitivity to community priorities, policies on parental consent, diverse funding structures, grade level, and site location (elementary, middle, or high school), it is difficult to find two identical SBHCs. That said, the aforementioned definition tends to hold true for the roughly 1,500 sites across the country (Juszczak et al., 2006; National Assembly on School-Based Health Care, 2002).

Relative to converting risk to resilience, SBHCs can be immensely helpful, particularly if children are economically challenged or live in regions under-served by the traditional medical establishment. In partnership with schools, health programs such as SBHCs could have a profound effect on learning outcomes as well, which include (but are not limited to) poor concentration in school, attendance, and disturbances of normal sequential cognitive development. These facilities located in schools are already beginning to prove their impact as attendance rates and seat time increase and children learn to manage their chronic illnesses (Lear, 2006, 2007). Citing the millions of school days missed annually for health reasons, findings from UNESCO confirm that good health is essential if children are to take advantage of formal learning. An ability to learn and even attend school is compromised by illness that could be mitigated if health services are accessible, and it is logical to consider schools as a location for not only learning but also implementing preventative health interventions (UNESCO, 2002).

Additional rationale for collaboration can be found in the similarities between schools and SBHCs—for example,

- predictors of poor health are also precursors to educational risk;
- both the school and the SBHC need community support and buy-in to optimize their potential as institutions; and
- relative to the EHD framework, both can contribute to resilience when they function as protective institutions.

Taking the potential power of school–SBHC partnerships further, Figure 24.2 reflects how SBHCs and school can serve as proactive factors to fiscally mitigate sensitive disadvantage. As noted earlier, Jenson and Fraser (2006) suggest that resilience be viewed on a continuum.

Children experiencing one or more risk factors manifest school-related difficulties in different ways, such as low test scores, struggles with reading, high dropout rates, minimal academic motivation, and disruptive behavior, to name a few examples. Sometimes, however, these academic markers are indicators of health-related problems.

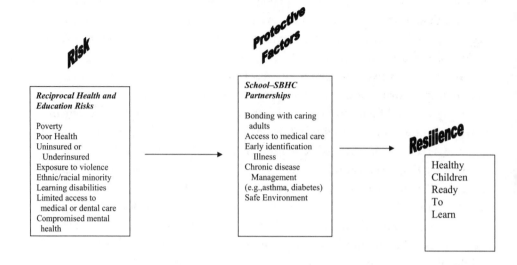

Note. Adapted from Geierstanger et al. (2004), Richardson (2007), and Rounds and Ormsby (2006).

Figure 24.2—From risk to resilience.

As it pertains to the nexus between health and poverty, again we see the tentacles of multiplied disadvantage. Low income increases the likelihood that youth will not be insured, see a dentist, and have to use emergency rooms as treatment sites. These same health issues trickle into schools and so manifest themselves in learning disabilities, short attention spans, poor attendance, and academic performance. Consider one childhood disease sensitive to income that has direct and indirect implications to school performance that SBHCs could mitigate. Over 6 million youth have been diagnosed with asthma in the United States. When income affects the treatment of asthma, youth are more apt to be seen in emergency rooms with severe attacks. Those who cannot control their asthma experience sleep disruption that deters attentiveness in school. Asthmatic children have rates of grade failure higher than those of nonasthmatics. When compared with children who are well, children who have asthma have almost twice the rate of learning disabilities (Diette et al., 2000; Fowler, Davenport, & Garg, 1992). Asthma, in addition to contributing to exorbitant health care costs (because preventative care is far less expensive than hospital treatment), causes over 6 million days of school absences (Wang, Zhong, & Wheeler, 2005). In just this example, the protective presence of an on-site SBHC would not only improve health outcomes but also influence learning readiness.

REFLECTIONS AND RECOMMENDATIONS

Numerous factors create risk in youth; however, if resilience is to be facilitated, careful attention should be paid to services and partnerships that can serve as buffers. According to Bronfenbrenner's EHD model (1976, 1979), systems can do much to alleviate the "dis-ease" that children face as they mature. Applying his theoretical framework further, interventions to mitigate risk and encourage resilience relative to child health and learning should rely more on systemic adjustments than on the individual characteristics or traits of children and their families.

Until now, much focus has been paid to risk as a predictor of child performance and potential. Concerted attention to risk and negative outcomes prompts a deficit-based intervention paradigm (Edwards et al., 2007). Although knowledge of risk and resilience do appear to have influenced educational and health practice, they do not appear to have prompted widespread integrated collaborative partnerships that foster resilience in children.

Coalitions between health (e.g., SBHCs and FRESH programs) and education have the potential to radically improve the lives of children. However, such partnerships and initiatives should not be construed as superficial measures, because in the short term they will not optimally support child development (Brooks, 2006). Protective strategies should include comprehensive services and sufficient dosages of interventions with sufficient intensity, and they should be socioculturally relevant and implemented by well-trained staff (Edwards et al., 2007; UNESCO, 2002).

Despite the proliferation of SBHCs across the United States and despite that of their international counterparts, the potential of the SBHC to meaningfully serve as a protective institution and its demonstrable impact on school accountability measures (such as attendance) are largely undocumented with quantified data. Intuitively and anecdotally, SBHC–school partnerships are an excellent model of a resilience partnership. The work of Dryfoos and others (Dryfoos, 2002, 2005; Kline, Silver, & Russell, 2001) indicate that locating SBHCs in schools is a more efficient and effective strategy to meet the health and mental health needs of little ones. FRESH was similarly founded on these principals. However, these calls are not yet grounded in replicated empirical studies. Many educational decision makers are unaware of SBHCs as a mode of health care, at least partially because of the need for more research. As such, I suggest the following areas be explored further: the relationships between and among dimensions of child health and learning in general and the efficacy of school–SBHC partnerships in particular. Shifting programmatic foci and empirical investigations to protective partnerships could quantify benefits of protective institutional interventions for economically challenged youth.

Even without pervasive quantified data, the proposed partnership is well grounded in intuition, anecdote, and theory. Healthy children are better prepared to learn and, as a result, are poised to grow into productive and healthy adults. The influence of health on learning—and education on health—is inseparable. Children do not leave stressors to well-being in their homes, and unwelcome classmates of hunger, illness, and disadvantage occupy seats in classrooms in wealthy nations such as the United States and emerging nations as well. In the absence of purposeful, integrated interventions, childhood potential languishes. Picture instead the power of a key unlocking the door of economically driven "dis-ease" in children—institutional alliances between schools and SBHCs or similar institutions. Perhaps this theme is best articulated by the UNICEF's Voices for Youth website: "Improving education [and, by inference, health] isn't just a question of getting more children into school. It's also about what happens to you while you're there."

REFERENCES

Annie E. Casey Foundation. (2007). *2007 kids count data book*. Baltimore: Author.

Arrington, E. G., & Wilson, M. N. (2000). A re-examination of risk and resilience during adolescence: Incorporating culture and diversity. *Journal of Child and Family Studies*, 9(2), 221–230.

Bellin, M. H., & Kovacs, P. J. (2006). Fostering resilience in siblings of youths with a chronic health condition: A review of the literature. *Health & Social Work*, 31(3), 209–216.

Bernard, B. (2004). *Resiliency: What we have learned*. San Francisco: WestEd.

Bloom, B., & Dey, A. N. (2006). *Summary health statistics for U.S. children: National Health Interview Survey, 2004*. Hyattsville, MD: National Center for Health Statistics.

Borman, G. D., & Overman, L. T. (2004). Academic resilience in mathematics among poor and minority students. *Elementary School Journal*, 104(3), 177–195.

Brendtro, L. K. (2006). The vision of Urie Bronfenbrenner: Adults who are crazy about kids. *Reclaiming Children and Youth*, 15(3), 162–166.

Brendtro, L. K., & Longhurst, J. E. (2005). The resilient brain. *Reclaiming Children and Youth*, 14(1), 52–60.

Bronfenbrenner, U. (1976). The experimental ecology of education. *Educational Researcher*, 5(9), 5–15.

Bronfenbrenner, U. (1979). *The ecology of human development.* Cambridge, MA: Harvard University Press.

Brooks, J. E. (2006). Strengthening resilience in children and youths: Maximizing opportunties through the schools. *Children and Schools,* 28(2), 69–76.

Children's Defense Fund. (2004). *The state of America's children 2004.* Washington, DC: Author.

Children's Defense Fund. (2006a). *Black child health fact sheet.* Retrieved September 24, 2007, from http://www.childrensdefense.org/site/PageServer?pagename=policy_ch_blackfact sheet.

Children's Defense Fund. (2006b). *Latino child health fact sheet.* Retrieved September 24, 2007, from http://www.childrensdefense.org/site/PageServer?pagename=policy_ch_latino factsheet.

Diette, G. B., Markson, L., Skinner, E. A., Nguyen, T. T., Algatt-Bergstrom, P., & Wu, A. W. (2000). Nocturnal asthma in children affects school attendance, school performance, and parents' work attendance. *Archives of Pediatrics and Adolescent Medicine,* 154(9), 923–928.

Dorn, S. (2007). *Eligible but not enrolled.* Retrieved September 29, 2007, from http://www.urban.org/url.cfm?ID=411549.

Douglas-Hall, A., & Koball, H. (2006). *Basic facts about low-income children: Birth to age 18.* Retrieved August 13, 2007, from http://www.nccp.org/pub_lic05.html.

Dryfoos, J. G. (2002). *Inside full-service community schools.* Thousand Oaks, CA: Corwin Press.

Dryfoos, J. G. (2005). Introduction. In J. F. Dryfoos, J. Quinn, & C. Barkin (Eds.), *Community schools in action: Lessons from a decade of practice* (pp. 3–26). Oxford, UK: Oxford University Press.

Dryfoos, J. G. (2006). Schools as places for health, mental health, and social services. In J. G. Lear, S. L. Isaacs, & J. R. Knickman (Eds.), *School health services and programs* (pp. 182–214). San Francisco: Jossey-Bass.

Edwards, O. W., Mumford, V. E., Shillingford, M. A., & Serra-Roldan, R. (2007). Developmental assets: A prevention framework for students considered at risk. *Children and Schools,* 29(3), 145–153.

Fass, S., & Cauthen, N. K. (2005). *Who are America's poor children?* Retrieved August 13, 2007, from http://www.nccp.org/pub_cpt05b.html.

Federal Interagency Forum on Child and Family Statistics. (2007). *America's children: Key national indicators of well-being 2007.* Washington, DC: U.S. Government Printing Office.

Fowler, M. G., Davenport, M. G., & Garg, R. (1992). School functioning of US children with asthma. *Pediatrics*, 90(6), 939–944.

Freudenberg, N., & Ruglis, J. (2007). Reframing school dropout as a public health issue. *Preventing Chronic Disease*, 4(4), 1–11.

Geierstanger, S. P., Amaral, G., Mansour, M., & Walters, S. R. (2004). School-based health centers and academic performance: Research, challenges, and recommendations. *Journal of School Health*, 74(9), 347–353.

Guo, G., & Harris, K. M. (2000). The mechanisms mediating the effects of poverty on children's intellectual development. *Demography*, 37(4), 431–447.

Hair, E., Halle, T., Terry-Humen, E., Lavell, B., & Calkins, J. (2006). Children's school readiness in the ECLS-K: Predictions to academic, health, and social outcomes in first grade. *Early Childhood Research Quarterly*, 21, 431–454.

Halterman, J. S., Montes, G., Aligne, A., Kaczorowski, J. M., Hightower, A. D., & Szilagyi, P. G. (2001). School readiness among urban children with asthma. *Ambulatory Pediatrics*, 1(4), 201–205.

Jenson, J. M. (2007). Research, advocacy, and social policy: Lessons from the risk and resilience model. *Social Work Research*, 31(1), 3–5.

Jenson, J. M., & Fraser, M. W. (2006). A risk and resilience framework for child, youth, and family policy. In J. M. Jenson & M. W. Fraser (Eds.), *Social policy for children and families: A risk and resilience perspective* (pp. 1–18). Thousand Oaks, CA: Sage.

Juszczak, L., Schlitt, J., Odum, M., Barangan, C., & Washington, D. (2006). School-based health centers: A blueprint for healthy learners—Data from the 2001–2002 school-based health center census. In J. G. Lear, S. L. Isaacs, & J. R. Knickman (Eds.), *School health services and programs* (pp. 294–307). San Francisco: Jossey-Bass.

Kitano, M. K., & Lewis, R. B. (2005). Resilience and coping: Implications for gifted children and youth. *Roeper Review*, 27(4), 200–205.

Kline, F. M., Silver, L. B., & Russell, S. C. (2001). *The educator's guide to medical issues in the classroom*. Baltimore: Brookes.

Lear, J. G. (2006). Children's health and children's schools: A collaborative approach to stengthening children's well-being. In J. G. Lear, S. L. Isaacs, & J. R. Knickman (Eds.), *School health services and programs* (pp. 3–38). San Francisco: Jossey-Bass.

Lear, J. G. (2007). Health at school: A hidden health care system emerges from the shadows. *Health Affairs*, 26(2), 409–419.

Lee-Bayha, J., & Harrison, T. (2002). *Using school–community partnerships to bolster student learning*. San Francisco: WestEd.

Mandleco, B. L., & Perry, J. C. (2000). An organizational framework for conceptualizing resilience in children. *Journal of Child and Adolescent Psychiatric Nursing*, 13(3), 99–111.

Mertensmeyer, C., & Fine, M. (2000). ParentLink: A model of integration and support for parents. *Family Relations*, 49(3), 257–265.

Mykota, D. B., & Muhajarine, N. (2005). Community resilience impact on child and youth health outcomes: A neighborhood case study. *Canadian Journal of School Psychology*, 20(5), 5–20.

National Assembly on School-Based Health Care. (2002). *School-based health centers: A national definition*. Washington, DC: Author.

National Center for Children in Poverty. (2007a). *Basic facts about low-income children: Birth to age 18*. New York: Columbia University, Mailman School of Public Health.

National Center for Children in Poverty. (2007b). *United States early childhood profile*. New York: Columbia University, Mailman School of Public Health.

National Center for Education Statistics. (2006). *The condition of education 2006* (NCES No. 2006-071). Washington, DC: U.S. Department of Education.

Orthner, D. K., Jones-Sanpei, H., & Williamson, S. (2004). The resilience and strengths of low-income families. *Family Relations*, 53(2), 159–167.

Reimer, M. S. (2002). Gender, risk, and resilience in the middle school context. *Children & Schools*, 24(1), 35–45.

Reiss, S. M., Colbert, R. D., & Hebert, T. P. (2005). Understanding resilience in diverse, talented students in an urban high school. *Roeper Review*, 27(2), 110–120.

Renn, K. A. (2003). Understanding the identities of mixed-race college students through a developmental ecology lens. *Journal of College Student Development*, 44(3), 383–399.

Richardson, J. W. (2005). *The cost of being poor: Poverty, lead poisoning, and policy implementation*. Westport, CT: Praeger.

Richardson, J. W. (2006). The health and cognitive consequences of international child poverty. In C. C. Yeakey, J. W. Richardson, & J. Brooks-Buck (Eds.), *Suffer the little children: National and international dimensions of child poverty and policy* (pp. 335–358). Oxford, UK: Elsevier.

Richardson, J. W. (2007). Building bridges between school-based health clinics and schools. *Journal of School Health*, 77(7), 337–343.

Rounds, K. A., & Ormsby, T. C. (2006). Health policy for children and youth. In J. M. Jensen & M. W. Fraser (Eds.), *Social policy for children and families: A risk and resilience perspective* (pp. 131–166). Thousand Oaks, CA: Sage.

Takanishi, R. (2004). *Leveling the playing field: Supporting immigrant children from birth to eight*. New York: Foundation for Child Development.

UNESCO. (2002). *Focusing resources on effective school health: A FRESH start to improving the quality and equity of education*. Paris: UNESCO.

UNESCO. (2007). *Educational for all by 20015: Will we make it?* Paris: UNESCO.

UNICEF. (2005). *The state of the world's children 2008*. New York: Author.

United Nations System Standing Committee on Nutrition. (2002). *SCN Working Group on Nutrition of School Age Children*. Retrieved February 13, 2008, from http://www.unsystem.org/scn/publications/AnnualMeeting/SCN29.

Vinson, J. A. (2002). Children with asthma: Initial development of the child resilience model. *Pediatric Nursing*, 28(228), 149–158.

Wang, L., Zhong, Y., & Wheeler, L. (2005). Direct and indirect costs of asthma in school-aged children. *Preventing Chronic Disease: Public Health Research, Practice, and Policy*, 2(1), 1–10.

About the Author

Jeanita W. Richardson, PhD, MEd – is an Associate Professor in the Department of Public Health Sciences at the University of Virginia School of Medicine. Her scholarship highlights the inextricable links between health and learning readiness particularly for disenfranchised children and youth. Her work has been published and presented in numerous national and international journals and conferences. Her consulting energies (Turpeau Consulting Group, LLC) are devoted to supporting healthy children who are ready to learn through the creation of health and educational policy bridges and include five years as a consultant to the W. K. Kellogg Foundation's School-Based Health Care Policy Program.

Expanding the Knowledge and Vision of School-Based Health Care: Engaging the Education Community

Joey Marie Horton and Jane Lima-Negron

INTRODUCTION

The school-based health center (SBHC) model can be described as a marriage between a school district and a health care facility interested in providing easily accessible health care to underserved students. Each partner has a role in planning, organizing, operating, evaluating, and supporting the SBHC. It is important to develop these partnerships early in the process of creating an SBHC program given the complexity of the partnership, which requires a mutual understanding of the roles and responsibilities associated with the establishment and operation of an SBHC. Both partners need to be engaged throughout the process to increase the effectiveness of the potential SBHC program in their community.

In 2009, the New York State Coalition for School-Based Health Care (referred to hereafter as the Coalition) rolled out a new programmatic initiative, the School-Based Health Centers Education and Assessment Project, as a strategic approach to educate school districts and charter school administrators in Western and Central New York on the SBHC model in the state. The program consisted of a toolkit, a series of customized informational presentations to school administrators, and consultation to school districts interested in assessing their readiness to develop a school-based health program. The Coalition's goal was to ensure that high-need school districts located within this region would have the resources necessary to understand and take advantage of the school-based health care model and thus become a more informed and prepared partner in the establishment of school-based health care programs.

This chapter describes the strategic efforts in engaging the educational community and the lessons learned from implementing the project in central New York.

The Coalition's work was supported by a grant from the Community Health Foundation of Western and Central New York (CHFWCNY). The CHFWCNY is a nonprofit private foundation, the mission of which is to improve the health and health care of the people of Western and Central New York.

SCHOOL-BASED HEALTH CENTERS IN NEW YORK STATE

Many students and families across New York State face significant barriers to accessing quality, comprehensive health care. SBHCs offer a unique opportunity for school districts to meet the health and mental health care needs of underserved students. SBHCs provide comprehensive primary and preventive health care. Enhancements to the basic school-based health model include onsite dental services, health education and promotion, and nutrition counseling, facilitated health insurance enrollment, family services, and community referrals.[1] SBHCs are defined and overseen by the New York State Department of Health, School Health Program.[2] The School Health Program services are provided at no out-of-pocket cost to the students or families who are enrolled. To have access to the services, parents/guardians must sign an enrollment form that acknowledges their consent for the SBHC to treat their child. SBHCs are staffed by a multidisciplinary team of licensed health care professionals and support staff. Currently, there are 230 approved SBHCs operating in New York State, serving nearly 200,000 students.[3] These SBHCs are located in areas with a high prevalence of unmet medical and psychological needs.[2]

The SBHC-sponsoring health care agency has the overall responsibility for the center's administration, operations, and oversight. School districts assist the SBHC by providing school space for the center at no cost to the sponsoring agency. The arrangement is documented by a memorandum of understanding signed by the school district and sponsoring agency. This shared-use agreement is typically used to outline and formalize the relationship between the sponsoring agency and the host school.[2]

Like other SBHCs throughout the United States, SBHCs in New York face limitations and challenges. The SBHCs' greatest limitation is their lack of financial sustainability. Their fundamental mission is to serve uninsured and medically underserved children and teens. As a result, a great deal of health and mental health care services are provided without reimbursement. As mentioned previously, SBHCs must provide all care at no cost to families; therefore, deductibles do not apply, and co-pays are not charged.[2] In addition, SBHCs are not recognized as a provider within New York State's Child Health Insurance Program also known as Child Health Plus (CHP). All SBHCs serve children enrolled in CHP; however,

SBHCs can only receive reimbursement for services provided to these children if one of the SBHC's physicians is designated as the child's primary care practitioner (PCP) or if the SBHC receives a referral from the child's PCP. In addition, school districts, in collaboration with sponsoring health care agencies, often have to make difficult decisions in determining which school building is most in need of the services offered by an SBHC given that, as per regulation, only students enrolled in the school building that houses the SBHCs are eligible to receive the services of the SBHC.[2] Limited resources and small student populations make it unlikely that every building in need will get an SBHC. Additionally, school districts interested in establishing a new SBHC must collaborate with a sponsoring health care agency to gain faculty, parent, and community support as well as significant financial contributions from foundations, individuals, and corporations to establish an SBHC, given high start-up costs and limited capacity to generate revenue. Without adequate stakeholder and financial support, a center, regardless of need, will not be able to open its doors.

Community support has been the driving force behind SBHCs for over twenty years in New York given the limitations and challenges they face. The Coalition began as a grassroots organization with a mission to engage communities in advocacy to increase awareness of the SBHC model and its benefits. SBHC funding is intimately tied to community awareness of the model. As an effective intervention, SBHCs not only provide direct health services but also empower children, adolescents, and families to overcome challenges that threaten their basic human right—quality, accessible health care. School districts can play a pivotal role in SBHC advocacy by encouraging and cultivating opportunities for youth, parents, faculty, and the community to advocate on behalf of SBHCs. Successful SBHCs are a partnership between sponsoring agencies and school districts which share the same common vision—all children will be healthy and ready to learn.

STRATEGIC APPROACH: ENGAGING THE EDUCATIONAL COMMUNITY

In early 2009, the Coalition began work on the first ever comprehensive SBHC report directed to school districts. With the support of the CHFWCNY, the Coalition compiled collective knowledge on SBHCs and their benefits and developed a resource tool that could be used to increase school districts awareness and knowledge of the school-based health model and to improve their ability to develop SBHCs in their districts. The final report, entitled "School-Based Health Centers: Expanding the Knowledge and Vision," was published in the summer of 2009. In the fall of 2009, the Coalition implemented the two-phase School-Based Health Center Education and Assessment Project. The first phase focused on providing direct education on the SBHC model, and the second phase centered on providing consultation to school administrators who were conducting a readiness assessment for an SBHC in their district.

The first phase focused on 19 high-need school districts in central New York that did not have an SBHC. The Coalition shared the aforementioned report with the 19 districts and informed them of an opportunity to participate in an informational forum on the school-based health care model. To engage the districts in the educational forums, several techniques were employed including mailings, phone calls, emails to school administrators, and collaboration with CHFWCNY consultants to contact local health care facilities to arrange meetings with school districts in their service area.

The Coalition then hosted a series of local educational presentations. The presentations were based on the aforementioned report and provided an in-depth overview of the nuts and bolts of the model. These local customized presentations were designed for school district administrators and faculty. Local health care agencies were also engaged throughout the presentations to encourage the development of partnerships between the two parties. In total, eight districts participated in educational forums. In an effort to expand the reach of this phase of the project, the Coalition was creative and flexible in terms of outreach and meeting dates and times. For example, the Coalition partnered with community organizations familiar to the school districts to coordinate the educational presentations in addition to seeking meeting forums where school district administrators already convened, such as monthly Board of Cooperative Educational Services' (BOCES') meetings or regional school superintendents' meetings.

In the second phase of this project, the Coalition acted as the readiness assessment coordinator for school districts interested in evaluating their readiness to open an SBHC. This assessment phase was scheduled to begin in March of 2010. However, in one school district it began concurrently with the first phase, given the district's eagerness to move forward with their readiness assessment as soon as possible.

The second phase was tailored to school districts who expressed a commitment to learning more about their readiness to open a new SBHC. Two districts provided commitment letters and letters of support to participate in this component. Each district received a face-to-face readiness assessment consultation that was tailored to their needs and included an overview of the project, a summary of their responsibilities, and an opportunity for planning and a question and answer session. In addition, each district received customized technical assistance throughout their readiness assessment phase. The Coalition provided a readiness assessment packet to each school district, which included items such as sample student, faculty, and parent surveys, focus group questions, and an assessment checklist. Regular follow-up calls and meetings were scheduled throughout the readiness assessment phase. Similar to phase one, local health care agencies were engaged during the process to further develop partnerships between districts and potential sponsoring organizations, as both are required to establish an SBHC.

To participate in this phase, the school district had to commit to providing a readiness assessment coordinator onsite to collaborate with the Coalition to complete the readiness assessment. The onsite coordinator was responsible for the day-to-day frontline management of the assessment, including distributing and collecting surveys, arranging meetings with focus groups and/or faculty, taking minutes during meetings or focus groups, and for entering data into the data templates provided by the Coalition. The onsite coordinators actively collaborated with the Coalition throughout this phase of the project. The Coalition provided the onsite coordinator with a $2,000 stipend for his/her work on this project, and the school district received $500 for expenses including copying, postage, and meeting costs associated with this assessment project.

The readiness assessment phase was extended, as it took more time than expected for the districts to begin the assessments, meet with stakeholders, and collect data. However, the districts had the advantage of being directly located in the school buildings, which greatly assisted them in the completion of data collection and convening stakeholders for the assessment. Lastly, as the final phase of the readiness assessment, the Coalition reviewed all quantitative and qualitative data collected by the district, including survey data, meeting notes, and community/school profiles and provided a written 5- to 10-page, objective assessment of the district's readiness to open an SBHC. At the time of writing, the two participating districts are moving forward with the Coalition's recommendations and continue to engage the Coalition in the development of an SBHC in their district.

LESSONS LEARNED

As this project reached its conclusion, the Coalition had a greater understanding of how to collaborate with the educational community to expand the knowledge and vision of the school-based health care model. One of the most important lessons learned was that this type of strategy cannot be completed by a district or an organization, such as the Coalition, in isolation. Districts needed a great deal of hands-on collaboration and consultation throughout this type of work. Multiple phone calls, emails, and meetings were needed to engage districts in the educational phase and throughout the readiness component. On the same note, the Coalition would not have been able to gain the type of quality information that was collected by the onsite readiness assessment coordinators. There was a great advantage in getting surveys and focus groups completed by district-based coordinators, as they were directly located in the schools and thus could manage an assessment strategy such as this on a day-to-day basis. As well, they could be more successful in gaining stakeholder buy-in than could external organizations.

An additional lesson learned was that strategies and plans must be customized to meet districts where they are. The project timeline had to be changed several times throughout the project. Some districts had to gain approval from their school boards or school building administrators to move forward, some districts were slow to respond, and others needed more time than originally anticipated to collect readiness data. Lastly, the Coalition learned that customizing the project's messages to meet the concerns and needs of the school districts was important as well. For example, the educational forums focused in greater detail on what the district's responsibilities would be in the establishment of an SBHC as opposed to an overview of the day-to-day operation of the SBHC, as this would be managed by a sponsoring health care agency.

In addition, the Coalition expressed excitement over the first-ever federal funding opportunity for SBHCs that was included in the 2010 Patient Protection and Accountable Care Act (PPACA). This was important as districts' main concern focused on how the establishment of an SBHC would be funded. The Coalition used this unique funding opportunity to engage offices within the New York State Department of Health. They requested that the department actively disseminate information about this funding opportunity and support and encourage high-need rural school districts and local health providers to seek funding from the PPACA to support the growth and financial sustainability of New York's SBHCs.

BARRIERS TO PARTICIPATION IN THE READINESS ASSESSMENT

The Coalition observed noteworthy barriers for school districts to participate in the readiness assessment phase of this project. First, the project occurred during a difficult economic climate. School districts were extremely concerned with their district's budgets and were experiencing severe budget cuts. One superintendent noted that this project was a great opportunity; however, as a result of budget cuts, he was dealing with staffing cuts and could not designate staff to coordinate the assessment. Similarly, it was difficult for districts to conceptualize expanding services when they were currently making tough decisions about what programs to cut, given their budgets and diminishing state funding. As well, several districts expressed concerns over participating in the readiness assessment component without knowing if funding would be available to open an SBHC once the readiness assessment was completed. In essence, some districts were resistant to learn the need without knowledge of an opportunity for funding to address the need.

Unexpectedly, the project revealed challenges in the regulatory environment for rural school districts to open SBHCs in communities with small student populations. As mentioned previously, per New York State regulation, SBHC services are made available only to the students enrolled in the school building with the SBHC. School districts were concerned about determining which of their school buildings were most in need, knowing that resource limitations would most likely prevent the school district or sponsoring agency from placing an SBHC in every building in need. Districts were also concerned about the students who would "age out" of having access to the SBHC if it was located in an elementary or middle school. Additionally, in many rural school districts the number of enrolled students is insufficient to support a dedicated SBHC in each school building.

The aforementioned regulatory restriction prohibited districts from establishing a center to serve students from two or more buildings or districts. The Coalition believes that students in need should not be denied SBHC services because they have "aged out" of the elementary or middle school that housed their SBHC or because the school building that they attend has a student population that is too small to support an SBHC. During these tough economic times, more and more children are in need of the type of services provided by SBHCs, and fewer sponsoring organizations can afford to open an SBHC in every school building in need. Modifying the New York State Department of Health regulation mandating that only students enrolled in the school building that houses the SBHC are eligible to receive the services of the SBHC[2] would help to provide greater access to high-need school-age children. This modification also would help to improve the financial sustainability of SBHCs as they could maximize the number of patients seen while minimizing operational costs.

As a result of this project, the Coalition met with the New York State Department of Health Rural Health Council and presented the SBHC model to several individuals from the department and rural health care organizations. The meeting, which was very well attended, resulted in a wealth of positive feedback. The Department of Health SBHC unit manager attended the meeting and was supportive despite previously expressed concern over the mention of requesting a change to the aforementioned regulation. The Coalition sent a formal letter to the Rural Health Council in the summer of 2010 recommending the waiver of the requirement that SBHCs should be based directly in a school and that SBHC services should be made available only to the students enrolled in that school,[2] at least on a demonstration or case-by-case basis. At the time of this writing, the aforementioned requirement has not yet been waived. Nonetheless, the Coalition is currently researching the policy to determine its impact on limiting the growth and financial sustainability of SBHCs in central New York.

CONCLUSION

Despite the fact that the Coalition reached only school districts in central New York via this education and assessment strategy, the Coalition was able to implement an engagement strategy that led to increased awareness and knowledge of the SBHC model by school districts in this region. In addition, the Coalition was able to develop a more thorough understanding of how to successfully engage the educational community and will utilize lessons learned throughout their work moving forward. Lastly, the Coalition was able to gain a more comprehensive understanding of the barriers that prevent the growth of the SBHC model, particularly in rural areas of the state. The Coalition and the education community have uncovered common ground in which they can advocate together to promote the growth and financial sustainability of SBHCs in New York so that a greater number of underserved children and youth are reached via this important model.

REFERENCES

1. New York State Coalition for School-Based Health Centers. School-based health centers: Expanding the knowledge and vision. 2009. Available at: http://www.nystatesbhc.org/joomla/images/sbhcs%20expanding%20the%20knowledge%20and%20vision%20-%20final%20report.pdf. Accessed April 4, 2011.

2. New York State Department of Health. *Principles and Guidelines for School-Based Health Centers in New York State.* Albany, NY: New York State Department of Health; 2006.

3. New York State Department of Health. School-based health centers fact sheet. 2011. Available at: http://www.health.state.ny.us/nysdoh/school/skfacts.htm. Accessed April 4, 2011.

About the Authors

Joey Marie Horton, MBA – holds a dual role of Co-Executive Director of the New York State Coalition for School-Based Health Centers and School-Based Health Program Coordinator for North Country Children's Clinic's six school-based health centers in Watertown in Northern New York. She holds a Master of Business Administration in Health Services Management from the School of Business at the State University of New York, Institute of Technology, and a Bachelor of Arts degree in Psychology and Health Studies from Queen's University in Kingston, Ontario. She is a member of the American College of Healthcare Executives and is a Board member of the Community Action Planning Council's Policy Council and the Greater Watertown Jaycees.

Jane Lima-Negron, MSW – has been the Co-Executive Director of the New York State Coalition for School-Based Health Centers since 2008. Ms. Lima-Negron has worked on major policy and grassroots initiatives for the Coalition by leading advocacy trainings to school-based health center staff, parents, and students. Her teaching experience includes community workshops on nutrition, reproductive health, and teen health rights. A native of New York City, she holds a Master of Social Work degree from Lehman College of the City University of New York City. She also holds a Bachelor of Arts degree in Anthropology from Lehman College. Ms. Lima-Negron is a member of the National Association of Social Workers and the Women's City Club of New York.

Rural School-Based Health Centers: Enhancing Access to Care by Eliminating Barriers

Stephen W. North and Chris Kjolhede

INTRODUCTION

The iconic yellow school bus is our nation's largest public transportation system, delivering students to approximately 21,680 rural public schools. For students at approximately 340 of these schools, the school bus provides access to both education and health care. Access to comprehensive medical services in rural areas of the United States continues to be a challenge for children and adolescents even in the second decade of this millennium. Rural school-based health centers (SBHCs) reduce many barriers that challenge rural communities' access to health care and are an effective method of providing students access to comprehensive health care.

The romanticized vision of life in a close-knit rural area is often translated into a perception, particularly by adolescents, of a lack of confidentiality in health care services. In our own rural communities this perception inhibits timely access to care by adolescents. We have seen this result in an unintended pregnancy or substance abuse that prevents high school graduation due to limited preventive care. The bucolic vision of rural communities should also be tempered by the reality of poverty that limits transportation and parents' availability to participate in visits. Rural SBHCs offer a means for delivering health care that address gaps in the safety net for children and adolescents in a confidential manner. SBHCs must be considered a valuable part of the health care reform discussions.

While federal and state governments focus on the barriers of inadequate insurance for children and adolescents, having an insurance card does not guarantee access to health care for rural youth. Two major barriers to rural pediatric and adolescent health care are the shortage of qualified health care providers and the limited availability of necessary services in a child's community. These factors make the promotion of the concept of the medical home, especially as one associated with a single primary care provider in a single setting, unrealistic in many rural areas.

Rates of health insurance for urban and rural adolescents are approximately the same[1]; however, finding a provider is a particularly significant challenge for rural adolescents. In the rural communities where we live and practice, there are shortages of primary care, mental health, and dental providers, reflecting national trends. Currently, there are 2,157 rural Health Professional Shortage Areas (HPSAs) and 910 urban HPSAs in the United States, and while approximately 25% of the US population lives in rural areas, only 10% of physicians practice in these areas.[2] In 1999, 87% of the 1,669 Mental Health Professional Shortage Areas in the United States were in nonmetropolitan counties.[2] This translates into 20% of nonmetropolitan counties that lack mental health services versus only five percent of metropolitan counties. The need for dental providers in rural communities is illustrated by the disproportion of dental providers in urban areas (60 per 100,000) versus rural areas (40 per 100,000).[3]

This provider shortage results in measurable shortfalls in the availability of comprehensive health care in rural communities. Significant evidence exists that children in rural communities have greater unmet health care needs than do children in urban areas. A recent study of food stamp recipients in Oregon[4] demonstrated that, compared to their urban counterparts, rural food stamp recipients were more likely to have unmet medical needs (odds ratio [OR]=1.48), difficulty obtaining dental care (OR=1.36), and visits to the emergency department in the past year (OR=1.42). Analysis of the 1999–2000 National Health Interview Survey revealed that rural adolescents are less likely to have a preventive visit compared to urban adolescents and that rural minority adolescents are less likely than their White peers to be insured, report a visit, or have a usual source of care.[1] An analysis of the National Ambulatory Medical Care Survey also found that rural children (ages 5–9 years old) were less likely than their urban peers to receive a routine well-child check.[5] In a rural Midwestern community, 44% of adolescents reported foregoing needed health care in the past year due to a lack of insurance, concerns about confidentiality, stigma surrounding depression, or not knowing where to access substance abuse treatment. This survey of nonurban adolescents (n=1,948) demonstrated that one half had not received needed health care services and identified two barriers: concerns about confidentiality and lack of access to services.[6] Child-focused social services, including case management and mental health support services, are more available in urban as opposed to rural counties.[7] For adolescents, rural residency is a factor associated with the emergency department being their only source for health care.[8]

It is difficult to say whether rural children and adolescents have higher rates of medical issues than do their nonrural peers. This literature illustrates that there are clearly defined needs to improve access to care in rural communities. Despite limited research it is clear that the ongoing rural provider shortage, combined with growing needs for preventive health care, provides an opportunity for rural SBHCs to meet the needs of students.

RURAL SCHOOL-BASED HEALTH CENTERS: AN OVERVIEW

SBHCs provide clinical services in a school or on school grounds as a means of improving attendance and academic outcomes. In an ideal setting an SBHC is able to provide comprehensive, multidisciplinary services; however, these may be limited by school and community resources and local perceptions of need. Qualified health care professionals work collaboratively with school personnel to meet the health care needs of individual students. Two key components of many SBHCs are a system for obtaining parental permission for children to receive health care services and an advisory board drawn from the entire school community. SBHCs not only improve access to health care services but also have been shown to reduce absenteeism, and emerging data demonstrate a positive impact on academic outcomes.[9]

Rural SBHCs account for 27% (n=339) of SBHCs in the United States.[10] Although these SBHCs are located in only 1.4% of rural schools, they provide a model for improving access to comprehensive health care. Table 26.1 describes the breadth of services offered in rural SBHCs.

THE BENEFITS OF SCHOOL-BASED HEALTH CARE

Rural SBHCs have been shown to improve the health-related quality of life for users compared to students who do not use those services.[11] In a study of Mississippi high school SBHCs, among respondents to the Child Health and Illness Profile—Adolescent Edition who rated their health status as "very poor," 60% identified the SBHC as their only source of health care.[12] In our experience, SBHCs also increased the connectedness of students to their schools. It is difficult to quantify the impact of a morning hug from the SBHC nurse or program manager, but this phenomenon clearly occurs in centers nationwide every day.

Ease of access is a strong incentive for the development of future rural SBHCs. The proportion of students who receive mental health services increased significantly with the presence of an SBHC. A three-year comparison of rates of utilization

TABLE 26.1 — RURAL SCHOOL-BASED HEALTH CENTERS, BY SELECTED CHARACTERISTICS

	No.	%
Type of Services Offered		
Primary care only	79	26.5
Primary care/Mental health	108	36.2
Primary care/Mental health/Plus	111	37.2
Total	298	100.0
Reproductive and sexual health services	264	88.6
Dental services	252	84.6
Grade Levels Served		
Elementary	11	4.0
Middle	20	7.2
High	76	27.5
Elementary–middle	17	6.2
Middle–high	19	6.9
Kindergarten to 12th grade	78	28.3
Other	55	19.9
Total	276	100.0
Missing	22	
Utilization of an Electronic Health Record		
Yes	83	29.6
No	197	70.4
Total	280	100.0
Missing	18	
Use Telemedicine System		
Yes	42	15.8
No	224	84.2
Total	266	100.0
Missing	32	

TABLE 26.1 — (CONTINUED)

	No.	%
Sponsoring Organization		
Local health department	44	14.8
Community health center	110	36.9
School system	35	11.7
Hospital/medical center	59	19.8
Mental health agency	1	0.3
University	5	1.7
Private nonprofit organization	13	4.4
Tribal government	3	1.0
Other	28	9.4
Total	298	100.0

Note. Data from the National Assembly on School-Based Health Care's 2007–2008 School Year Census.[15] Total number of school-based health centers responding was N=298.

at rural and urban SBHCs found higher rates of utilization at the rural clinics.[13] Additionally, the authors found that the visits to the rural SBHCs were more likely to be for acute health issues and mental health issues than were visits to the urban clinics. Based upon these findings Wade et al. concluded that "supporting and expanding their use in rural districts may provide a viable policy solution for lawmakers who are looking to increase access in rural, medically underserved communities."[14] The utilization of the rural SBHCs for acute care and mental health services clearly supports the argument that these centers can have a direct impact on the ease of access for students. As we examine the strength of the rural SBHCs, it is important to remember that the vast majority of rural family medicine and pediatric practices do not provide integrated mental health services or health education.

A critique of SBHCs that both authors have heard from community physicians, potential funders, and insurers is that SBHCs cannot serve as a true primary care facility because of the perceived inability to provide after-hours care for their patients. However, few modern outpatient medical practices provide true 24/7 care. After-hours phone calls are sent to the on-call physician, who may be part of a community call pool and may not provide direct care to the patient. Frequently a contracted telephone nurse service responds to all but the most serious of medical issues. In most states SBHCs are required to have backup coverage 24/7. This coverage most frequently comes from a larger medical organization that sponsors the SBHC and follows a model similar to those medical practices just described. Since we have few doctors making house calls for febrile second graders regardless of where they receive their health care, the argument that SBHCs lack around-the-clock care and therefore cannot serve as primary care providers lacks validity.

RURAL SCHOOL-BASED HEALTH CENTERS AS THE MEDICAL HOME

The phrase "medical home" has become a buzzword in pediatrics and family medicine, gaining steam over the course of the past decade. First introduced by the American Academy of Pediatrics in 1967 as a central location for a child's medical record, the concept has grown into a new definition of a practice that focuses on the doctor–patient relationship. The "Patient-Centered Medical Home," as promoted by the American Academy of Family Physicians, the American Academy of Pediatrics, the American College of Physicians, and the American Osteopathic Association, "facilitates partnerships between individual patients and their personal physicians."[16] These organizations have collectively established a series of principles that describe this model (see Table 26.2).

As we have established, rural SBHCs, though small in number, provide an important service for the students at their schools. In addition to the statistics presented earlier, we believe that the SBHC may provide a better medical home for rural children than the office of their pediatrician or family physician due to decreased distance and increased potential for continuity of care. A comparison of the principles defining the Patient-Centered Medical Home and the services provided by SBHCs illustrates this point.

TABLE 26.2 — CHARACTERISTICS OF THE PATIENT-CENTERED MEDICAL HOME

Personal physician
Physician-directed medical practice
Whole person orientation
Coordinated and/or integrated care
Focus on quality and safety
Enhanced access

Note. Adapted from the Joint Principles of the Patient-Centered Medical Home.[16]

The *Joint Principles of the Patient-Centered Medical Home*[16] makes multiple statements that place a physician at the center of the medical home. In many rural communities, where the recruitment and retention of primary care physicians is becoming more difficult, defining a medical home as requiring a physician at the center may not be practical. In the majority of SBHCs, nurse practitioners with training in family medicine or pediatrics provide the care. In these settings they lead the health care team, coordinate care with specialty providers, and ensure care that meets professional and community standards. Collaborating physicians oversee the work of SBHC nurse practitioners providing chart reviews, emergency backup, and consultations.

An advantage of nurse practitioners serving as the center of the medical home is their understanding of the community. It is our observation that nurse practitioners in rural communities frequently grew up where they now practice and, due to their family and community ties, are less likely to move. Having been raised in the community and continuing to have strong roots often leads to improved continuity of care. Additionally, cultural competence of the care and the potential to work closely with the community is enhanced by pre-existing relationships.

SBHCs provide "whole person orientation" and coordinate integrated care in a way that most freestanding practices cannot because the SBHCs' relationship with the school is enhanced by proximity and predefined methods of collaboration. Multidisciplinary care is a cornerstone of SBHCs. Being integrated with the school allows for improved access to occupational, physical, and speech therapy; observation of students in their classrooms and working directly with teachers to address identified needs; collaboration with the exceptional children's program to write individualized education plans; and direct input into the school's meal and exercise programs. This level of integration and collaboration between educators and health care providers is unique to SBHCs regardless of community size.

These illustrations demonstrate how rural SBHCs have all of the characteristics of the Patient-Centered Medical Home and have potential to provide more comprehensive care and develop more patient-focused partnerships than do traditional rural practices. In addition, rural SBHCs have potential to impact public health and community investments in rural schools. Direct access to students provides rural SBHCs the ability to collaborate with the schools and public health officials on population and individual health interventions. These may include distributing the H1N1 vaccine, addressing obesity through a combination of changes in the school lunch program and a walking program, or schoolwide smoking prevention programs. Additionally, SBHCs have the potential to serve as sentinels for communicable disease outbreaks and emerging risk-taking behaviors and can contribute this service to the larger medical community.

Rural schools have traditionally served as community centers; however, their role has decreased in many communities. Co-locating comprehensive health care services in schools may provide the benefit of bringing more parents to the school. This in turn may allow for improved communication between families, health care providers, and teachers. Taking advantage of the increased parental traffic should allow schools to increase their exposure to the community and the community to focus on education.

FUTURE STEPS

Rural SBHCs currently provide high-quality, comprehensive care, and in many instances serve as the de facto medical home for students. As our nation moves toward comprehensive health care for all, adopting the SBHC model, especially in rural areas, will improve early intervention and prevention in ways that more traditional models find difficult. We believe that discussions of the medical home concept in rural communities, and perhaps all communities, must include the SBHC as a Patient-Focused Medical Home.

Financial sustainability is a distinct challenge for all SBHCs and the majority of school districts in the United States. In rural communities, limited public and private financial resources amplify this strain. Solutions to these challenges must be explored, including cost sharing among regional SBHCs, increased reimbursement from public and private insurance for preventive care and mental health services, and funding streams based on the added value that SBHCs bring to school settings.

As attempts are made to improve the comprehensive health services available in rural schools, it is essential to consider the growing field of telemedicine. Currently, there are approximately 15 school-based telemedicine projects in rural communities in the United States. These school-based networks provide a variety of services including acute care, chronic disease management, health education, and obesity prevention, although no single network is currently providing the full scope of services available in a comprehensive rural SBHC. Embracing this technology will allow the enhancement of existing rural SBHC services and the expansion of high-quality health care services to other rural schools.

Political support for SBHCs and growing recognition of the rural provider shortage has created the opportunity for expansion of rural SBHCs and their role as medical homes. Continued adoption and growth of this model is essential in meeting the health care needs of rural students and must not be overlooked in the next decade.

REFERENCES

1. Probst JC, Moore CG, Baxley EG. Update: health insurance and utilization of care among rural adolescents. *J Rural Health*. 2005;21(4):279–287.

2. Gamm LD, Hutchinson LL, Dabney BJ, Dorsey AM, eds. *Rural Healthy People 2010: A Companion Document to Healthy People 2010*. Vol. 1. College Station: The Texas A&M University System Health Science Center, School of Rural Public Health, Southwest Rural Health Research Center; 2003.

3. National Rural Health Association. What's different about rural health care? 2011. Available at: http://www.ruralhealthweb.org/go/left/about-rural-health/what-s-different-about-rural-health-care. Accessed April 15, 2011.

4. DeVoe JE, Krois L, Stenger R. Do children in rural areas still have different access to health care? Results from a statewide survey of Oregon's food stamp population. *J Rural Health*. 2009;25(1):1–7.

5. Cayce KA, Krowchuk DP, Feldman SR, Camacho FT, Balkrishnan R, Fleischer AB. Healthcare utilization for acute and chronic diseases of young, school-age children in the rural and non-rural setting. *Clin Pediatr (Phila)*. 2005;44(6):491–498.

6. Elliott BA, Larson JT. Adolescents in mid-sized and rural communities: foregone care, perceived barriers, and risk factors. *J Adolesc Health*. 2004;35(4):303–309.

7. Belanger K, Stone W. The social service divide: service availability and accessibility in rural versus urban counties and impact on child welfare outcomes. *Child Welfare*. 2008;87(4):101–124.

8. Wilson KM, Klein JD. Adolescents who use the emergency department as their usual source of care. *Arch Pediatr Adolesc Med*. 2000;154(4):361–365.

9. Walker SC, Kerns SE, Lyon AR, Bruns EJ, Cosgrove TJ. Impact of School-Based Health Center use on academic outcomes. *J Adolesc Health*. 2010;46(3):251–257.

10. National Assembly on School-Based Health Care. *2004–2005 Annual Census*. Washington, DC: National Assembly on School-Based Health Care; 2005.

11. Wade TM, Mansour ME, Line K, Huentelman T, Keller KN. Improvements in health-related quality of life among school-based health center users in elementary and middle school. *Ambul Pediatr*. 2008;8(4):241–249.

12. Bradford JY, O'Sullivan PS. The relationship between the use of health clinics in rural Mississippi schools and the CHIP-AE adolescent health profile. *J Sch Nurs*. 2007;23(5):293–298.

13. Guo JJ, Wade TJ, Keller KN. Impact of school-based health centers on students with mental health problems. *Public Health Rep*. 2008;123(6):768–780.

14. Wade TJ, Mansour ME, Guo JJ, Huentelman MA, Line K, Keller KN. Access and utilization patterns of school-based health centers at urban and rural elementary and middle schools. *Public Health Rep.* 2008:123(6);739–750. Available at: http://www.ncbi.nlm.nih.gov/pmc/articles/PMC2556719. Accessed August 14, 2011.

15. Strozer J, Juszczak L, Ammerman A. *2007–2008 National School-Based Health Care Census.* Washington, D.C: National Assembly on School-Based Health Care; 2010.

16. American Academy of Family Physicians, American Academy of Pediatrics, American College of Physicians, American Osteopathic Association. *Joint Principles of the Patient-Centered Medical Home.* 2007. Available at: http://www.aafp.org/online/etc/medialib/aafp_org/documents/policy/fed/jointprinciplespcmh0207.Par.0001.File.dat/022107medicalhome.pdf. Accessed July 23, 2011.

About the Authors

Stephen W. North, MD, MPH – is a Family Physician and Adolescent Medicine Specialist in the Appalachian Mountains of western North Carolina. He developed the MY Health-e-Schools school-based telemedicine program to provide comprehensive school-based health services in small rural schools. The network launched in three schools in April 2011 and will expand to 11 schools by 2013. Dr. North founded the Center for Rural Health Innovation to explore multiple ways to improve access to quality health care in rural communities. Dr. North and his wife, Jennifer Larson, MD, are both second-generation rural physicians and live in Dr. Larson's hometown with their two sons.

Chris Kjolhede, MD, MPH – is an Attending Pediatrician and Research Scientist at Bassett Medical Center in Cooperstown, New York. He is currently focusing his research on addressing the problem of childhood obesity, on the relationship between maternal obesity and lactation success, and on the evaluation of school-based health care. His clinical practice includes a primary care clinic with part-time hospital coverage, and he is the Director of a School-Based Health Program that has 18 school-based health centers in 13 school districts. He fulfills the role of school physician for five school districts. He is also the primary investigator for a four-year, New York State Department of Health project providing resources and technical assistance to assist schools in establishing a healthier environment. He serves as the Past-Chairman of the Board of Directors for the New York State Coalition for School-Based Primary Care. He is also an Associate Professor of Clinical Pediatrics for the College of Physicians and Surgeons, Columbia University, New York.

Toward a Healthy High Schools Movement: Strategies for Mobilizing Public Health for Educational Reform*

Jessica Ruglis and Nicholas Freudenberg

Although research shows that education and health are closely intertwined, health professionals have difficulty using this evidence to improve health and educational outcomes and reduce inequities. We call for a social movement for healthy high schools in the United States that would improve school achievement and graduation rates; create school environments that promote lifelong individual, family, and community health and prevent chronic illness, violence, and problems of sexual health; and engage youths in creating health-promoting environments. Achieving these goals will require strengthening and better linking often uncoordinated efforts to improve child health and education. Only a broad social movement has the power and vision to mobilize the forces that can transform educational and health systems to better achieve health and educational equity.

In 1997, the World Health Organization noted, "Schools could do more than any other single institution to improve the well-being and competence of children and youth."[1(p1)] Yet in the United States, more young Black men move from high schools to prison than to higher education[2] and more pregnant young women drop out of high school than graduate.[3] In 2007, more than 6 million students in the United States between the ages of 16 and 24 years dropped out of high school,[4] putting them at risk for lifetime economic, social, and health disadvantage.[5]

In this commentary, we call on public health professionals to contribute to an emerging social movement for healthy high schools that can reverse these dismal

---

* This chapter previously appeared in the September 2010 issue of the *American Journal of Public Health* and is reprinted with permission in its entirety. Ruglis J, Freudenberg N. Toward a healthy high schools movement: strategies for mobilizing public health for educational reform. *Am J Public Health.* 2010;100(9);1565–1571.

statistics, thus offering millions of young people a safer path to healthy and productive adulthood and our nation a road to ending the health and educational inequities that continue to shame us. A healthy high schools movement would seek to improve school achievement and graduation rates; create school environments that promote lifelong individual, family, and community health; and focus on prevention of chronic illness, violence, and problems of sexual and mental health. It would also work to engage youths in creating health-promoting school and community environments.

RATIONALE FOR A HEALTHY HIGH SCHOOLS MOVEMENT

Higher educational attainment leads to better health throughout the lifespan; at the same time, healthier students, families, and communities have higher levels of educational achievement.[6-9] As Sen has observed,[10] better health and education enable people to realize their capabilities to be free and productive members of democratic societies. Unfortunately, our nation's limited support and sectoral approach to education and health care have often prevented us from realizing the benefits of this reciprocal relationship, thus missing an important opportunity to improve school achievement, promote health, and reduce socioeconomic and racial/ethnic disparities in health and education. Moreover, the correct insight that parents also have responsibility for health and education has often led policymakers to focus on individual rather than systemic change.

We call for a revitalized social movement for healthy schools. Our commentary is based on prior reviews and syntheses of the literature from education, public health, and school health[4,11-23] and on our experiences working in schools and youth programs as researchers and practitioners. With influence from the World Health Organization and other researchers,[15,16,24] we define healthy schools as educational institutions that are committed to creating curricula, social and physical environments, and social relationships that promote healthy life trajectories for students, families, staff, and communities. We call for a social movement because only such a force can transform schools and health institutions to move beyond their current limitations to advance a vision that can mobilize the diverse constituencies needed to change policies and practices. Although all levels of education, from preschool to universities, could benefit from a healthy schools movement, our focus is on high schools because most youths are now lost to further schooling at this level[25,26] and high schools offer high potential for population health benefits.

The public health rationale for healthy high schools is straightforward. First, adolescence is a critical time for the prevention of chronic diseases such as heart disease, cancer, and diabetes.[27,28] These conditions impose a growing burden on the American population and drive health inequities. Helping young people to develop healthy behaviors and create social conditions that prevent chronic disease could bring lifetime health and economic benefits.[29]

Second, US high schools face a graduation rate crisis. Nationally, 70.6% of students graduate from high school.[26] Although more than three quarters of Asian and White students graduate from high school, American Indians, Blacks, and Latinos all have graduation rates around 50%.[26,30] Many of the nation's lowest graduation rates are in the largest urban school districts.[26] Young people who do not attain high school diplomas suffer a wide range of negative social, economic, political, health, and criminal justice outcomes,[17-19] setting them up for a lifetime of further disadvantage. Moreover, even young people who graduate often lack the skills to prosper in a changing economy,[31] showing the importance of considering both the quality and quantity of education.

Third, young people spend more waking hours in school than anywhere else, making the school environment an important influence on health. Among school conditions that have been associated with poor health and educational outcomes are bullying,[32] discriminatory policing and disciplinary procedures,[33,34] high-stakes testing in which a single test leads to being left back a year,[35] promotion of unhealthy food,[36] decaying school infrastructures,[37] and lack of opportunity for physical activity.[38] Low-income and Black and Latino young people are much more likely to experience these adverse conditions, making the experience of schooling a contributor to health inequalities.

BUILDING BLOCKS FOR HEALTHY SCHOOLS

Although healthy schools require a transformation of current approaches to education and health, fortunately, the elements of more comprehensive approaches are well established and have been implemented in a variety of settings. As listed in Table 27.1, these elements include comprehensive school health programs,[39,40] school-based health clinics,[41,42] school food programs,[43] sexuality education and pregnancy prevention,[44,45] special programs for pregnant and parenting adolescents,[46] substance abuse prevention and treatment programs,[47,48] violence prevention programs,[49] mental health programs,[50,51] and school–community programs.[52,53] An achievable first step in creating healthier schools is to focus on expanding the reach, quality, and coordination of existing services. Although almost every high school has some of these components, few have all and rarely are they sufficiently integrated to achieve potential synergies.

TABLE 27.1—HEALTH INTERVENTIONS THAT MAY CONTRIBUTE TO IMPROVED SCHOOL COMPLETION RATES

Type of Intervention	Program Activities	How the Intervention Contributes to Goals
Coordinated school health program	Health education; physical education; health services; nutrition services; counseling, psychological, and social services; healthy school environment; health promotion for the staff, family, and community; partnerships	Teaches decision-making skills for better life choices; reduces absenteeism; offers early intervention and referrals for problems involving learning, psychological factors, substance abuse, and mental health; makes schools more engaging; connects students to caring adults; engages families and communities in lives of young people.
School-based health clinic	Primary and preventive health care; referrals; assistance in finding health insurance and health care for family; reproductive health services; mental health counseling	Reduces family health problems; offers early intervention and treatment of psychological and physical health problems that can interrupt schooling; reduces adolescent pregnancy.
Dental, vision, and hearing program	Dental, vision, and hearing screenings, services, and products	Enhances educational ability of students so they can see, hear, and not be distracted by toothaches.
School food program	Provision of healthy, affordable food; removal of unhealthy food from vending machines and cafeterias; may include community gardens, farm-to-school activities	Contributes to healthier eating, prevents obesity, reduces future risk for chronic diseases.
Mental health program	Assessment and early intervention for young people with psychological, learning, or behavioral problems; referrals for children and families; counseling; staff training	Prevents problems that can interfere with school from becoming more serious; connects young people to caring adults; makes school more engaging; provides counseling or referrals for family mental health problems.
Substance abuse prevention and treatment program	Alcohol, tobacco, and drug use prevention education; peer education; early intervention for drug users; support for young people with substance-abusing parents; referrals for drug treatment or counseling	Reduces or delays onset of heavy alcohol or marijuana use; offers young people with a drug-using parent a source of support; makes school more engaging.

TABLE 27.1 — (CONTINUED)

Type of Intervention	Program Activities	How the Intervention Contributes to Goals
Sex, HIV infection, and pregnancy prevention programs	Sex education; HIV infection prevention services; referrals for reproductive and sex health services; birth control; peer education; sexually transmitted infection prevention	Reduces or delays adolescent pregnancy; connects young people to caring adults or peers who encourage healthy behavior.
Services for pregnant and parenting adolescents	Child care; parenting education; reproductive health services; continued participation in high school academics and courses	Encourages and supports adolescent mothers to continue schooling; delays second pregnancy.
Violence prevention program	Peer education and mediation; anger management; conflict resolution; violence prevention education; psychosocial services; individual and group counseling	Makes young people feel safer in school; makes school more engaging; connects young people to caring adults or peers who encourage healthy behavior.
School climate	Policy changes to reduce stigmatization, bullying, aggressive policing, or punitive disciplinary measures; peer education; increased opportunities for close adult–student interactions	Improves student engagement in school activities; connects young people to caring adults; reduces bullying, stigmatization, and distrust of authority.

Source. Modified from Freudenberg and Ruglis.[19(p11)]

NEW DIRECTIONS AND PROMISING PRACTICES

A second step in creating healthier schools is to identify new directions and promising practices. We propose a few actions related to each of the broad goals of a movement.

Improvement of School Achievement and Graduation Rates

Because completing high school is increasingly a prerequisite for good health and full participation in society, finding new ways to improve school achievement and reduce socioeconomic and racial/ethnic inequities in graduation rates is a key strategy for improving our nation's health. Among the factors that have been consistently associated with school completion are engagement in school, connection to caring adults, disciplinary procedures that are perceived as fair, and school organization.[20,21,54–56] Each provides opportunities for health intervention.

School curricula that engage young people in analyzing the issues that matter to them—family, relationships, health and sexuality, social justice, paths to adulthood, and options for food, health care, and employment—can be used to develop the academic skills that young people need and avoid the boredom that drives so many young people from school.[22] School health programs, especially those staffed by community-based adults, can offer students the connections to other caring adults that are associated with better school achievement.

In their understandable desire to ensure that schools are safe, many school systems have developed disciplinary procedures that rely on metal detectors, mandatory arrests, routine drug testing, and "zero tolerance" for infractions.[57] In some cases, these procedures discourage young people from attending school or lead to the expulsion of students who could succeed in a more nurturing environment.[58,59] At the same time, few schools have successfully implemented programs to reduce the bullying or discrimination based on gender, race/ethnicity, or sexual orientation that can discourage school completion.[60] Through their experience in violence prevention and mediation, health and mental health professionals can help schools to develop more balanced and effective disciplinary approaches.

Finally, research shows that most students who do not complete high school drop out in the 9th or 10th grade.[25,26] Thirteen of the nation's 50 largest school districts lose at least half of all noncompleters in the 9th grade,[26] an astonishing rate of school failure. Developmentally, young people entering high school are striving for independence, choosing the peers who will become primary in their life, making sense of their sexualities and gender norms, and often traveling to and from school through unsafe neighborhoods. Small learning communities[61,62] or "freshmen families" are one model for reducing freshman dropout. In these small communities, students become responsible for one another, fostering the development of trust; communal responsibility; safety; social, emotional, and academic support; and healthy communication and relationships. Repositioning absenteeism, truancy, and missed school work from being solely a disciplinary problem to an issue of care can encourage support networks, problem solving, and opportunities to focus on social, sexuality, and emotional needs that are often barriers to the ability to engage in classroom activities.[63] Health professionals can serve as key members of these learning communities.

Creation of Schools That Promote Individual, Family, and Community Health

As enduring institutions that serve most young people and their families in every community, schools have great potential for health promotion. Given the importance of adolescence as a time for shaping lifetime health, especially for disadvantaged youths, schools can play a lead role in reducing health inequities.

Some approaches that warrant examination are to use schools as sites for identifying family health problems, to link schools with community health care networks, to use schools as catalysts for creating healthier community environments, and to make schools centers for psychological and reproductive health and comprehensive sexuality education. Several innovative programs have demonstrated success in bringing together services, linking schools and communities, and engaging parents.[64-66] These warrant further attention and replication.

With their ongoing relationships with young people, high schools are a place where adults can identify youths and families with such diverse problems as learning disorders, obesity, pregnancy, mental health and substance abuse problems, chronic diseases such as asthma and diabetes, and vision and hearing problems. Although adolescents are healthier than other age groups, many young people fail to get treatment for health problems.[67] Finding better ways for schools to focus on underlying health problems while still protecting confidentiality and privacy are daunting challenges. School-based health centers already play this role, but to fully realize this potential, they need to expand to more schools, move beyond serving only those who walk through their doors, and better link with community health providers.[68] Expanding the role of the school nurse is another option that builds on existing resources.[69]

To have an impact on population health, schools need to connect young people with identified problems to services. Establishing or expanding existing partnerships among schools and community health centers,[52] linking schools more systematically to community health care resources, and creating systematic electronic and other information exchanges between schools and health care institutions can help schools to play a stronger role in prevention.

The nation's more than 23 000 public high schools can become a resource for health promotion. Most high schools have fitness facilities or sports fields that are idle during evenings, weekends, and summers. Recent innovations in school food programs such as school-based farmers markets, school–community agriculture projects, farm-to-school programs, and community cooking classes show that schools can become centers for community change.[38] Similarly, many schools already provide sexuality education and adolescent parenting services and dispense contraceptives, but these programs are often uncoordinated, embattled, and lack the resources to reach all young people.[70] Expanding the scope and improving the quality of these services can help to improve women's health and reproductive health.

Engagement of Young People in Creating Healthier Schools

The largest untapped resource for improving school and community environments is the energy, imagination, and expertise of young people themselves. Engaging youths in improving education, health care, and health promotion provides new opportunities for experiential education and the preparation of citizens who can contribute to solving the nation's social problems. Linking schools, families, and communities can create new momentum for social and political change. Among the approaches that have been tried are service learning,[71] participatory action research,[72] peer education and counseling,[73] and youth advisory boards or councils. By weaving these strategies into the fabric of healthy schools, it may be possible to reimagine schools that are youth friendly as well as educationally sound. Among the school policies and programs that could benefit from investigation by young people are disciplinary rules, student services, health and sexuality education, substance use services, and promotion policies. Although adults need to make final policy decisions on many of these issues, bringing the voices of youths into the decision-making process benefits all.

TOWARD A SOCIAL MOVEMENT

Schools—and other social institutions—change in at least two ways. First, the daily practice of policymakers, teachers and staff, young people, and parents yield ongoing incremental reforms. As we have seen, thousands of schools, health institutions, and professionals are now working to improve school health services and better link educational and health systems. Although it needs better coordination, more systematic evaluation, and more financial support,[23,74] this work is necessary but not sufficient for realizing the potential for creating healthier schools.

In our view, to achieve that aim also requires a movement for healthy high schools. Social movements are groups of individuals and organizations that work inside and outside established political institutions to redress grievances, change policies, and achieve justice.[75] In the last century, many significant advances in public health resulted from the civil rights, women's, environmental, and AIDS movements.[75]

Both education and health are the responsibility of established systems that have a stake in the status quo, few linkages for policy coordination, and difficulty in articulating or implementing transformative changes. In the United States, both systems are under attack for failing to achieve their stated goals and costing too much, despite the chronic underfunding of schools and communities most in need. To expect these embattled systems to define and implement a vision of healthier schools seems unrealistic. But if creation of a movement is needed to play this role, from where will such a movement emerge? And how can public health professionals play a role in its birthing? Table 27.2 lists some specific actions health professionals can consider, as described in this commentary.

TABLE 27.2—ROLES FOR HEALTH PROFESSIONALS IN A HEALTHY HIGH SCHOOLS MOVEMENT

Goal	Possible Activities
Improve school achievement and graduation rates.	1. Join local and regional dropout prevention councils. 2. Create forums in which local and state educational and health professionals and officials can identify and solve problems. 3. Document impact of various health problems such as adolescent pregnancy, substance use, and mental health problems on school achievement and completion. 4. Synthesize and summarize existing research findings on school achievement and health for political and educational policymakers. 5. Document impact of disciplinary procedures and policing strategies on health and school achievement. 6. Evaluate dropout prevention interventions to identify successful models and pathways by which they achieve results. 7. Support parent, community, and youth organizations working to improve school achievement and completion.
Create schools that promote individual, family, and community health.	1. Develop and evaluate innovative policy and programmatic approaches to school health and sexuality education. 2. Support and advocate for increased and more stable funding for school-based health centers. 3. Establish and evaluate improved services for parenting adolescents and for students with family members with chronic conditions. 4. Develop health, community, and school food councils that advocate for healthier school food. 5. Train health professionals who can work across health and education systems. 6. Defend sexuality education and reproductive health services against ideological attacks and aid in the development of comprehensive health and sexuality education curricula. 7. Advocate for policies that remove unhealthy commercial interests (e.g., beverage companies) from schools. 8. Establish and evaluate partnerships to bring students and their families into community health services. 9. Oppose local, state, and federal budget cuts that endanger the well-being of young people or exacerbate educational or health inequities.
Engage young people in creating healthier school and community environments.	1. Establish youth leadership development programs in health facilities and universities. 2. Train young people to be community-based health researchers. 3. Create or support youth participatory action research projects on school—health nexus. 4. Develop work, study, internship, and apprenticeship options for young people in school and community health programs. 5. Expand, strengthen, and evaluate peer health programs. 6. Assist young people to bring policy agenda on schools and health into political arena.

Movements emerge from existing mobilizations of people when grievances are perceived, windows of policy opportunity are open, an infrastructure to sustain a movement is in place, and issues are framed to attract attention. A movement for healthy schools has as its foundations current campaigns for educational and health care reform, especially those focusing on equity issues. School dropout is a particularly salient issue to mobilize the civil rights, educational, business, health, and other sectors.[19] In these sectors, the movement's base already exists in the hundreds of thousands of current school and community health programs, students, professionals, and activists engaged in healthy youth development.

Framing the issues in a way that can move diverse sectors into action is a key task. Several factors seem critical. First, to win the support of educators, any transformation must better link health and educational outcomes. Some evidence shows that healthy students learn better than unhealthy ones,[76] but to convince schools to assume a role in students' health will require showing them that doing so will improve outcomes that matter to them: school attendance (a source of funding), disciplinary actions, academic achievement, and school completion. Public health researchers need to do a better job of explicating these pathways.

Second, a movement for healthy schools needs to expand the time frame in which policymakers consider the benefits of healthier schools. Reducing dropout rates, preventing chronic diseases, and improving the environment of schools cost money in the short run, but the benefits are returned over several decades in the form of better health, more productive citizens, and lower health care costs. Convincing decisionmakers to make these investments will require overcoming the current demand for short-term returns. A movement can teach funders and policymakers that the time it takes to improve adolescent outcomes and to make organizational changes in schools is often longer than grant, budget, or political cycles.

Furthermore, throughout history, young people have often been involved in mobilizing major social movements and creating policy change. Health professionals can prepare young people to play these leadership roles, advocate for their voices in relevant policy processes, and help them to do the research needed to make their case.

Advocates of improved school health also need to make clear that the goal is not simply to outpost more health programs in more schools. With schools increasingly strapped with mandates and sanctions focusing on accountability and testing, it would be a mistake to view health as one more unfunded mandate to impose on schools. Moreover, bringing a new sector into schools can have unintended consequences. For example, outsourcing school safety to police departments has, among other things, criminalized low-income youths and youths of color and contributed to what some have labeled the school-to-prison pipeline.[77] Rather, our goal is to encourage the health and educational systems to engage in a dialogue on how they can better meet their mandates together than separately. Mobilized constituencies of young people, parents, and advocates can help to persuade reluctant bureaucrats in both systems that new, more integrated approaches are needed.

CONCLUSIONS

A healthy high schools movement can contribute to improved population health in 3 ways. First, it can help to increase school achievement and graduation rates. Second, it can assist in the creation of schools that promote individual, family, and community health; prevent the onset of chronic diseases; and reduce risks from substance use, sexual behavior, unhealthy diet, and violence. Finally, it can engage young people in creating healthier environments, policies, and institutions, thus tapping the unrealized social and human capital that young people offer. Such a movement would also serve as a pipeline to future occupations in the human and health services. By achieving these goals, a healthy high schools movement has the potential to contribute to reductions in educational and health inequities—enduring problems that undermine democracy, economic development, and social justice.

REFERENCES

1. WHO Global School Health Initiative. *Primary School Physical Environment and Health*. Geneva, Switzerland: World Health Organization; 1997.

2. Petti B, Western B. *Mass Imprisonment in the Life Course: Race and Class Inequality in US Incarceration*. Princeton, NJ: Princeton University; 2003.

3. Hoffman SD. *By the Numbers: The Public Costs of Teen Childbearing*. Washington, DC: National Campaign to Prevent Teen Pregnancy; 2006.

4. Center for Labor Market Studies, Northeastern University, and the Chicago Alternative Schools Network. *Left Behind in America: The Nation's Dropout Crisis, Boston, Massachusetts and Chicago, Illinois*. Boston, MA: Center for Labor Market Studies; April 2009.

5. Belfield C, Levin HM, eds. *The Price We Pay: Economic and Social Consequences of Inadequate Education*. Washington, DC: Brookings Institution Press; 2007.

6. Woolf SH, Johnson RE, Phillips RL Jr, Philipsen M. Giving everyone the health of the educated: an examination of whether social change would save more lives than medical advances. *Am J Public Health*. 2007;97(4):679–683.

7. Jemal A, Thun MJ, Ward EE, Henley SJ, Cokkinides VE, Murray TE. Mortality from leading causes by education and race in the United States, 2001. *Am J Prev Med.* 2008;34(1):1–8.

8. Ross C, Wu C. The links between education and health. *Am Sociol Rev.* 1995;60:719–745.

9. Novello AC, Degraw C, Kleinman D. Healthy children ready to learn: an essential collaboration between health and education. *Public Health Rep.* 1992;107(1):3–15.

10. Sen A. *Development as Freedom.* 2nd ed. New York, NY: Anchor; 2000.

11. *When Girls Don't Graduate, We All Fail.* Washington, DC: National Women's Law Center; 2007. Available at: http://www.nwlc.org/pdf/DropoutReport.pdf. Accessed March 2, 2010.

12. Bridgeland JM, DiIulio J Jr, Morison KB. *The Silent Epidemic Perspectives of High School Dropouts.* Washington, DC: Civic Enterprises; 2006.

13. Lear JG, Isaacs SL, Knickman JR, eds. *School Health Services and Programs.* San Francisco, CA: Jossey-Bass; 2006.

14. Orfield G, ed. *Dropouts in America: Confronting the Graduation Rate Crisis.* Cambridge, MA: Harvard Education Press; 2004.

15. Waters SK, Cross DS, Runions K. Social and ecological structures supporting adolescent connectedness to school: a theoretical model. *J Sch Health.* 2009;79(11):516–524.

16. Tang KC, Nutbeam D, Aldinger C, et al. Schools for health, education and development: a call for action. *Health Promot Int.* 2009;24(1):68–77.

17. Fine M, Ruglis J. Circuits and consequences of dispossession: the racialized realignment of the public sphere for US youth. *Transforming Anthropol.* 2009;17(1):20–36.

18. Muennig P. Consequences in health status and costs. In: Belfield C, Levin HM, eds. *The Price We Pay: Economic and Social Consequences of Inadequate Education.* Washington, DC: Brookings Institution Press; 2007:125–141.

19. Freudenberg N, Ruglis J. Reframing school dropout as a public health issue. *Prev Chronic Dis.* 2007;4(4):1–11. Available at: http://www.cdc.gov/PCD/issues/2007/oct/07_0063.htm. Accessed December 12, 2009.

20. Ekstrom RB, Goertz ME, Pollack JM, Rock DA. Who drops out of high school and why? Findings from a national study. *Teach Coll Rec.* 1986;87(3):356–373.

21. Rothstein R. *Class and schools: Using Social, Economic and Educational Reform to Close the Black–White Achievement Gap.* Washington, DC: Economic Policy Institute; 2004.

22. National Research Council and Institute of Medicine. *Engaging Schools: Fostering High School Students' Motivation to Learn.* Washington, DC: National Academies Press; 2004.

23. Institute of Medicine. *Schools and Health: Our Nation's Investment*. Washington, DC: National Academy Press; 1997.

24. *WHO Expert Committee on Comprehensive School Health Education and Promotion*. Geneva, Switzerland: World Health Organization; 1995.

25. Abrams L, Haney W. Accountability and the grade 9 to 10 transition: the impact on attrition and retention rates. In: Orfield G, ed. *Dropouts in America: Confronting the Graduation Rate Crisis*. Cambridge, MA: Harvard Education Press; 2004:181–205.

26. Swanson C. *Cities in Crisis 2009: Closing the Graduation Gap*. Bethesda, MD: Editorial Projects in Education Inc; 2009. Available at: http://www.edweek.org/rc/articles/2009/04/22/cities_in_crisis.html. Accessed December 12, 2009.

27. Harris KM, Gordon-Larsen P, Chantala K, Udry JR. Longitudinal trends in race/ethnic disparities in leading health indicators from adolescence to young adulthood. *Arch Pediatr Adolesc Med*. 2006;160(1):74–81.

28. Mulye TP, Park MJ, Nelson CD, Adams SH, Irwin CE Jr, Brindis CD. Trends in adolescent and young adult health in the United States. *J Adolesc Health*. 2009;45(1):8–24.

29. Burt MR. Reasons to invest in adolescents. *J Adolesc Health*. 2002;31(6 suppl):136–152.

30. Swanson C. *Who Graduates? Who Doesn't? A Statistical Portrait of Public High School Graduation, Class of 2001*. Washington, DC: Urban Institute; 2004.

31. Casner-Lotto J, Rosenblum E, Wright M. *The Ill-Prepared US Workforce Exploring the Challenges of Employer-Provided Workforce Readiness Training*. New York, NY: The Conference Board; 2009.

32. Gruber JE, Fineran S. The impact of bullying and sexual harassment on middle and high school girls. *Violence Against Women*. 2007;13(6):627–643.

33. Sullivan L. *Deprived of Dignity: Degrading Treatment and Abusive Discipline in New York City and Los Angeles Public Schools*. New York, NY: National Economic and Social Rights Initiative; 2007.

34. Bear GG. School discipline in the United States: prevention, correction and long term social development. *School Psychol Rev*. 1998;27(1):14–32.

35. Orfield G, Kornhaber ML, eds. *Raising Standards or Raising Barriers? Inequality and High-Stakes Testing in Public Education*. New York, NY: Century Foundation Press; 2001.

36. Finkelstein DM, Hill EL, Whitaker RC. School food environments and policies in US public schools. *Pediatrics*. 2008;122(1):e251–e259.

37. *School Facilities: American's Schools Not Designed or Equipped for the Twenty-First Century*. Washington, DC: General Accounting Office; 1995. Publication GAO ED383056.

38. Story M, Nanney MS, Schwartz MB. Schools and obesity prevention: creating school environments and policies to promote healthy eating and physical activity. *Milbank Q.* 2009;87(1):71–100.

39. *Coordinated School Health Programs.* Atlanta, GA: National Center for Chronic Disease Prevention and Health Promotion; n.d.

40. Symons CW, Cinelli B, James TC, Groff P. Bridging student health risks and academic achievement through comprehensive school health programs. *J Sch Health.* 1997;67(6): 220–227.

41. Morone J, Kilbreth E, Langwell K. Back to school: a health care strategy for youth. *Health Aff.* 2001;20(1–2):122–136.

42. McCord M, Klein J, Foy J, Fothergill K. School-based clinic use and school performance. *J Adolesc Health.* 1993;14(2):91–98.

43. O'Toole TP, Anderson S, Miller C, Guthrie J. Nutrition services and foods and beverages available at school: results from the School Health Policies and Programs Study 2006. *J Sch Health.* 2007;77(8):500–521.

44. Kirby D. The impact of schools and school programs upon adolescent sexual behavior. *J Sex Res.* 2002;39(1):27–33.

45. Card JJ. Teen pregnancy prevention: do any programs work? *Annu Rev Public Health.* 1999;20:257–285.

46. Sadler L, Swartz M, Ryan-Krause P. Supporting adolescent mothers and their children through a high school-based child care center and parent support program. *J Pediatr Health Care.* 2003;17(3):109–117.

47. Gottfredson D, Wilson D. Characteristics of effective school-based substance abuse prevention. *Prev Sci.* 2003;4(1):27–38.

48. Elliott L, Orr L, Watson L, Jackson A. Secondary prevention interventions for young drug users: a systematic review of the evidence. *Adolescence.* 2005;40(157):1–22.

49. Mytton J, DiGuiseppi C, Gough D, Taylor R, Logan S. School-based violence prevention programs: systematic review of secondary prevention trials. *Arch Pediatr Adolesc Med.* 2002;156(8):752–762.

50. Haynes NM. Addressing students' social and emotional needs: the role of mental health teams in schools. *J Health Soc Policy.* 2002;16(1–2):109–123.

51. Jennings J, Pearson G, Harris M. Implementing and maintaining school-based mental health services in a large, urban school district. *J Sch Health.* 2000;70(5):201–205.

52. Fothergill K, Ballard E. The school-linked health center: a promising model of community-based care for adolescents. *J Adolesc Health.* 1998;23(1):29–38.

53. Dryfoos J. Full-service community schools: a strategy—not a program. *New Dir Youth Dev.* 2005;(107):7–14.

54. Resnick MD, Bearman PS, Blum RW, et al. Protecting adolescents from harm: findings from the National Longitudinal Study on Adolescent Health. *JAMA.* 1997;278(10): 823–832.

55. McNeely CA, Nonnemaker JM, Blum RW. Promoting school connectedness: evidence from the National Longitudinal Study of Adolescent Health. *J Sch Health.* 2002;72(4): 138–146.

56. Rumberger RW. Why students drop out of school. In: Orfield G, ed. *Dropouts in America: Confronting the Graduation Rate Crisis.* Cambridge, MA: Harvard Education Press; 2004:131–156.

57. Noguera P. Schools, prisons, and social implications of punishment: rethinking disciplinary practices. *Theory Pract.* 2003;42(4):341–350.

58. Browne J, Losen D, Wald J. Zero tolerance: unfair, with little recourse. *New Dir Youth Dev.* 2001;92:73–99.

59. *Test, Punish, and Push Out: How "Zero Tolerance" and High-Stakes Testing Funnel Youth Into the School-to-Prison-Pipeline.* Washington, DC: Advancement Project; 2010. Available at: http://www.advancementproject.org/sites/default/files/publications/01-EducationReport-2009v8-HiRes.pdf. Accessed April 2, 2010.

60. Srabstein J, Piazza T. Public health, safety and educational risks associated with bullying behaviors in American adolescents. *Int J Adolesc Med Health.* 2008;20(2):223–233.

61. Oxley D. *Small Learning Communities.* Philadelphia, PA: Laboratory for Student Success at Temple University Center for Research in Human Development and Education; 2005.

62. National High School Center. *Easing the Transition to High School: Research and Best Practices Designed to Support High School Learning.* Washington, DC: American Institutes for Research; 2007. Available at: http://www.betterhighschools.org/docs/NHSC_TransitionsReport.pdf. Accessed October 28, 2009.

63. Ofer U, Jones A, Miller J, et al. *Safety With Dignity: Alternatives to the Over-Policing of Schools.* New York, NY: Annenberg Institute for School Reform, New York Civil Liberties Union, and Make the Road New York; 2009. Available at: http://www.nyclu.org/content/safety-with-dignity-alternatives-over-policing-of-schools-2009. Accessed March 10, 2010.

64. Philliber S, Kaye JW, Herrling S, West E. Preventing pregnancy and improving health care access among teenagers: an evaluation of the children's aid society-Carrera program. *Perspect Sex Reprod Health.* 2002;34(5):244–251.

65. Schwartz SE, Petersen SB. A new developmentalist role: connecting youth development, mental health, and education. *New Dir Youth Dev.* 2008;(120):57–77.

66. Kriechman A, Salvador M, Adelsheim S. Expanding the vision: the strengths-based, community-oriented child and adolescent psychiatrist working in schools. *Child Adolesc Psychiatr Clin N Am*. 2010;19(1):149–162.

67. Park MJ, Brindis CD, Chang F, Irwin CE Jr. A midcourse review of the healthy people 2010: 21 critical health objectives for adolescents and young adults. *J Adolesc Health*. 2008;42(4):329–334.

68. Silberberg M, Cantor JC. Making the case for school-based health: where do we stand? *J Health Polit Policy Law*. 2008;33(1):3–37.

69. Whitehead D. The health-promoting school: what role for nursing? *J Clin Nurs*. 2006;15(3):264–271.

70. Ott MA, Santelli JS. Approaches to adolescent sexuality education. *Adolesc Med State Art Rev*. 2007;18(3):558–570.

71. Fox M, Mediratta K, Ruglis J, Stoudt B, Shah S, Fine M. Critical youth engagement: participatory action research and organizing. In: Sherrod LR, Torney-Purta J, Flanagan CA, eds. *Handbook of Research and Policy on Civic Engagement in Youth*. New York, NY: Wiley. In press.

72. Denner J, Coyle K, Robin L, Banspach S. Integrating service learning into a curriculum to reduce health risks at alternative high schools. *J Sch Health*. 2005;75(5):151–156.

73. Pearlman DN, Camberg L, Wallace LJ, Symons P, Finison L. Tapping youth as agents for change: evaluation of a peer leadership HIV/AIDS intervention. *J Adolesc Health*. 2002;31(1):31–39.

74. Peters LW, Kok G, Ten Dam GT, Buijs GJ, Paulussen TG. Effective elements of school health promotion across behavioral domains: a systematic review of reviews. *BMC Public Health*. 2009;12(9):182.

75. Brown P, Zavestoski S, eds. *Social Movements in Health*. San Francisco, CA: Wiley-Blackwell; 2005.

76. Murray NG, Low BJ, Hollis C, Cross AW, Davis SM. Coordinated school health programs and academic achievement: a systematic review of the literature. *J Sch Health*. 2007;77(9):589–600.

77. Edelman MW. The Cradle to Prison Pipeline: an American health crisis. *Prev Chronic Dis*. 2007;4(3):A43.

About the Authors

Jessica Ruglis, PhD, MPH, MAT – is Assistant Professor of Human Development at McGill University. A former W. K. Kellogg Health Scholar and urban educator, she is a founding member of the Public Science Project. She conducts mixed-methods, interdisciplinary, community-based participatory action research. Her research, writing, advocacy, and legal consultation focuses on the impact of education, health, social, and juvenile justice policy to health and human development across the life course; relationships between schooling, education, health disparities, and intergenerational inequality; social determinants of health; health equity; early school leaving and school dis/engagement; child and adolescent health; school-based health; and youth development, activism, and organizing.

Nicholas Freudenberg – is Distinguished Professor of Public Health at City University of New York School of Public Health at Hunter College, where he directs its doctoral program. For the past 30 years he has worked with community organizations, schools, advocacy groups, and government agencies to develop, implement, and evaluate policies and program to promote health and reduce inequalities in health. He has published six books and dozens of scientific articles on urban health, public health policy, the links between education and health, incarceration and health, and other topics.

The Vital Role of School-Based Health Centers in Creating a Violence-Free School Environment

Terri D. Wright

In April 2009, after being constantly taunted and harassed at school, 11 year-old Carl Joseph Walker-Hoover ended his life. That same month, 11 year-old Jaheem Herrera hung himself because he was tired of being bullied. In the fall of 2009, honor roll student Derrion Albert was brutally beaten to death by a group of teens while walking home from school, and 15 year-old Michael Brewer was burned on more than three quarters of his body after a group of five teenagers doused him in rubbing alcohol and set him on fire. And after three months of unrelenting verbal assaults and physical threats, 15 year-old Phoebe Prince took her life early in 2010. Have we failed our youth?

Every day 160,000 students in grades K–12 miss school or leave early due to bullying and violence.[1] Half of students responding to the Ethics of American Youth Survey in 2010 admitted that they bullied someone in the past year, and nearly half say they were bullied, teased, or taunted in a way that seriously upset them.[2] Students who are repeatedly bullied receive poorer grades and participate less in class discussions.[3] One third of all high school students say that violence is a big problem at their school, and one in four say they do not feel very safe at school.[3]

According to the Centers for Disease Control and Prevention (CDC), **youth violence** is the intentional use of physical force or power by a young person between the ages of 10 and 24 years against another person, group, or community, with the youth's behavior likely to cause physical and psychological harm. The young person can be a victim, an offender, or a witness to the violence, or a combination of all three. Youth violence includes various behaviors, such as bullying, fighting (e.g., slapping, hitting, kicking), electronic aggression (also referred to as cyber-bullying), weapons use, and gang violence.[4] **School violence** is a subset of youth violence that occurs on school property, on the way to and from school, during a school-sponsored event, and/or on the way to and from a school-sponsored event.[4]

During the 2005–2006 school year, 38% of public schools reported at least one incident of violence to police, and in the following year, 32% of students reported being bullied during the school year, with 4% being cyber bullied.[4] Bullying and fear of being bullied impairs the student's ability to engage in a positive and affirming educational experience. For example, 6% of students aged 12 to 18 years reported that they were afraid of attack or harm at school, and 6% avoided a school activity or certain spaces at school in the previous 6 months due to fear of harm or attack.[5]

School violence and particularly bullying can result in depression, anxiety, and even suicide. Exposure to violence often causes more emotional harm than physical harm for young people. Whether real or perceived, violence or the threat of it can lead young people to feel tense, anxious, and afraid, and it can breed feelings of hopelessness and despair.

Suicide, or self-directed violence, encompasses a range of violent behaviors, including acts of fatal and nonfatal suicidal behavior, and nonsuicidal intentional self-harm (i.e., behaviors where the intention is not to kill oneself, as in self-mutilation). Though not a behavior, suicidal ideation, for example, thinking about, considering, or planning for suicide, is included.[6] In a recent study on bullying in one state, the CDC published that, compared with students who were neither bullies nor bullying victims, both middle and high school bully-victims (defined as those who were both bullies and have been bullied) were more than three times as likely to report seriously considering suicide as well as intentionally injuring themselves.[7] Among 15 to 24 year olds, suicide accounts for 12.2% of all deaths annually. In 2009, almost 14% of students in grades 9–12 considered suicide in the previous 12 months, and 6.3% made at least one suicide attempt.[8]

Carl Joseph, Jaheem, Derrion, Michael, and Phoebe are some of the faces behind these statistics. This mental distress may foster unhealthy behaviors, including aggression, substance abuse, eating disorders, and suicide. It can also affect students' ability to succeed in school and can contribute to dropout rates. Educational success is compromised when young people feel anxious, unsafe, or depressed. Students who report being victims of violent crime are twice as likely to receive mostly C's as to receive mostly A's or mostly B's.[9]

Additionally, violence as depicted in war has an adverse impact on young people. In research conducted by the US Department of Defense, six out of 10 military families said that their children have increased levels of fear and anxiety when a parent is sent to war. One third of these families report that the child's grades and behavior in school have suffered as a result.[10]

THE ROLE OF SCHOOL-BASED HEALTH CENTERS IN CREATING A SAFE ENVIRONMENT FOR SCHOOL SUCCESS

Fear and violence clearly disrupt the learning environment and student success. Fortunately, school-based health centers (SBHCs) can play a catalytic role in averting school violence, mitigating exposure to violence, and facilitating overall school wellness. They are also essential partners in the school and community response to violent events through the provision of early intervention programs and services. They are critical allies in restoring safety and calm for school-aged children who have been victimized or have witnessed violence. However, their contributions as key partners with schools' efforts to create safe environments are often overlooked. In order to change this trend, school-based health care must be reframed so that educators understand the critical role that SBHCs can play in the prevention of school violence and school dropout. By providing vital health and mental health services in schools, SBHCs help young people mediate violence, manage the emotional impact of violence, and connect troubled youth to the resources needed to help them heal. They can partner with students and school personnel to identify the issues and offer strategies, policies, and programs to resolve them before they adversely impact students and affect learning and school retention. For example, SBHCs could have led the schoolwide anti-bullying and anti-violence programs that may have saved the lives of Jaheem, Carl Joseph, Michael, Derrion, and Phoebe by virtue of identifying their suffering early enough to change the ultimate cost of ignoring their plight.

SBHCs are ideally positioned to be a catalyst for creating a healthy school for young people and are much more likely to begin mental health services for adolescents than are any other types of providers. Students with access to an SBHC are more likely to receive mental health and wellness screenings and counseling than are those enrolled in Medicaid or with private insurance, and students report that they trust the confidentiality afforded by SBHCs.

THE ROLE FOR SCHOOL-BASED HEALTH CENTERS IN PREVENTING SCHOOL VIOLENCE

In addition to providing health services, SBHCs can make a number of valuable contributions toward the goal of making schools violence free, including:

- Introduce and implement evidenced-based programs that have a proven and positive impact on the school climate (see the list of resources in Table 28.1).

TABLE 28.1—RESOURCES FOR SCHOOL-BASED HEALTH CENTERS

The following resources are available to support school-based health centers in addressing youth violence and creating healthy school environments

Centers for Disease Control and Prevention, *Preventing Youth Violence: Program Activities Guide*—strategies for prevention and early intervention. www.cdc.gov/violenceprevention

Center for Effective Collaboration and Practice, *Early Warning, Timely Response: A Guide to Safe Schools*—a guide to violence prevention and intervention and crisis response in schools. cecp.air.org/guide

Safe Schools Ambassadors Program—a national program to reduce bullying, improve student–adult engagement at school and improve the school climate. www.community-matters.org/safe-school-ambassadors

Stop Bullying Now Campaign (Health Resources Services Administration)—resources to help children and adults address bullying. www.stopbullyingnow.hrsa.gov

Safe Schools/Healthy Students Initiative—a discretionary grant program from the US Departments of Education, Justice, and Health and Human Services that provides students, schools, and communities with federal funding to implement an enhanced, coordinated, comprehensive plan of activities, programs, and services that focus on promoting healthy childhood development and preventing violence and alcohol and other drug abuse. www.sshs.samhsa.gov/initiative/default.aspx

National School Safety Center—information and resources highlighting school safety research, practice, strategies and trends. www.schoolsafety.us

After School.gov—connects after-school providers to federal resources that support children and youth during out-of-school hours. www.afterschool.gov

Be Safe and Sound in School, National Crime Prevention Council— a program model that addresses school safety problems by evaluating physical conditions as well as cultural and social variables such as bullying, violence, and vandalism that may promote an unsafe environment. www.ncpc.org/programs/be-safe-and-sound-campaign

National Youth Violence Prevention Resource Center—a central source of information on prevention and intervention programs, publications, research, and statistics on youth violence. www.safeyouth.org

National Youth Gang Center (NYGC)—provides resources for addressing community gang problems. www.iir.com.nygc

- Partner with school staff to develop and implement a school safety plan, including incorporating safety into school wellness plans, developing safe routes to school, and establishing school discipline policies that affirm students and aren't detrimental to students' education.
- Engage students in improving the physical and emotional school environment and implementing peer-to-peer prevention and intervention programs that help students address school violence and mental distress.
- Provide support services and programs such as mediation and conflict resolution, bullying, gang and suicide intervention and prevention, and after-school programs and activities that provide students with safe places to play.
- Advocate for safe school legislation at the school district, tribal, state, and federal levels.

SBHCs *must* be the catalysts for healthy and safe schools. Through their schoolwide programs, physical and mental health services, and policy advocacy, SBHCs can enhance the safety, school success, and overall well-being of all students. Let's not have another Jaheem, Carl Joseph, Derrion, Michael, or Phoebe.

REFERENCES

1. Centers for Disease Control and Prevention. Understanding school violence fact sheet 2010. 2010. Available at: http://www.cdc.gov/violenceprevention/pdf/SchoolViolence_FactSheet-a.pdf. Accessed May 3, 2011.

2. Josephson Institute Center for Youth Ethics. Ethics of American Youth Survey. 2010. Available at: http://www.charactercounts.org/programs/reportcard/2010/index.html. Accessed April 19, 2011.

3. Juvonen J, Wang Y, Espinoza G. Bullying experiences and compromised academic performance across middle school grades. *J Early Adolesc.* 2011;31(1);152–173.

4. Centers for Disease Control and Prevention. About school violence. 2011. Available at http://www.cdc.gov/ViolencePrevention/youthviolence/schoolviolence/index.html. Accessed April 19, 2011.

5. National Center for Education Statistics, Institute of Education Sciences. Indicators of school crime and safety: 2007. 2007. Available at: http://nces.ed.gov/programs/crimeindicators/crimeindicators2007. Accessed April 19, 2011.

6. Crosby AE, Ortega L, Melanson C. *Self-Directed Violence Surveillance: Uniform Definitions and Recommended Data Elements, Version 1.0.* Atlanta, GA: Centers for Disease Control and Prevention, National Center for Injury Prevention and Control; 2011.

7. Centers for Disease Control and Prevention. Bullying among middle school and high school students—Massachusetts, 2009. *MMWR* 2011;60(15):465–471.

8. Centers for Disease Control and Prevention. Suicide: facts at a glance. 2010. Available at: http://www.cdc.gov/violenceprevention/pdf/Suicide_DataSheet-a.pdf. Accessed April 19, 2011.

9. Bauer L, Guerino P, Nolle KL, Tang S-W, Chandler K. *Student Victimization in US Schools: Results From the 2005 School Crime Supplement to the National Crime Victimization Survey* (NCES 2009-306). Washington, DC: National Center for Education Statistics, Institute of Education Sciences, US Department of Education; 2008.

10. Zoroya G. Troops' kids feel war toll. *USA Today.* June 25,2009. Available at: http://www.usatoday.com/news/military/2009-06-24-military-kids_N.htm. Accessed July 23, 2011.

About the Author

Terri D. Wright, MPH, ABD – is the Director of the newly established Center for School, Health, and Education at the American Public Health Association. She provides leadership to the strategic development of school-based health programming and policy to avert school dropout. Formerly, she served for 12 years as a Program Director for Health Policy at the W. K. Kellogg Foundation and provided leadership for Foundation's school-based health care policy program. Terri was Maternal and Child Health Director and Bureau Chief for Child and Family Services at the Michigan Department of Community Health where she managed policy, programs, and resources with the goal of reducing preventable maternal, infant, and child morbidity and mortality. She has her Bachelor's degree in Community and School Health and Master's degree in Public Health. She is currently a doctoral candidate in Public Health at the University of Michigan. Terri takes an active leadership role in several professional and community organizations including the Institute of Medicine Roundtable on the Promotion of Health Equity and the Elimination of Health Disparities.

School-Based Health Centers: Cost–Benefit Analysis and Impact on Health Care Disparities[*]

*Jeff J. Guo, Terrance J. Wade,
Wei Pan, and Kathryn N. Keller*

Racial or ethnic health care disparities are a social phenomenon that reveals differences in utilization and quality of health care because of accessibility, operation of health care systems, cultural or socioeconomic status, and discrimination at the individual and patient–provider level.[1–5] Recent literature has documented ethnic and racial disparities in the health care system across a wide range of diseases. According to the Centers for Disease Control and Prevention,[6] African Americans had higher prevalence rates across many chronic diseases, including perinatal diseases, diabetes mellitus, hypertension, and obesity. Health care disparities can lead to decreased quality of life, loss of economic opportunities, and perceptions of injustice.[7] Twenty-two percent of African American children and adolescents were classified as overweight or obese and 68% were fully vaccinated, compared with White children and adolescents, who were less likely to be overweight or obese (12%) and more likely to be fully vaccinated (78%).[6,8]

For some illnesses, health care disparities are manifested through the underuse of treatments and procedures.[9–11] School-aged children and adolescents have high prevalence rates of some chronic diseases including asthma (estimated at 7%) and attention deficit/hyperactivity disorder (estimated at between 3% and 6%).[7,12,13] However, African American children and adolescents with asthma had more hospitalizations, disability, and a higher mortality rate compared with that of White

* This chapter previously appeared in the September 2010 issue of the *American Journal of Public Health* and is reprinted with permission in its entirety. Guo JJ, Wade TJ, Pan W, Keller K. School-based health centers: cost–benefit analysis and impact on health care disparities. *Am J Public Health.* 2010;100(9);1604–1610.

children and adolescents with asthma.[14,15] Moreover, African American children and adolescents were also less likely to access mental health services.[16–19]

School-based health centers (SBHCs) are thought to be 1 solution to reduce these health status and health care disparities across groups. SBHCs provide essential primary care (e.g., mental health treatment, dental care, well-child check-ups) for students. SBHCs, by their location in schools, are designed to overcome many health care access barriers, including transportation, lack of providers, lack of insurance coverage, and inconvenient appointment times because of parents working. By 2008, more than 1980 SBHCs nationwide had been established with partial support from the federal government, foundations, Medicaid, health insurance companies, and other programs such as "Healthy Schools Healthy Communities."[20–22] In many SBHCs, the majority of enrolled students are uninsured or low income, ranging from 50% to 90% of the patient load.

Numerous studies have documented that SBHCs can effectively reduce health care access barriers and emergency room visits in children and adolescents.[23–31] These in-school services can also alleviate barriers such as nonadherence and inadequate access to mental health services for youths.[23,32–34] With the SBHC, students received more mental health care services,[23] less hospitalization,[24,26] fewer urgent or emergency visits,[25–28] and fewer transportation and pharmacy costs.[26]

Although SBHCs have demonstrated their value to school-aged children and adolescents, their impact on addressing health care disparities has not been evaluated. Moreover, it is unclear whether the SBHC is cost-beneficial. With these considerations in mind, we sought to measure the impact of SBHCs on addressing health care disparities among students in schools with SBHCs compared with students in comparable schools without SBHCs. The central hypotheses were that increased accessibility to primary care services with SBHCs would reduce the gaps of health care disparities over time by increasing needed primary care. Second, by providing timely and essential primary care, the SBHC program would have a positive net social benefit to the population.

METHODS

We used a longitudinal quasi-experimental repeated-measures design. Four school districts (7 schools in total) with newly implemented SBHCs were matched with 2 other school districts (6 schools in total), based on urban or rural status, percentage of non-White students, and percentage of students in the free or reduced-price school lunch program. The target population was school-aged students (kindergarten through 12th grade) enrolled in schools in the Greater Cincinnati, Ohio, area who were also enrolled in Ohio Medicaid or the State Children's Health Insurance Program (SCHIP) from academic years 1997 through 2003. All students in the SBHC had parental approval to participate. The written consents for evaluation were documented in each SBHC. Because of the nature of retrospective data analysis, researchers did not modify or alter any medical treatment or services for student participants. There was little risk to study participants.

The SBHCs were established in September 2000 and provided for students in kindergarten through eighth grade. All enrolled students were eligible to use the SBHC. The SBHCs were open on weekdays during the school academic quarters and closed in the summer quarter. Each SBHC was equipped with basic medical instruments (examination bed, blood pressure meter, weight and height scale, urgent medications) and the Welligent version 5.0 Web-based computerized medical record system (Welligent Inc, Norfolk, VA) to track SBHC encounters. The SBHC was managed by a medical partner (e.g., nurse practitioner and health worker) related to primary care and specialist physicians (e.g., pediatrician). Each SBHC was typically staffed by 1 nurse practitioner and 1 nurse technician. A part-time pediatrician was present in some schools for 3 hours per week. A licensed mental health therapist was in service in some schools 1 or more days per week. Among these school districts, a large number of students (ranging from 50% to 88%) was enrolled in the free or reduced-price school lunch program because of their low family incomes.[35]

Data Sources

Four primary data sources were used for this study: school enrollment files, Ohio Medicaid claims, SBHC encounter records, and parents' and SBHC coordinators' survey data. First, schools provided student enrollment databases identifying student names and demographics for each school year from the 2000–2001 school year to the 2002–2003 school year. There were 9240 unique students.

Second, school enrollment data were linked with the Ohio Medicaid claim database, which is an automated database that includes Medicaid enrollment records, as well as patients' pharmacy, medical, hospital inpatient, and outpatient institutional claims from September 1997 to February 2003. This totaled 5069 unique students based on matched name, sex, race, date of birth, and county code. Thirteen students who switched between an SBHC and non-SBHC comparison school were excluded. Because of the implementation of the Health Insurance Portability and Accountability Act and other regulation changes, we were unable to collect and use the completed Medicaid claims data from March 2003 to August 2003.

Third, SBHC encounter data from the 4 intervention schools that documented students' visits in SBHCs were retrieved from the Welligent database. During the study period, 4136 students were enrolled in the SBHC program, of which 2314 students used the service, generating a total of 7572 SBHC encounters.

Fourth, surveys of both parents and SBHC coordinators were conducted to collect data regarding cost and benefit information (such as travel distance from home to the hospital or clinic), hours spent for students' physician visits, facility utility and space cost, and health care grants received as a result of local SBHC programs.

Outcome Measures and Covariates

The primary outcome measure for our study was quarterly total health care cost per student, as a proxy for health care utilization, which was defined as the total dollar amount that Medicaid paid for inpatient and outpatient care, physician encounters, mental health services, pharmacy, procedures, and diagnoses. For each claim reimbursement, total health care reimbursement was adjusted by using the medical component of the Consumer Price Index (MCPI) as the dollar value in 2002. The annual MCPI rates of change were 4.6% in 2002, 4.7% in 2001, 4.2% in 2000, 3.7% in 1999, 3.4% in 1998, and 2.8% in 1997.[36-38]

The covariates included the student's age as of September 30, 2000. Sex and race were dichotomous variables. The number of enrollment months was defined for each child enrolled in the Medicaid program during the study period. Enrollment categories included aid for disabled or blind, Temporary Assistance for Needy Families (TANF), SCHIP, and managed care organizations (MCOs).

Cost–Benefit Analysis

Cost–benefit analysis (CBA) is a method to compare the value of resources consumed (costs) in providing a program or intervention to the value of the consequence (benefit) from that program or intervention.[36] Two major components for CBA are costs and consequences. This view of CBA assumes that the SBHC is being compared with a non-SBHC alternative. A CBA requires health outcomes of the SBHC to be valued in monetary units, thus enabling us to compare the program's incremental cost with its incremental outcomes.

We looked at the costs of (or resources consumed by) the SBHCs from 3 sectors: (1) the health care sector (e.g., SBHC operation costs, such as prescription drugs, medical equipment, and physician and nurse hours), (2) the patient and family sector (e.g, out-of-pocket expenses in traveling to get medical care, copayments, and lost work time), and (3) other sectors (e.g., essential start-up funds [not including SBHC operational costs] and costs for school facility use).

We considered certain activities that would not have occurred without a SBHC to be incremental benefits from the program, including (1) the students' health status change, which can be measured in terms of equivalent value of clinical effects; (2) other sector savings, including other value or grants created by the SBHCs; (3) resources saved by the SBHCs or costs not spent on an alternative, which mirror the costs and were measured according to the 3 cost sectors: health care savings, patient and family savings, and other sector savings such as the community multiplier effect (R. Greenbaum, PhD and A. Desai, PhD, Ohio State University, written communication, April 30, 2003); and (4) unquantifiable benefits, such as healthy students having better attendance and better learning performance, and increased access to care for racial/ethnic minorities.

The net social benefit[36] from implementing the SBHC was calculated as total benefits minus the total costs based on the previously defined components. To measure and estimate the cost–benefit variables, we constructed 2 sets of questionnaires. The first was administered to a random sample of parents through phone interviews,[23] including the frequency of child sick visits and hospitalizations, distance from home to physician offices and hospitals, and number of days off for child sick leave. Study samples were randomly selected from SBHC and non-SBHC schools and, as such, we assume the results from questionnaires to be representative of all parents in the specific schools. The second survey was administered through self-report to the SBHC administrative staff or coordinators in each SBHC about their working hours, facility and equipment costs, and other operational costs.

Data Analysis

To test equivalency between SBHC and non-SBHC comparison schools on demographic characteristics, we used the t test for continuous data including age, months enrolled, and percentages of enrollment categories; we used the χ^2 test for dichotomous variables.

We employed hierarchical linear modeling using HLM version 5.05 (Scientific Software International Inc, Lincolnwood, IL)[39] on a repeated-measures basis, allowing for the control of unbalanced observations with time-series quarterly data because of student attrition in different schools or different enrollment periods in Medicaid programs. The multiple observations are properly originated as nested within students. The quarterly total Medicaid costs (adjusted 2002 dollar value) per student were measured as time-related variables for all eligible students to analyze growth trends including linear, quadratic, and cubic growth trends.[39] The nested-structure growth analysis allows for examination of students' health care utilization changes over time. Unlike other repeated measures analyses, HLM can examine the fit of data with an unequal number of repeated observations for each individual student. Two levels of HLM models were involved in the analysis: a level-1 polynomial model of the repeated observations for the effect of time including 22 quarters from fall 1997 to winter 2003 on the outcome variable of the quarterly health care cost, and level-2 linear models of the individual student-level measures for the effects of the individual differences (such as sex, race, age, SBHC intervention, SCHIP, aid for disabled or blind, and MCO) on the linear, quadratic, and cubic growth trends.

RESULTS

Of 5056 students (45% African American and 49% female), there were 3673 students enrolled in SBHC schools and 1383 students enrolled in schools without SBHCs (Table 29.1). The students in the non-SBHC comparison group were younger, had fewer enrollment months, were enrolled in the SCHIP program at greater proportions, and were enrolled in an MCO in smaller proportions compared with that of students in the SBHC group. Medicaid spent a total of $30 million dollars on all 5056 students during the 5.5 years. The major cost components included mental health services ($8.9 million, 29.7%), outpatient care ($7.3 million, 24.3%), hospitalization and emergency room visits ($5.7 million, 19%), physician encounters ($3.3 million, 11%), and prescription drugs ($2.8 million, 9.3%).

Health Care Disparities

Table 29.2 summarizes the final least-squares estimates of fixed effects with robust standard errors for quarterly total Medicaid costs under the HLM analysis. African American students had lower health care costs than did other students ($P = .061$) in Fall 2000, indicating some health care disparities at the beginning of the SBHC program. The gap was closed after the implementation of the SBHC according to the growth curves displayed in Figure 29.1.

Cost–Benefit Analysis

Figure 29.2 summarizes both costs and benefits that were estimated based on 3 years of SBHC operation. The CBA was based on all students enrolled in each SBHC school regardless of different medical insurance or noninsurance. There were a total of 7608 students enrolled in 4 schools or districts with SBHCs.

COSTS

For health care sector costs, we used total funding of $1 382 260 for the first 3 years of operation as a proxy for the costs of SBHC operation because the funding enabled SBHCs to initiate and maintain personnel, equipment, and space for SBHC

TABLE 29.1 — DEMOGRAPHICS AND CHARACTERISTICS FOR STUDENTS ENROLLED IN BOTH MEDICAID AND SCHOOLS WITH SCHOOL-BASED HEALTH CENTERS (SBHCS) AND FOR STUDENTS ENROLLED IN SCHOOLS WITHOUT SBHCS: GREATER CINCINNATI, OH, 1997–2003

	Students Enrolled in Schools With SBHCs (n=3673)	Students Enrolled in Schools Without SBHCs (n=1383)	P [a]
Male, no. (%)	1906 (51.9)	697 (50.4)	.315
Age,[b] y, mean (range)	8.41 (3–15)	8.04 (3–15)	<.001
Race, no. (%)			
White	1947 (53)	732 (52.9)	.917
Black	1664 (45.3)	613 (44.3)	.508
Hispanic	18 (0.5)	4 (0.3)	
Asian	4 (0.1)	0	
American Indians	4 (0.1)	0	
Other	37 (1.0)	35 (2.5)	
No. of months enrolled in Medicaid program,[c] mean (SD)	40.3 (18.1)	38.4 (18.0)	<.001
Enrollment,[c] % (SD)			
SCHIP	32.5 (0.35)	37.3 (0.37)	<.001
Aid to disabled or blind	4.2 (0.18)	4.5 (0.18)	.613
MCO	24.8 (0.27)	14.6 (0.27)	<.001
TANF	94.5 (0.20)	93.5 (0.21)	.144
Quarterly total cost 1997–1998 academic year, mean $			
Black	173.9	208.9	
Non-Black	158.8	230.3	
Quarterly total cost 1998–1999 academic year, mean $			
Black	198.6	250.7	
Non-Black	152.1	245.0	
Quarterly total cost 1999–2000 academic year, mean $			
Black	210.5	289.9	
Non-Black	214.5	321.2	

TABLE 29.1 — (CONTINUED)

	Students Enrolled in Schools With SBHCs (n=3673)	Students Enrolled in Schools Without SBHCs (n=1383)	P [a]
Quarterly total cost 2000–2001 academic year, mean $			
Black	293.7	364.2	
Non-Black	276.7	340.3	
Quarterly total cost 2001–2002 academic year, mean $			
Black	401.8	343.6	
Non-Black	348.3	423.0	
Quarterly total cost 2002–2003 academic year, mean $			
Black	394.5	341.6	
Non-Black	374.2	334.2	

Note. MCO = managed care organization; SCHIP = State Children Health Insurance Plan; TANF = Temporary Assistance for Needy Families. The total sample size was n = 5056.

[a] Students in schools with SBHCs compared with students in schools without SBHCs, by the t test for age and months enrolled, and by the χ^2 test for other variables.

[b] Age was calculated as (September 30, 2000 minus the student's date of birth) divided by 365.25.

[c] Enrollment category is not mutually exclusive. As recipients could have been in multiple enrollment categories during the study period, the recipient's aid category was defined by the percentage of enrollment months for which the recipient was enrolled in each program.

activities. We estimated the 7572 SBHC encounters as $479 929 by using Medicaid reimbursement value. For patient and family sector costs, we estimated a copayment total of $75 720 with $10 per SBHC encounter. Also, although each school donated space to the SBHCs, we estimated $60 750 for the market value of the space over the 3 years in the schools with SBHCs.

BENEFITS

We estimated total value of health state changes to be $954 387 on the basis of Medicaid claims, including (1) the total value of the additional mental health care for students was $771 840 over 3 years, (2) the increased dental care benefit was $38 568 over the first 3 years, and (3) that nurse practitioners spent 30% to 50% of their time on nonbillable activities such as services for teachers and staff, student

TABLE 29.2—FINAL ESTIMATION OF EFFECTS OF THE SCHOOL-BASED HEALTH CENTER (SBHC) PROGRAM ON THE GROWTH TRENDS OF THE QUARTERLY TOTAL MEDICAL COSTS: GREATER CINCINNATI, OH, 1997–2003

Fixed Effect[a]	Growth Trend Variable[b]	b (SE)	t	P
Initial status[c]	B_0			
Intercept[2]	G_{00}	193.270 (50.31)	3.842	<.001
Sex	G_{01}	48.979 (32.81)	1.493	.135
Race	G_{02}	−86.095 (46.01)	−1.871	.061
Age	G_{03}	13.190 (5.97)	2.210	.027
SBHC	G_{04}	−48.477 (37.82)	−1.282	.200
MCO	G_{05}	−12.987 (47.55)	−0.273	.785
SCHIP	G_{06}	10.520 (38.26)	0.275	.783
Disabled	G_{07}	1825.471 (290.68)	6.280	<.001
Linear growth[d]	B_1			
Intercept[2]	G_{10}	−9.859 (9.69)	−1.018	.309
Sex	G_{11}	5.373 (5.24)	1.025	.306
Race	G_{12}	−0.148 (6.71)	−0.022	.983
Age	G_{13}	2.482 (1.05)	2.363	.018
SBHC	G_{14}	8.338 (5.96)	1.398	.162
MCO	G_{15}	−8.412 (8.16)	−1.030	.303
SCHIP	G_{16}	−3.020 (6.04)	−0.500	.616
Disabled	G_{17}	−9.771 (34.61)	−0.282	.778
Quadratic growth[d]	B_2			
Intercept[2]	G_{20}	−0.615 (0.66)	−0.931	.352
Sex	G_{21}	−0.084 (0.40)	−0.208	.835
Race	G_{22}	0.732 (0.55)	1.325	.185
Age	G_{23}	0.044 (0.08)	0.521	.602
SBHC	G_{24}	0.711 (0.50)	1.411	.158
MCO	G_{25}	−0.553 (0.77)	−0.720	.471
SCHIP	G_{26}	−0.127 (0.57)	−0.222	.824
Disabled	G_{27}	−7.969 (2.28)	−3.500	.001

(CONTINUED ON NEXT PAGE)

TABLE 29.2—(CONTINUED)

Fixed Effect[a]	Growth Trend Variable[b]	b (SE)	t	P
Cubic growth[d]	B_3			
Intercept[c]	G_{30}	−0.004 (0.10)	−0.042	.967
Sex	G_{31}	−0.010 (0.06)	−0.174	.863
Race	G_{32}	0.057 (0.08)	0.755	.450
Age	G_{33}	−0.008 (0.01)	−0.620	.535
SBHC	G_{34}	−0.010 (0.07)	−0.140	.889
MCO	G_{35}	−0.004 (0.10)	−0.035	.972
SCHIP	G_{36}	−0.089 (0.08)	−1.159	.247
Disabled	G_{37}	−0.067 (0.30)	−0.224	.823

Note. MCO = managed care organization; SCHIP = State Children Health Insurance Plan. Final estimation of variance component: level 1 = 1 537 702.88; degrees of freedom = 5048; χ^2 = 33 762; P < .001. The total sample size of eligible students was n = 5056.

[a]*Linear model of quarterly Medicaid cost was regressed on race, sex, age, SBHC, SCHIP, aid for disabled or blind, and MCO for their growth trends.*

[b]G_{00}, G_{10}, G_{20}, and G_{30} are for the intercepts; G_{01}, G_{11}, G_{21}, and G_{31} are for the effects of gender (male = 1 and female = 0) on the growth trends; G_{02}, G_{12}, G_{22}, and G_{32} are for the effects of race (Black = 1 and others = 0) on the growth trends; G_{03}, G_{13}, G_{23}, and G_{33} are for the effects of age (years in September 2000) on the growth trends; G_{04}, G_{14}, G_{24}, and G_{34} are for the effects of SBHC (SBHC = 1 and non-SBHC = 0) on the growth trends; G_{05}, G_{15}, G_{25}, and G_{35} are for the effects of MCO enrollment on the growth trends; G_{06}, G_{16}, G_{26}, and G_{36} are for the effects of SCHIP enrollment on the growth trends; and G_{07}, G_{17}, G_{27}, and G_{37} are for the effects of disabled enrollment on the growth trends.*

[c]*Degrees of freedom for initial status are 5048.*

[d]*Degrees of freedom for linear growth, quadratic growth, and cubic growth are 74 565.*

smoking cessation programs, student health status consultations, and staff meetings. The value of nonbillable health care activities was estimated as 30% of SBHC office visits with a total cost of $143 979. Other created value was estimated to be $457 598 from the additional funding attracted by SBHCs from local children's hospitals and Healthy School Healthy Community grants.

Resources saved from the health care sector included potential cost-savings for hospitalization, estimated as $228 144 or $970 per student with asthma,[24] and, according to Medicaid claims, potential savings for prescription drugs were estimated to be $443 532. From the patient and family sector, SBHCs prevented productivity losses of $542 761 by parents who would otherwise have had to take their children to other sources of care. We estimated the value of the parent's time in the Cincinnati metropolitan region as equal to the blue- and white-collar combined average hourly rate of $17.92. Over the 7572 SBHC encounters, the SBHCs

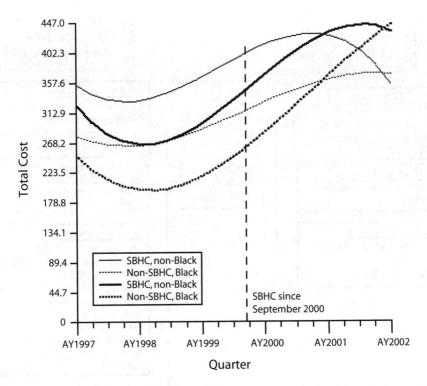

Note. AY = academic year. The sample size for eligible students enrolled in a participating school and enrolled in Medicaid was n = 5056. Total cost equals the quarterly total Medicaid reimbursement amount per student.

FIGURE 29.1 — Growth trends of quarterly total Medicaid costs by school-based health center (SBHC) and race: Greater Cincinnati, OH, 1997–2003.

saved parents between $542 761 (4 hours work time per parent) and $1 085 522 (8 hours work time per parent). Also, because students received care in the SBHCs, their parents saved a substantial amount of travel expenses. From parent survey data, the average time to a physician's office was 28 minutes round trip in an urban area and 46 minutes round trip in a rural area. With the rate of $0.35 per mile, we estimated total travel expenses to be $42 956.

Regarding resources saved from other sectors, SBHC staff identified and referred students to additional primary care. With a Medicaid reimbursement rate of $69 per visit, we estimated Medicaid spent $42 642 for the 618 documented referrals. We also estimated the community multiplier effect as $638 726 from a societal perspective, which was related to $1.00 Medicaid spent for a $3.15 multiplier effect in Ohio (written communication with Professors R. Greenbaum, PhD and A. Desai, PhD, Ohio State University, written communication, April 30, 2003).

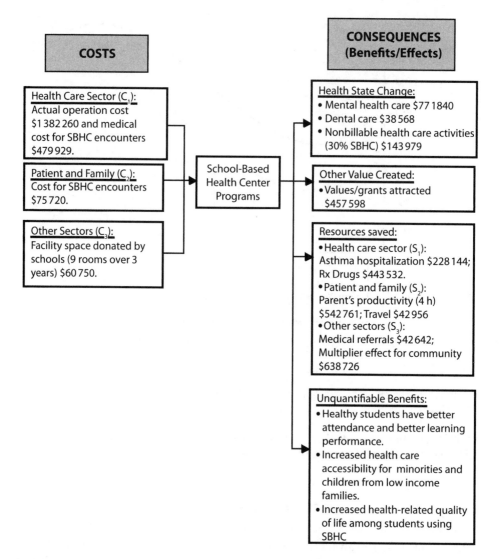

FIGURE 29.2—Estimated net social benefits of school-based health centers (SBHCs), with components of costs and benefits over the 3-year period: Greater Cincinnati, OH, 2001–2003.

For the 42.25% of students with Medicaid, the community multiplier effect was estimated as:

$$\$479\,929 \times 42.25\% \times 3.15 = \$638\,726. \qquad \text{(Eq. 29.1)}$$

Finally, the unquantifiable benefits included at least 5 aspects. First, SBHCs helped African American children and adolescents from low-income families get health care they may not have otherwise received, closing the gap in potential health care disparities (Figure 29.1). Second, about 80% of students in schools with SBHCs returned to class after SBHC encounters. We believe that students with better attendance are more successful at school. However, because this was beyond our study scope, we were unable to quantify this benefit. Third, increased early mental health services received by students in SBHC schools may reduce costly future treatment of those students. Because of the limited time frame of this study, we were unable to quantify this impact. Fourth, increased dental care received by students in SBHC schools might prevent or reduce costly future dental treatment. Fifth, we found that students with asthma in schools with SBHCs had a lower risk of hospitalization and emergency room visits compared with that of students with asthma in schools without SBHCs. It is possible that students with asthma in schools with SBHCs had better asthma management. However, we were unable to quantify the benefit related to quality of life and future health care savings.

Net Social Benefit Estimation

On the basis of the assumptions made and the calculations performed, as described previously, we estimated the net social benefit of the SBHCs over the 3 years to be $1.35 million. This is a low-end estimation that is based on total costs of $1 998 659 and total benefits of $3 350 746.

DISCUSSION

In the urban areas within Cincinnati, increased attention has been paid to racial and ethnic health disparities in an effort to increase the accessibility to health care services for African Americans and low-income families. When one considers that nearly 50% of the population in urban areas within Cincinnati is African American, it is very meaningful that SBHCs provide essential health care for these students and aim at eliminating barriers to health care.

SBHCs appear to have a significant ability to reduce health care access disparities among African Americans and disabled students, as these groups received more primary care since SBHCs opened in September 2000. This suggests that having access to an SBHC can help reduce or eliminate access barriers to care and reduce health care disparities for these vulnerable populations—a matter of equity in utilization and not excess utilization. This finding should be robust because the time-series HLM analysis was employed to control for some variations in students' ages and Medicaid enrollments.

The cost–benefit analysis showed that a net social benefit of the SBHC program in the 4 Ohio school districts was about $1.35 million over 3 years. Because Medicaid was the primary payer of services to children and adolescents, we also looked at the cost benefits to Ohio Medicaid. In our previously published studies and final report,[24,25,40] students in SBHC schools benefited from more dental services, less prescription drug use, more mental health services, and fewer hospitalizations. Increased Medicaid costs of $1 179 264 (increased dental care of $121 344 plus increased mental health services of $1 057 920) were offset by the total savings of $1 713 228 (savings of $1 395 456 from prescription drugs and savings of $317 772 from hospitalization for students with asthma). Net 3-year Medicaid savings was $533 964, which equals roughly $35.20 savings per child per year.

Our study does not account for the reported increase in health-related quality of life among students participating in SBHCs compared with students in schools without SBHCs.[41] These unquantifiable benefits of SBHCs may also exceed any extra costs to the Medicaid program. Although we can only speculate as to how much benefit there is to Medicaid, we still believe it is important for Medicaid to foster improved access to health care for minorities and children from low-income families, and to increase access to children's mental health services, dental care, and other health care.

Our study also has relevance to broader health policy issues. SBHCs provide important primary care for children and adolescents, indicating benefits to federal and state governments for improving coordination between the SBHCs and state Medicaid and managed care organizations.[42–44] The SBHC schools in Greater Cincinnati have a large proportion of children and adolescents who are African American students from lower-income families. If one considers concerns about racial disparities and acknowledged barriers to care for the poor and uninsured, the SBHC program is particularly well suited to address these disparities, especially among students with chronic disease such as mental health conditions and asthma.

The SBHC is a model for providing quality health care services for children and adolescents that eliminates most barriers students face when they are trying to access health care. SBHCs address problems regarding transportation, lack of nearby providers, lack of providers accepting public insurance, and parental difficulties getting time away from work to take a child to the doctor, which in turn helps parents retain employment and helps employers increase worker productivity. Moreover, they are in a unique position to reduce financial, language, familial, and cultural barriers in providing care for children and adolescents in the community in which they live. By providing services on-site, SBHCs help return students to the classroom more quickly, meaning they miss less instruction time.

Our study was limited to school-aged children and adolescents in the Greater Cincinnati area. We were unable to assess students with other insurance plans or no insurance because the primary data source used was retrospective Medicaid claims database. We also did not differentiate between students who were treated by the SBHCs and students in the SBHC schools who were not treated. Finally, during the 5.5-year study period, the natural history of disease epidemics among school-age children and adolescents varies along with maturation of students, which may influence the time trends.

In conclusion, SBHCs were cost beneficial to the society. The health care utilization for African American and disabled students increased after the SBHC program and closed the gaps of health care disparities. SBHCs should be seen as a health service delivery model to help address a lack of accessing timely care for disadvantaged students.

REFERENCES

1. Institute of Medicine. *Unequal Treatment. Confronting Racial and Ethnic Disparities: View Health Care.* Washington, DC: The National Academies Press; 2003.

2. Cook BL. Effect of Medicaid managed care on racial disparities in health care access. *Health Serv Res.* 2007;42(1 pt 1):124–145.

3. Smedley BD, Stith AY, Nelson AR, eds. *Board on Health Sciences Policy. Unequal Treatment: Confronting Racial and Ethnic Disparities in Health Care. Executive Summary.* Washington, DC: Institute of Medicine, National Academy Press; 2002.

4. Lillie-Blanton M, Parsons P, Gayle H, Dievler A. Racial differences in health: not just black and white but shades of gray. *Annu Rev Public Health.* 1996;17:411–448.

5. Weinick RM, Zuvekas SH, Cohen JW. Racial and ethnic differences in access to and use of health services, 1977–1996. *Med Care Res Rev.* 2000;57(suppl 1):36–54.

6. Centers for Disease Control and Prevention, Office of Minority Health. Health disparities experienced by Black or African Americans—United States. *MMWR Morb Mortal Wkly Rep.* 2005;54(1)1–3.

7. Centers for Disease Control and Prevention. *Health, United States, 2004; With Chartbook on Trends in the Health of Americans.* Table 30. Hyattsville, MD: National Center for Health Statistics; 2004. Available at: http://www.cdc.gov/nchs/data/hus/hus04trend.pdf#03. Accessed June 30, 2006.

8. McKinnon J. The Black population 2000. Census 2000 brief. Washington, DC: US Dept of Commerce, US Census Bureau; 2001. Available at: http://www.census.gov/prod/2001pubs/c2kbr01-5.pdf. Accessed June 30, 2006.

9. Cooper GS, Koroukian SM. Geographic variation among Medicare beneficiaries in the use of colorectal carcinoma screening procedures. *Am J Gastroenterol.* 2004;99(8):1544–1550.

10. Cooper GS, Yuan Z, Landefeld CS, Rimm AA. Surgery for colorectal cancer: race-related differences in rates and survival among Medicare beneficiaries. *Am J Public Health.* 1996;86(4):582–586.

11. Bernabei R, Gambassi G, Lapane K, et al. Management of pain in elderly patients with cancer. Systematic assessment of geriatric drug use via epidemiology. *JAMA.* 1998;279(23):1877–1882.

12. Richters JE, Arnold LE, Jensen PS, et al. NIMH collaborative multisite multimodal treatment study of children with ADHD: I. Background and rationale. *J Am Acad Child Adolesc Psychiatry.* 1995;34(8):987–1000.

13. Goldman LS, Genel M, Bezman RJ, Slanetz PJ. Diagnosis and treatment of attention-deficit/hyperactivity disorder in children and adolescents. Council on Scientific Affairs, American Medical Association. *JAMA.* 1998;279(14):1100–1107.

14. Akinbami LJ, LaFleur BJ, Schoendorf KC. Racial and income disparities in childhood asthma in the United States. *Ambul Pediatr.* 2002;2(5):382–387.

15. Newacheck PW, Halfon N. Prevalence, impact, and trends in childhood disability due to asthma. *Arch Pediatr Adolesc Med.* 2000;154(3):287–293.

16. Wells R, Hillemeier MM, Bai Y, Belue R. Health service access across racial/ethnic groups of children in the child welfare system. *Child Abuse Negl.* 2009;33(5):282–292.

17. Coker TR, Elliott MN, Kataoka S, et al. Racial/ethnic disparities in the mental health care utilization of fifth grade children. *Acad Pediatr.* 2009;9(2):89–96.

18. Howell E, McFeeters J. Children's mental health care: differences by race/ethnicity in urban/rural areas. *J Health Care Poor Underserved.* 2008;19(1):237–247.

19. US Surgeon General. Mental health: a report of the surgeon general. Washington, DC: US Dept of Health and Human Services; 1999. Available at: http://www.surgeongeneral.gov/library/index.html. Accessed June 30, 2006.

20. Schilitt J, Santelli J, Juszczak L, et al. Creating access to care: school-based health center census 1998–1999. Washington, DC: National Assembly on School-Based Health Care; 2000. Available at: http://www.nasbhc.org/site. Accessed June 30, 2006.

21. Dryfoos JG. School-based health centers in the context of education reform. *J Sch Health.* 1998;68(10):404–408.

22. Lear JG. Health at school: a hidden health care system emerges from the shadows. *Health Aff (Millwood).* 2007;26(2):409–419.

23. Guo JJ, Wade TJ, Keller KN. Impact of school-based health centers on students with mental health problems. *Public Health Rep.* 2008;123(6):768–780.

24. Guo JJ, Jang R, Keller KK, McCracken A, Pan W, Cluxton RJ. Impact of school-based health centers on children with asthma. *J Adolesc Health.* 2005;37(4):266–274.

25. Young TL, D'angelo SL, Davis J. Impact of a school-based health center on emergency department use by elementary school student. *J Sch Health.* 2001;71(5):196–198.

26. Adams EK, Johnson V. An elementary school-based health clinic: can it reduce Medicaid costs? *Pediatrics.* 2000;105(4 pt 1):780–788.

27. Kaplan DW, Brindis CD, Phibbs SL, Melinkovich P, Naylor K, Ahlstrand K. A comparison study of an elementary school-based health center: effects on health care access and use. *Arch Pediatr Adolesc Med.* 1999;153(3):235–243.

28. Kaplan DW, Calonge BN, Guernsey BP, Hanrahan MB. Managed care and school-based health centers. Use of health services. *Arch Pediatr Adolesc Med.* 1998;152(1):25–33.

29. Meeker RJ, DeAngelis C, Berman B, Freeman HE, Oda D. A comprehensive school health initiative. *Image J Nurs Sch.* 1986;18(3):86–91.

30. Fisher M, Juszczak L, Friedman SB, Schneider M, Chapar G. School-based adolescent health care. Review of a clinical service. *Am J Dis Child.* 1992;146(5):615–621.

31. Balassone ML, Bell M, Peterfreund N. A comparison of users and nonusers of a school-based health and mental health clinic. *J Adolesc Health.* 1991;12(3):240–246.

32. Walter HJ, Vaughan RD, Armstrong B, Krakoff RY, Tiezzi L, McCarthy JF. School-based health care for urban minority junior high school students. *Arch Pediatr Adolesc Med.* 1995;149(11):1221–1225.

33. Weist MD, Paskewitz DA, Warner BS, Flaherty LT. Treatment outcome of school-based mental health services for urban teenagers. *Community Ment Health J.* 1996;32(2):149–157.

34. Anglin TM, Naylor KE, Kaplan DW. Comprehensive school-based health care: high school students' use of medical, mental health, and substance abuse services. *Pediatrics.* 1996;97(3):318–330.

35. Wade TJ, Keller KN, Guo JJ, Huentelman T, Line K, Mansour ME. Access and utilization patterns across the first three years of implementation of elementary and middle school school-based health centers. *Public Health Rep.* 2008;123(6):739–750.

36. Drummond MF, O'Brien B, Stoddart GL, et al. *Methods for the Economic Evaluation of Health Care Programs.* New York, NY: Oxford University Press; 1999:52–96.

37. Bureau of Labor Statistics. Consumer Price Index for all urban consumers 1997, 1998, 1999, 2000, 2001, 2002. Washington DC: US Dept of Labor. Available at: http://www.bls.gov. Accessed June 1, 2003.

38. Bureau of Labor Statistics. Medical care inflation continues to rise. Washington DC: US Dept of Labor; 2001. Available at: http://www.bls.gov/opub/ted. Accessed June 1, 2003.

39. Raudenbush SW, Bryk AS. *Hierarchical Linear Models: Applications and Data Analysis Methods*. 2nd ed. Thousand Oaks, CA: Sage; 2002.

40. Guo JJ, Jang R, Cluxton RJ. Evaluation of health outcomes and costs among Medicaid recipients enrolled in school-based health centers. A prescription for success. Cincinnati, OH: Health Foundation for Greater Cincinnati; 2004. Available at http://www.health foundation.org/publications.html. Accessed June 30, 2006.

41. Wade TJ, Mansour M, Line K, Huentelman T, Keller KE. Improvements in health-related quality of life among school-based health center users in elementary and middle school. *Ambul Pediatr*. 2008;8(4):241–249.

42. Health care: school-based health centers can expand access for children. Washington DC: US Government Accounting Office; 1994. GAO publication GAO/HEHS 95-35.

43. Leonard M. GAO: Health reform could help school-based health centers. *Nations Health*. 1994;24(6):3–4.

44. Waxman HA. Juvenile detention centers: warehousing children with mental illness? The House Committee on Government Reform. Washington, DC: US Congress; 2004. Available at: http://oversight.house.gov. Accessed June 30, 2006.

About the Authors

Jianfei (Jeff) J. Guo PhD BPharm – is a tenured professor at the University of Cincinnati (UC) Medical Center College of Pharmacy and Department of Public Health Sciences. He has been teaching graduate courses and has served as graduate student advisor. He has extensive research experience on child health outcome research, school-based health center evaluation, drug safety and Pharmacoepidemiology, orphan drug policy, drug utilization review, drug-induced hepatotoxicity, cost–benefit analysis, cost-effectiveness analysis, and more. He sits on editorial boards for five journals. He has published over 60 peer-reviewed research papers in different journals, as well as book chapters and editorials, book reviews, letters to the editor, or commentaries.

Terrance J. Wade, PhD – is the Canada Research Chair in Youth and Wellness and Professor and Chair of the Departments of Community Health Sciences at Brock University. His research employs a multidisciplinary, population-focused perspective to investigate the social and structural determinants of child health and development, examining life trajectories that lead to a variety of childhood and adult health outcomes. He is currently the principal investigator on a Heart and Stroke Foundation of Ontario (HSFO) study that is examining the social determinants of child hypertension.

Wei Pan, PhD – is an Associate Professor of Quantitative Research Methodology in the Educational Studies Program at the University of Cincinnati. He received his PhD in Measurement and Quantitative Methods from Michigan State University. He has been involved in many research projects funded by federal agencies, such as the National Institutes of Health, the US Department of Education, and the National Science Foundation. His current research interests are causal inference, propensity score analysis, resampling, multilevel modeling, structural equation modeling, meta-analysis, and their applications in the social, behavioral, and health sciences.

Kathryn N. Keller – is the Senior Program Officer for School-Aged Children's Healthcare at The Health Foundation of Greater Cincinnati. She implemented initiatives totaling over $22 million related to school-based health care services throughout Greater Cincinnati, including 24 SBHCs. She received the degree of MPA from University of Cincinnati. She has served as a board member for the National Assembly on School-Based Health Care and has published several high impact articles about school-age health care issues.

Making the Business Case for School-Based Health Centers

Whitney Brimfield, Adrienne Ammerman,
and Linda Juszczak

School-based health centers (SBHCs) are a "disruptive innovation"—defined by Clayton Christopher as "an innovation that allows a whole new population of consumers access to a product or service that was historically only accessible to consumers with a lot of money or a lot of skill."[1] SBHCs bring equity to access to health care for children and adolescents by providing high-quality, comprehensive, culturally sensitive health, mental health, and oral health care to children and adolescents where they are: in school.

With that equity comes significant opportunity. Studies repeatedly show that a primary determinant of a child's ability to succeed in school is access to health care.[2] And, over the course of life, the strongest predictor of an individual's health and socioeconomic status is academic achievement.[3] Thus, it follows that the presence of an SBHC in a school can have an impact on students' academic achievement and future success. In fact, studies have proven this impact, showing that SBHCs improve attendance,[4] increase grade-point average,[2] and decrease dropout rates.[5] Given these proven positive effects of SBHCs on the future workforce, it stands to reason that the private sector should have a vested interest in expanding access to SBHCs.

Currently, the private sector investment in SBHCs is limited—only 28% of SBHCs receive funding from corporations or businesses.[6] However, there is a strong argument for a greater investment given the facts. As outlined in this chapter, SBHCs:

- Have a significant social impact
- Address problems before they become costly crises
- Are sustainable when designed and managed well
- Are supported by leaders in the private sector

These favorable characteristics make SBHCs a wise and forward-looking investment. Right now, there are more than 1,900 SBHCs providing access to services for 1.7 million students.[6] Although SBHCs reach across social, economic, and geographic divides, the demand for SBHC services is far greater than the capacity to provide those services. There are 21 million adolescents in the United States,[7] 20 million children in poverty,[8] and 15 million children with mental health challenges.[9]

There is clear evidence of demand for SBHCs in more communities. According to the 2004–2005 SBHC Census conducted by the National Assembly on School-Based Health Care (NASBHC), an additional 5,808 SBHCs are required to meet the unmet health care needs of all children aged 6 to 17 years.[10] The NASBHC hopes for a near future when there are 4,000 SBHCs serving nearly four million students—getting us close to the total number that will meet the need. Investments from the private sector in SBHC programs that are designed and managed for sustainability will be critical to meeting this goal.

The return on investment for the private sector is a healthier, better prepared, and stronger workforce.

SCHOOL-BASED HEALTH CENTERS HAVE A SIGNIFICANT SOCIAL IMPACT

There are severe inequities in educational achievement and health care access among children and adolescents in this country.[2] The unifying force behind these gaps is poverty. Poverty is cyclical and difficult to get out of; those in poverty have hampered access to resources and greater barriers to success. SBHCs can help break the cycle by improving child and adolescent health (Figure 30.1).

Poverty affects a child's IQ, home environment, parental health and mental health, and physical environment, resulting in great barriers to success and achievement. Right now the United States has a large population—almost 16 million children (aged 18 and under)—living below the poverty level.[8] Unless the cycle of poverty is broken, those numbers will increase.

It seems clear that interventions to increase academic achievement and improve health, thereby decreasing poverty, would mitigate some of these effects. However, despite well-intentioned efforts and pockets of success, these problems persist. Recent research on global adolescent health indicates that adolescent morbidity is at its height right now and that "what distinguishes the causes of death of young people is that most deaths have behavioral causes exacerbated by national policy or failures of health-service delivery systems, or both."[11(p853)]

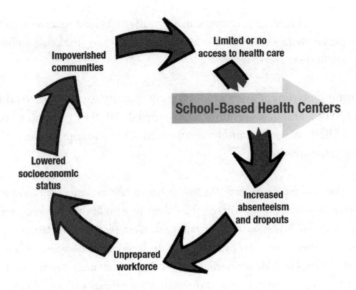

Figure 30.1 — Impact of school-based health centers on the cycle of poverty.

These problems seem insurmountable, and the cycle of disparity and lessened opportunity that results seems endless. That is, until you walk into an SBHC. SBHCs are a proven, common-sense model for addressing these gaps. Recent research draws a correlation between SBHC services, improved health, increased attendance, and improvements in grade-point average over time.[2]

SBHCs exist at the intersection of education and health and are the caulk that prevents children and adolescents from falling through the cracks. They provide care—primary health, mental health and counseling, family outreach, and chronic illness management—without concern for students' ability to pay and in a location that meets students where they are: at school. And, *because* of their location in the school building, SBHCs are firsthand witnesses to social determinants of health and academic achievement—bullying, school violence, depression, stress, poor eating habits, and so on—that health providers outside of a school setting may miss. Staff in SBHCs have the time and the insight to address these social determinants, making them uniquely attuned to the needs of the students.

For an example of a community that has recognized the potential of SBHCs to address long-term problems, one need look only as far as Erie County, Pennsylvania. Mike Batchelor, MPP, President of Erie Community Foundation (April 6, 2011, phone conversation), explains,

> Erie City has the highest poverty rate of anywhere in Pennsylvania. As a
> community foundation we decided to increase access to predecessors of

poverty—workforce opportunities, quality early childhood education, and health care. We landed on SBHCs as a potential solution that could address all three of these areas.

Erie Community Foundation held open community forums to introduce the concept of SBHCs, and it was embraced. In April 2010, they released a request for proposal for SBHC planning, and have awarded three planning grants.

Mr. Batchelor concludes:

> Our goal is to reduce poverty. We know that certain indicators contribute to poverty, including the percentage of children with no health insurance, teen pregnancy, and low educational attainment. We want to use SBHCs as a tool to address these indicators by improving the health and education of young people. SBHCs provide measurable access that we can use when we reach out to the donor community and prove that these things make a difference in fighting poverty.

It is clear that the presence of more SBHCs with greater sustainability will improve child and adolescent health outcomes and lead to improved educational achievement, thus breaking the cycle of poverty. A testimonial from Nidia Escobar, now 20 years old, a passionate student SBHC advocate is the best evidence of this:

> When I was in ninth grade I ditched school a lot and got bad grades. I knew that I didn't want to be another statistic—getting pregnant and dropping out—but I wasn't sure what I wanted to do with my life. That changed a lot when I started getting involved at the health center at my school. I had problems that were so personal and so big . . . if the health center wasn't there for me it would have been too much of an obstacle to overcome on my own (personal communication, January 12, 2010).

SBHCs are transforming the front line of health and mental health care for children and adolescents like Nidia by removing financial, emotional, and procedural barriers to accessing care.

An increase in the number of SBHCs can have the following results:

- Increased health quality for children and adolescents with access to SBHCs versus the general population
- Principals reporting improvements in the school climate and overall demeanor of students
- Increased recognition by community leaders that SBHCs are indispensable

As long-term impact is measured, communities with SBHCs will have:

- Students with lower dropout rates, increased grade-point averages, and higher graduation rates
- Reduced emergency room visits, lower hospitalization costs, and decreased insurance expenditures
- Active and engaged families that use and advocate for SBHCs
- A stronger, better prepared workforce

The social impact of SBHCs is impressive, and is growing as they expand to more communities across the country.

SBHCs address problems before they become costly crises. In addition to being a common sense approach to ensuring that all children and adolescents are healthy and achieving to their fullest potential, SBHCs reduce health care costs, making them a wise investment. For example, a study of Medicaid-enrolled children served by an SBHC in Atlanta, Georgia, found that SBHCs reduced Medicaid expenses by almost $1,500 annually for their patients in comparison to children on Medicaid but attending a school without an SBHC. Savings were realized by significantly lower inpatient, transportation, drug, and emergency department expenses.[12]

In a later interview, Dr. Veda Johnson, Assistant Professor of Pediatrics at Emory University School of Medicine and an author of the Medicaid study,[12] says:

> We've demonstrated in a very practical way that SBHCs decrease the cost of transportation because children are right there. SBHCs also reduce the cost of medication and drug use because we don't prescribe as many medications as in a routine physicians' office because we can monitor them more closely.[13(p103)]

Additional studies have found:

- SBHCs reduced inappropriate emergency room use, increased use of primary care, and resulted in fewer hospitalizations among regular users.[14]
- The number of hospitalizations and emergency department visits decreased for children with SBHCs in Cincinnati schools (2.4-fold and 33.5%, respectively)—with an estimated savings of nearly $1,000 per child.[15]
- A nationwide SBHC program to manage childhood asthma would have an estimated total savings for opportunity costs of work loss and premature death at $23.13 billion.[16]
- SBHC patients cost Medicaid an average of $30.40 less than comparable, non-SBHC patients.[17]

The above studies—and others—demonstrate that SBHCs are cost-effective. Yet still there are many that operate on shoestring budgets, limiting their impact. As with any social enterprise, sustainability is a challenge and a responsibility for

- Stable health care provider sponsors, including being part of a health care system such as the Indian Health Service, Tribal 638 clinic, federally qualified health center, or hospital
- Ability to get the funds generated from Medicaid and the Children's Health Insurance Program (CHIP) and third-party billing returned to the operating budget of the individual SBHC
- Maximized Medicaid outreach and enrollment of all eligible youth
- Payer mix—high Medicaid-eligible population of users
- Ability to maximize visits by properly coding them
- Fully integrated practice management system where electronic health records are linked with billing accounts receivable/accounts payable
- Improve billing systems
- Use a nurse case manager to more efficiently coordinate and deliver care
- Having support staff that increase productivity
- Implementation of electronic health records
- Increasing capacity to enroll kids in public insurance programs (Medicaid or CHIP)

Adapted from New Mexico Alliance for School-Based Health Care.[22]

Figure 30.2—Blueprint for a financially sustainable school-based health center (SBHC).

SBHCs. More and more, SBHCs are implementing business plans and seeking opportunities to generate revenue to remain a sustainable solution for their communities and our nation.

SBHCs are sustainable when well designed, managed, and maintained (Figure 30.2). For the private sector to invest significantly in SBHCs they want to see that SBHCs are going to be around for the long term. In fact, the movement is making great strides in transitioning from a marginal, passion-driven "cause" to a federally authorized model of health care that is nationally recognized and respected.[18]

In part, this success is due to an organized national movement to bring SBHCs to the forefront of the federal policy debate, led by the NASBHC. However, the more critical component of SBHCs' increasing longevity is strategic business planning—serving the community around the school, improving billing systems, and diversifying revenue. Often this work is supported by funders that want to protect their community investments by enabling SBHCs to engage in strategic planning for long-term sustainability.

According to the NASBHC's 2007–2008 National Census, SBHCs are maturing; 72% are five years or older, up from 41% in 1998.[5] This illustrates the increasing sustainability of the model. At the same time, 287 SBHCs opened between 2003 and 2007, indicating a growth in demand.[5]

In addition, a growing number of SBHCs see patient populations beyond the schools they serve,[5] further entrenching them in the communities where they reside and allowing them to maximize their outreach and potential reimbursement.

Health Information Technology (HIT) is another critical piece in the sustainability equation. More SHBCs are adopting HIT to enhance their work. More than half use electronic billing systems (56%) and online management informa-tion systems (53%).[5] A smaller number use electronic medical records (32%) and electronic prescribing (22%).[5] This is a critical development because HIT enables SBHCs to make their billing and collection practices more efficient. These changes can be largely credited to the increasing sophistication of the SBHC field—learning from experience and responding to funders that reward SBHCs that plan for the long term.

Two organizations that are currently working on increasing SBHC sustain-ability are the Health Foundation of Greater Cincinnati and the Colorado Health Foundation.

Kate Keller, MPA, Senior Program Officer at the Health Foundation of Greater Cincinnati, runs the Foundation's SBHC funding program, which provides grants for SBHC planning, operations, and sustainability. The Foundation currently has three grantees that serve four schools. The Foundation previously funded 11 other SBHCs that are now no longer reliant on their grants.

"When we first started supporting SBHCs, we didn't put a lot of thought into sustainability—we focused on opening the centers and getting services to kids," Ms. Keller says. "A few years later it became more important to us that we come up with a financially sustainable model without losing the essence of the SBHC" (phone conversation, March 30, 2011).

The Foundation now has each grantee start with a year of planning that includes designing an SBHC that will meet the needs of the community while also creating a realistic plan that will keep it open for the long run. This includes a business model and financial projections based on population, insurance, and payer mix, and how they plan on keeping the SBHC going beyond the grant funding. In addition, the Foundation requires that grantees locate sources of matching funds after the first year of their award.

The Foundation also works with new and older grantees on practice manage-ment work, including how to look at patient flows, how to get patients in the door, and how to project reimbursement based on well-child visits. "SBHCs really need to figure out the best way to provide care to bring in money—for example, by hav-ing the least expensive providers provide the least expensive services" (Kate Keller, phone conversation, March 30, 2011).

Ms. Keller believes that the Foundation's model has contributed to more of an awareness of the investment that it takes to keep an SBHC open for the long haul. "When people get in to these programs they are starry eyed about them, but there's a reality to keeping those doors open. When grant funding ends they go into it aware of that reality and they're prepared for it" (phone conversation, March 30, 2011).

The Colorado Health Foundation (CHF) is another organization that has supported the SBHC model in their state for several years, but has more recently focused on the sustainability of the model. In June 2009, CHF launched a four-year initiative that helps SBHCs strategize to become as profitable as possible while also addressing policy barriers to sustainability.

Under this initiative, communities that want to start or expand SBHCs complete a readiness assessment and then apply for a planning grant to create a business plan. The plan includes a narrative that outlines products, services, markets, and communications strategies as well as financial templates that walk through a series of projections, including payer mix and reimbursement rates. Amy Latham, MPA, Senior Program Officer with CHF, notes: "The business plan shows the gap between projected revenue and expenses, and that's where Colorado Health Foundation's funding comes in—we help figure out strategies to shrink that gap" (phone conversation, March 30, 2011).

SBHCs have learned to be creative in using financial and in-kind support to address some of these funding gaps (Figure 30.3). Sponsors (organizations that serve as the primary administrative home) of SBHCs are most typically a local health care organization, such as a community health center, a hospital, or a local health department.[5] SBHCs often receive additional support from schools and

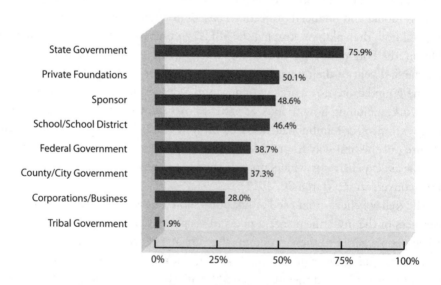

Figure 30.3—Sources of school-based health center funding.

others through in-kind donations of space and services.[5] The majority indicate that they do not have financial responsibility for construction, renovation, maintenance and/or janitorial services, utilities, or rent.[5]

The majority of SBHCs bill public insurance for health center visits, including Medicaid and the Children's Health Insurance Program (CHIP). Fifty-nine percent of SBHCs bill private insurance; 38% bill students or families directly.[5] A majority of SBHCs also assist children and families with enrollment in public insurance programs.

SBHCs also receive support from revenue sources not related to billing, including state government, private foundations, sponsor organizations, and schools or school districts.[5] Thirty-nine percent of SBHCs receive funding from the federal government,[5] and—thanks to health care reform—this number is likely to increase dramatically in the next few years. The Patient Protection and Affordable Care Act (PPACA; P.L.111-148), signed into law by President Barack Obama on March 23, 2010, mandates $200 million over four years for capital improvements and equipment purchases. The PPACA also created a new federal program for SBHCs— thereby recognizing SBHCs as part of the national health care safety net.

The hard reality is that—although the SBHC movement is strengthened by a diverse range of financial sources—the continuity of services provided for vulnerable populations is also put at risk because of insufficient reimbursement for covered and uncovered services, slashed funding from local and state governments, and a lack of federal funding for operations. The NASBHC, with support from its state affiliates, is working at the national level to find solutions to these issues.

When SBHCs are sustainable, the possibilities are endless for their community impact. The private sector is increasingly recognizing the value of SBHCs and the value in making long-term investments in the model.

SCHOOL-BASED HEALTH CENTERS ARE SUPPORTED BY LEADERS IN THE PRIVATE SECTOR

With funding challenges abounding, SBHCs have to seek creative solutions to maintain their critical services. As is true with many community-based services in this time of economic stress, demand for SBHC services is growing. In fact, an increasing number of SBHCs are seeing members of the community beyond the students at their school. As of 2007, just 36% of SBHCs reported serving *only* children who attend the schools they serve.[5] With this in mind, the SBHC field is increasingly reaching out to leaders in the private sector to help support the important services they provide to the community.[5]

The avenues through which connections are made between SBHCs and the private sector take many forms. As is to be expected, private sector investments in SBHCs, while always altruistic, are not always philanthropic. For example, some corporate relationships with SBHCs are built for marketing purposes, still others connect to work force development, and many are related to reducing the tax burden for profitable enterprises. The following are several case studies on various approaches to private sector investment in SBHCs.

Market-Driven Investment—Welch Allyn

Like many corporations that provide philanthropic support to social ventures, Welch Allyn sees SBHCs as a growing market for their products, particularly with the recent federal investment of funds for construction and equipment grants, which will infuse SBHCs with capital to purchase many of the products that Welch Allyn manufactures and distributes. As a result, Welch Allyn has gone above and beyond the typical corporate partner by:

- Working closely with the NASBHC and other national SBHC advocates to educate policymakers and regulators about SBHCs;
- Providing insight into how the federal grant program could be structured to best benefit SBHCs; and
- Offering SBHC-specific product bundles and pricing to assist the federal grant applicants.

Workforce-Driven Investment—CVS/Caremark

CVS/Caremark is a leader in the retail pharmacy industry and is well-known for their commitment to workforce development (Figure 30.4).[19] They have adopted SBHCs as a part of their workforce development strategy. As such, they

---

"As CVS Caremark looks toward the future and to securing the needs of our workforce, our employees, and their families, we understand that the capacity of America's children to achieve their education and successfully pursue meaningful careers is fundamental. We also understand that, far too often, these achievements are endangered by a lack of access to preventative and primary health care.

The data is compelling. School-based health centers are the most cost effective and efficient solution to these challenges, and they lead to improved student attendance, test scores, and graduation rates."

Ernie Dupont
Director
CVS Caremark Workforce Initiatives

Figure 30.4—CVS Caremark workforce initiatives.[19]

are promoting the role SBHCs play in creating a healthy, well-prepared, and well-trained workforce.

Community-Driven Investment—Metropolitan Sewer District of Cincinnati

The Health Foundation of Greater Cincinnati is funding an SBHC at the Oyler school for a five-year commitment—the first two years they are providing $200,000, and then up to $150,000 over the next three years. However, Oyler must locate matching funds for the final $150,000. Oyler is partnering with the Metropolitan Sewer District of Greater Cincinnati, which held two fundraisers for the SBHC. Ms. Keller says that "These events raised $37,000 towards keeping the SBHC operational, and they built community awareness. This is a great example of different city divisions supporting each other and supporting kids" (phone conversation, March 30, 2011).

Investment Through New Market Tax Credits—Financial Institutions

The New Market Tax Credit (NMTC) Program is a federal program designed to attract investment capital to projects serving low-income populations. Financial institutions are eligible to apply through this program administered by the Community Development Financial Institutions (CDFI) Fund of the US Department of Treasury for authority to allocate NMTC funds to designated Community Development Entities (CDEs). They become the administrators of the allocation, empowering the CDEs to make investments in the community they serve. Although the CDE must have a mission of serving low-income areas, it can have a wide range of organizational structures including nonprofit, government affiliate, financial institution, or for-profit developer. As a result of their investment in the fund, the financial institution receives tax credits equal to 39% of the allocation over a seven-year period. Thus, the program is an attractive opportunity for entities with large tax burdens, like financial institutions, to alleviate some of their tax liabilities.

Traditionally the NMTC Program has funded large construction projects like community health centers, tracts of affordable housing, and charter schools. Several financial institutions are currently investigating opportunities to use these credits to fund capital investments in SBHCs. The feasibility of investing in SBHCs through NMTCs hinges on the fact that the results of the investment must be maintained for seven years beyond the date of the initial capital investment. Thus, any SBHC that received NMTC funds would have to be able to maintain operations for at least 7 years. While this might not be difficult for well-established programs, it could be a greater challenge for new programs, which are the ones most likely to benefit from NMTCs.

Investment Driven by Tax Status—Nonprofit Hospitals and Health Care Agencies

Large hospital systems are required by law to reinvest in community benefit in order to maintain their tax exempt 501 (c)(3) status. Many hospital systems (25%)[5] sponsor SBHCs in order to fulfill this requirement. As a result of a recent study by the Internal Revenue Service (IRS) that determined a lack of uniformity in how hospitals are meeting the requirement, the PPACA created a new form—Schedule H[20]—that all nonprofit hospitals are now required to submit along with their 990 tax statements.

The form requests detailed information on how investments are made in community benefit. Most often, hospitals' community benefit involves covering care to the uninsured, also known as uncompensated care—56% of hospitals included in the IRS study reported uncompensated care as one of their community benefit investments.[21] Medical education and training (23%), research (15%), and community programs (6%) were the next largest community benefit investments.

Most often, SBHC programs fit under the community program line item. In addition, the IRS is challenging the varied definitions that hospitals have of "uncompensated care" and, according to anecdotal reports, is considering eliminating that as an option for community benefit investments. Thus, there is a likely opportunity for SBHCs to garner greater support from hospitals as these rules evolve.

One of the largest and most committed community benefit investments in SBHCs is from Kaiser Permanente. In addition to supporting SBHCs in Oakland, California, where they are headquartered, with a $10 million investment in 2009, Kaiser Permanente Community Benefit recently chose to invest a portion of its employees' Take and Give Campaign in SBHCs. More than 22,500 eligible Kaiser Permanente employees, dentists, and physicians took the Total Health Assessment, designed to help people better understand how their health is affected by lifestyle habits and behavior. Kaiser Permanente's workforce was encouraged to "take" the Total Health Assessment, and in return, Kaiser Permanente would "give" $50 as a matching contribution for each person's participation. The campaign raised more than $1 million, a portion of which was invested in a grant to the NASBHC to expand the number of SBHCs providing much-needed oral health care to public school students across the country.

Given what we know from the case studies just mentioned about the numerous avenues and opportunities for private sector investment in SBHCs, a number of which have bottom-line benefits to the investor, it is clear that there is room to increase the percentage of SBHCs that receive support from the private sector well beyond the 28% mark. The greatest challenge to increasing private sector investment is the limits on available time and energy from SBHC staff to build relationships with the private sector. However, as the tax implications of investing in SBHCs continue to gain prominence, there will be more incentive for the private sector to seek out relationships with SBHCs. This is an area with significant growth potential.

Partnerships between SBHCs and the private sector can help realize the full social impact of the model. We know that the current need for SBHC services far outstrips their availability, and we know that the potential social impact of SBHCs is far greater than what is currently being realized. The gap between the current reality and the potential lies in wiser investments. The responsibility for these investments lies in part with the SBHC movement and in part with the private sector.

The SBHC movement must advocate for better stewardship of the cost savings realized by SBHCs in the form of reinvestment of those savings back into the model. This reinvestment can happen at the federal level through improved Medicaid and CHIP reimbursement and through appropriation of federal funds for SBHC operations. This reinvestment can happen at the state and local level. NASBHC is proud to be the national voice for the SBHC movement in leading this work at the federal level.

Along with strong advocacy, the field can bridge the gap by continuing to incorporate sustainability practices in their work. Business planning, financial projections, and improved billing practices are critical to the future success of the SBHC model.

The private sector must consider SBHCs an opportunity for investment, not just an opportunity for philanthropy. We know that numerous such opportunities exist, and those that are leading the way will bring others along with them. These investments will result in short-term financial benefits in terms of tax credits and other returns and long-term benefits when it comes to a healthy and successful future workforce.

The result of these new and strengthened partnerships will be innovative ways of sustaining this uniquely "disruptive innovation." If we do all this, we'll be able to realize the true social impact of SBHCs—leading to healthier, more successful children, adolescents, and communities.

REFERENCES
1. Christensen C. Key concepts: disruptive innovation. Clayton Christenson Web Site. Available at: http://www.claytonchristensen.com/disruptive_innovation.html. Accessed April 4, 2011.

2. Basch CE. *Healthier Students Are Better Learners: A Missing Link in School Reforms to Close the Achievement Gap*. Research Review No. 6. New York, NY: Campaign for Educational Equity, Teachers College, Columbia University. 2010.

3. Winkelby MA, Jatulis DE, Frank E, Fortmann SP. Socioeconomic status and health: how education, income, and occupation contribute to risk factors for cardiovascular disease. *Am J Public Health*. 1992;82(6):816–820.

4. Walker SC, Kerns SE, Lyon AR, Bruns EJ, Cosgrove TJ. Impact of school-based health center use on academic outcomes. *J Adolesc Health*. 2010;46(3):251–257.

5. Kerns SE, Pullmann MD, Walker SC, Lyon AR, Cosgrove TJ, Bruns EJ. Adolescent use of school-based health centers and high school dropout. *Arch Pediatr Adolesc Med*. 2011;165(7):617–623.

6. Strozer J, Juszczak L, and Ammerman A. *2007–2008 National School-Based Health Center Census*. Washington, DC: National Assembly on School-Based Health Care; 2010.

7. US Census Bureau. *Population Estimates Program*. Available at: http://factfinder. census.gov/servlet/DTTable?_bm=y&-geo_id=01000US&-ds_name=PEP_2009_ EST&-_lang=en&-_caller=geoselect&-state=dt&-mt_name=PEP_2009_EST_G2009_ T006_2009&-format=. Accessed April 11, 2011.

8. US Census Bureau. *Current Population Survey, 2010 Annual Social and Economic Supplements. POV01: Age and Sex of All People, Family Members and Unrelated Individuals Iterated by Income-to-Poverty Ratio and Race: 2009*. Available at: http:// www.census.gov/hhes/www/cpstables/032010/pov/new01_100_01.htm. Accessed July 26, 2011.

9. US Department of Health and Human Services. *Achieving the Promise: Transforming Mental Health Care in America*. Rockville, MD: Substance Abuse and Mental Health Services Administration, New Freedom Commission on Mental Health; 2003. DHHS Pub. No. SMA-03-3832.

10. Juszczak L, Moore A, Schlitt J. *School-Based Health Centers National Census School Year 2004–2005*. Washington, DC: National Assembly on School-Based Health Care; 2007.

11. Blum RW. Young people: not as healthy as they seem. *Lancet*. 2009;374(9693):853–854.

12. Adams EK, Johnson V. An elementary SBHC: can it reduce Medicaid costs? *Pediatrics*. 2000;105(4 pt 1):780–788.

13. Ammerman A. School-based health care: how it is funded. *SEEN Magazine*. 2010. Available at: http://www.seenmagazine.us/Sections/ArticleDetail/tabid/79/ArticleID/864/ smid/403/reftab/326/Default.aspx. Accessed April 7, 2011.

14. Santelli J, Kouzis A, Newcomer S. SBHCs and adolescent use of primary care and hospital care. *J Adolesc Health*. 1996;19(4):267–275.

15. Guo JJ, Jan R, Keller KN, McCracken AL, Pan W, Cluxton RJ. Impact of SBHCs on children with asthma. *J Adolesc Health*. 2005;37(4): 266–274.

16. Tai T, Bame SI. Cost-benefit analysis of childhood asthma management through school-based clinic programs. *J Community Health*. 2011;36(2):253–260.

17. Wade TJ, Guo JJ. Linking improvements in health-related quality of life to reductions in Medicaid costs among students who use school-based health centers. *Am J Public Health*. 2010;100(9):1611–1616.

18. United States Senate Democrats. Patient Protection and Affordable Care Act as passed. H.R. 3590. Available at: http://democrats.senate.gov/reform/patient-protection-affordable-care-act-as-passed.pdf. Accessed May 3, 2011.

19. CVS/Caremark Web site. CVS/Caremark Workforce Initiatives page. Available at: http://info.cvscaremark.com/our-company/corporate-responsibility/workplace/workforce-initiatives. Accessed May 3, 2011.

20. Internal Revenue Service. Schedule H. Available at: http://www.irs.gov/pub/irs-pdf/f990sh.pdf. Accessed April 7, 2011.

21. Internal Revenue Service. *Hospital Compliance Project Interim Report*. Available at: http://www.irs.gov/pub/irs-tege/eo_interim_hospital_report_072007.pdf. Accessed April 7, 2011.

22. New Mexico Alliance for School-Based Health Care. *Core Characteristics of Sustainable SBHC. Executive Summary—August 2010*. Available at: http://www.nmassembly.org/pdfs/CORE%20CHARACTERISTICS%20OF%20SUSTAINABLE%20SBHC%20Summary%202010Aug.pdf. Accessed April 7, 2011.

About the Authors

Whitney Brimfield – is Director of Engagement at the National Assembly on School-Based Health Care (NASBHC) where she leads the Outreach and Engagement team. She works with the Executive Director and Executive Board to achieve resource development goals; supervises the communications, membership, and state relations; and assists with business development for NASBHC's professional services. Whitney's background is in reproductive and adolescent health and health communications. In 2004, she received her Master's in Health Science from Johns Hopkins Bloomberg School of Public Health. Prior to her graduate degree, Whitney was Development Director at the DC Campaign to Prevent Teen Pregnancy. Whitney has a Bachelor's in Biology from Haverford College.

Adrienne Ammerman – is Communications Director at the NASBHC. Prior to joining NASBHC, Adrienne managed press communications for the National Women's Law Center and was responsible for marketing and communications at Bread for the City, a nonprofit that provides direct services to low-income Washington, DC, residents. Adrienne first became passionate about the potential to use communications to promote and enhance health and well-being of young people while a fellow at an adolescent health nonprofit in New Delhi, India, where she worked with Indian media to raise awareness about child marriage and teen pregnancy. Adrienne graduated with a Bachelor's in Gender and Sexuality from the New School in New York City and is currently a master's candidate in Health Communication at Johns Hopkins University.

Linda Juszczak – is President of the NASBHC. Her 35 years of professional experience includes work as a nurse practitioner and a director for hospital, community, and school-based programs for adolescents. She has also held responsibilities as a faculty member and for developing policies impacting adolescents and school-based health centers. She was the founding President of the New York Coalition for School-Based Primary Care and is a founding member of the NASBHC. Linda's faculty appointments have been at Yale University, New York University, Cornell University, and Albert Einstein College of Medicine. She received her undergraduate degree from Skidmore College, a Master's in Nursing at the University of Colorado, a Pediatric Nurse Associate certificate and Master's in Public Health from the University of Minnesota, and a Doctorate in Nursing from Yale University. Linda has published extensively on adolescent health and school-based health care. She continues to maintain a practice as a pediatric nurse practitioner in adolescent medicine.

School-Based Health Centers: Adapting to Health Care Reform and the Utilization of Health Information Technology*

Denise Holmes

BACKGROUND

Students perform better when they show up for class, healthy and ready to learn. School-based health centers (SBHCs) bring the doctor's office to the school so students can avoid health-related absences and get support to succeed in the classroom. SBHCs may vary based on community need and resources. An SBHC provides comprehensive preventive and primary health care services to students on or near a school campus. While SBHCs vary to meet the community's needs, there are general characteristics shared by all SBHCs.

- They are designed to serve all students with a focus on the uninsured and underserved.
- An advisory board of community representatives, parents, youth, and family organizations participate in planning and oversight of the health center.
- They are staffed by a multidisciplinary team of health care professionals. The staff may include a physician/medical director, nurse practitioner or physician's assistant, registered nurse, school nurse, social worker, psychologist, licensed professional counselor, and receptionist. Some SBHCs also employ dental providers including dentists, dental hygienists, and dental assistants.
- The SBHC may have linkages with a hospital and/or other providers to accept referrals for complex health problems and to provide services to students during hours when the SBHC is not open.

*Commissioned by the School Community Health Alliance of Michigan and presented at the National Data and reporting Workshop on November 17, 2010 with funding from the Kresge Foundation.

SCHOOL-BASED HEALTH CARE   433

- The SBHC works cooperatively with school nurses, coaches, counselors, classroom teachers, and school principals and their staff to ensure that it is an integral part of the life of the school.
- Written consents signed by parents are required for children before services can be provided.
- Clinical services are the responsibility of a qualified health provider (hospital, community health center, health department, group medical practice, and so on).

The SBHC provides a comprehensive range of services that specifically meet the serious health problems of young people as well as provides general medical care.

There are many benefits provided by the SBHC:

- Attends to unmet health care needs by placing health care where the kids are and when they need it.
- Supports students by providing a safe place to talk about sensitive issues such as depression, family problems, relationships, and substance abuse.
- Supports the school environment by helping children stay in school and by identifying and addressing health problems that may intervene in the learning process.
- Supports families by attending to a child's routine health care needs, which allows parents to stay at work.
- Saves money by keeping children out of hospitals and emergency rooms.
- Teaches students to be better health care consumers.
- Strengthens the connection between the community and the school.[1]

The services range from preventive services to chronic illnesses to primary care, including:

- Routine checkups/physical exams
- Health education
- Immunizations
- Referral and follow-up for specialty care
- Laboratory testing
- Reproductive health care
- Diagnosis and treatment of sexually transmitted diseases
- Mental health services
- Crisis intervention
- Individual, family, and group counseling
- Prescription and dispensing of medications
- Treatment of acute injuries and illnesses
- Nutrition counseling and weight management
- Dental care (selected sites only)

The most commonly reported staffing models are:

- Primary Care (PC)—The primary care model is typically staffed by a nurse practitioner or physician assistant with medical supervision by a physician. Although 25% of SBHCs with a PC model have physicians on staff, their role is largely administrative: 61% of those physicians report providing four or less hours of clinical services per week. Clinical support to primary care providers is offered by a registered or licensed practical nurse with assistance from a medical assistant or health aide. In a small percentage of these SBHCs, primary care staff may be augmented by social service, health education, or dental professionals. Mental health services are not offered in this model.
- Primary Care Mental Health (PCMH)—The largest group of SBHCs is staffed by primary care providers in partnership with a mental health professional, whether a licensed clinical social worker, psychologist, or substance abuse counselor. Clinical and administrative support is similar to the PC model.
- Primary Care Mental Health Plus (PCMH+)—This model is the most comprehensive; primary care and mental health staff are joined by other disciplines to complement the health care team. The most common addition is a health educator, followed by social services case manager and nutritionist.[2]

Today, there are approximately 1,700 centers across the country located in 45 states plus the District of Columbia. A majority (96%) of the SBHCs are located in the school building, while 3% are in a separate facility on school property. Only 1% are mobile, or nonfixed. SBHCs are located in geographically diverse communities, with the majority (57%) in urban communities. More than one quarter (27%) of SBHCs are in rural areas. The following table (Table 31.1) shows the number of SBHCs in each state.[2]

Settings for SBHCs are as varied as the types of schools in the United States. A large majority (80%) of the programs report serving at least one grade of adolescents (sixth grade or higher). A national trend over the last few years has been to redesign schools to create nontraditional grade combinations as a way to improve students' academic success. The 2007–2008 National SBHC Census (hereafter Census) shows a similar change in the number of SBHCs located in "other" schools with nontraditional grade combinations such as grades seven through twelve (20%). Sponsors (organizations that serve as the primary administrative home) of SBHCs are most typically a local health care organization, such as a community health center (28%), a hospital (25%), or local health department (15%). Other community sponsors include nonprofit organizations, universities, and mental health agencies. Twelve percent of SBHCs are sponsored by a school system.

TABLE 31.1—NATIONAL DISTRIBUTION OF SCHOOL-BASED HEALTH CENTERS

Alabama: 5	Indiana: 87	Nebraska: 1	Rhode Island: 2
Alaska: 3	Iowa: 16	Nevada: 6	South Carolina: 7
Arizona: 81	Kansas: 2	New Hampshire: 1	South Dakota: 6
Arkansas: 4	Kentucky: 20	New Jersey: 40	Tennessee: 21
California: 160	Louisiana: 64	New Mexico: 79	Texas: 70
Colorado: 45	Maine: 26	New York: 206	Utah: 5
Connecticut: 79	Maryland: 71	North Carolina: 49	Vermont: 5
Delaware: 28	Massachusetts: 59	Ohio: 17	Virgin Islands: 1
District of Columbia: 4	Michigan: 90	Oklahoma: 11	Virginia: 19
Florida: 245	Minnesota: 16	Oregon: 51	Washington: 20
Georgia: 3	Mississippi: 31	Pennsylvania: 28	West Virginia: 50
Illinois: 62	Montana: 3	Puerto Rico: 2	Wisconsin: 8

SBHCs are often supported by schools and others through in-kind donations of space and services. The majority indicate that they do not have financial responsibility for construction and renovation (66%); maintenance and/or janitorial services (77%); utilities (82%); or rent (93%). School health services and SBHCs partner to provide care for students. Census data show that over three quarters (78%) of schools in which SBHCs are located has a school nurse. Where both are present, 40% are located in separate facilities while 38% are co-located within the same health suite. Eighty-two percent of schools in which SBHCs are located have a school-employed mental health provider in the building—of these 67% are separate from the health center, and 15% are co-located with the health center. Thirty percent of SBHCs partner with the school to support students with special health care needs (students with health issues that affect their ability to learn and/or attend school). SBHCs support the academic success of these students in several ways: monitor medications (95%); review medical records (94%); assist in implementing the Individualized Health Plan (IHP; 75%); and serve on the Individualized Education Plan (IEP) development committee (70%).[2]

Students in schools with SBHCs are predominantly members of minority and ethnic populations who have historically experienced under-insurance, uninsured, or other health care access disparities. Thirty-six percent of SBHCs report serving only children who attend the schools they serve, a decrease from the 2004–2005 Census, where 45% reported serving only the student population. This trend indicates that SBHCs are expanding their ability to provide access to care to others in the community. Factors that may have influenced this trend are increased budgetary constraints and a weak economy, coupled with greater need for affordable health care in the community. Patient populations seen by SBHCs that open their doors beyond their school's students include: students from other schools in the community (58%); out-of-school youth (34%); faculty and school personnel (42%); family members of students (42%); and other community members (24%).[2]

The majority of SBHCs (95%) are open during normal school hours. Beyond the school day, the Census shows that 60% are open after school, 49% before school, and 36% during the summer. SBHCs are typically open for more than 30 hours per week. Sixty-seven percent report a pre-arranged source of after-hours care to assist students outside of normal SBHC operating hours through an on-call service.[2]

FUNDING

State funding has been a leading factor in the growth of SBHCs over the past decade primarily through state general funds and the Maternal and Child Health Block Grant under Title V of the Social Security Act. In recent years, states have tapped into other resources such as tobacco taxes and funds from tobacco settlement dollars to fund SBHCs. In addition, many states have recognized the need and advantages to billing third-party resources, such as Medicaid, for their services.

The majority of SBHCs bill public insurance for health center visits, including Medicaid (81%), the Children's Health Insurance Program (68%), and Tri-Care (41%, the health care program serving active duty service members, National Guard and Reserve members, retirees, their families, and survivors). Fifty-nine percent of SBHCs bill private insurance; 38% bill students or families directly. A majority of SBHCs (85%) also assist children and families with enrollment in public insurance programs. Improving the effectiveness of billing and collection practices and enrolling children and families in public insurance has been a major focus of sustainability efforts for SBHCs.

SBHCs also report receiving support from a variety of revenue sources not related to billing, including state government (76%), private foundations (50%), sponsor organizations (49%), and school or school district (46%). Thirty-nine percent of SBHCs receive funding from the federal government.

Managed care organizations (MCOs) play a large role in an SBHC's ability to get reimbursed for services. Critical to being reimbursed for care is whether an MCO recognizes services delivered in an SBHC and whether the provider is considered to be a primary care provider or part of the recognized or approved primary care network. The census showed that 35% of MCOs recognize SBHC staff as primary care providers or preferred providers, while 30% of SBHCs indicate that MCOs do not recognize them as such.[2]

A closer look at federal and state funding sources indicates support from a diverse base of federal programs. Almost a quarter (23%) of SBHCs receive Section 330 monies through the Public Health Service Act for community, migrant, and rural health centers; these SBHCS are mainly sponsored by Community Health Centers. State Departments of Public Health are the most common source of state funds—almost half of SBHCs report receiving funds from these state entities—while the departments of human or social services and education fund about 11% of programs. In 21 states, the state funds or sponsors a grant program specifically dedicated to SBHCs.[3]

NATIONAL DEVELOPMENTS

Recent federal legislation has changed the face of health care and health care delivery. The Patient Protection and Affordable Care Act (PPACA; aka the "health care reform act") mandates health insurance coverage to all eligible individuals. The "Health Information Technology for Economic and Clinical Health (HITECH)" Act, (part of the American Recovery and Reinvestment Act of 2009 [ARRA], or the "stimulus package") promotes the adoption of health information technology (HIT) to improve efficiency, quality, and safety. HITECH contains funds for financial incentives for eligible professionals and hospitals to adopt electronic health records and for their meaningful use, state Health Information Exchange (HIE) projects, support for "HIT extension services," demonstration projects such as "Beacon Communities," education and workforce training programs; standards for IT interoperability.

THE PATIENT PROTECTION AND AFFORDABLE CARE ACT

School-Based Health Care–Specific Provisions

PPACA includes two specific provisions related to SBHCs: language authorizing a federal SBHC grant program and an emergency appropriation that would provide $200 million for SBHCs over four years.

Individual Health Coverage

The PPACA requires US Citizens and legal residents to have qualifying health coverage or face a tax penalty. The penalty will be phased in beginning in 2014 and will reach the greater of $695 ($2,085 maximum for a family) or 2.5% of household income in 2016. After 2016, the penalty will be increased by the cost of living.

The federal mandate for individuals to have qualifying health coverage is important to SBHCs because some parents do not seek out coverage for their children, even if it is available at little or no cost, and studies have shown that children of uninsured parents are less likely to use health services even when the children have health coverage.

Employer-Based Health Coverage

The PPACA does not mandate that employers must offer insurance to their employees. However, the PPACA does provide for the following:

- Employers of 50 or more fulltime employees (30 hours per week) who do not offer insurance must pay a fee (equal to the tax credit received by employees or $400 per employee receiving a tax credit, whichever is less).
- Employers of 200 or more employees must automatically enroll employees into plans offered by the employer (employees may opt out if they have insurance from another source).
- Small Business Tax Credits of up to 35% of the employer's contribution would be available in 2011 and 2012 (less than 25 employees with an average wage of $40,000 or less and employers of 10 or fewer employees with an average wage of $20,000 or less would receive full credit); in 2013 and beyond the percentage would increase to 50% for employers of fewer than 25 employees. The credit will be available for two years.

General Mandates

Effective September 2010, the PPACA changes many long-held policies for all insurers: Coverage is extended to dependent children to age 26 years, insurers cannot exclude children from coverage due to pre-existing conditions, there are no lifetime limits on coverage, insurers are prohibited from rescissions of coverage except for cases of fraud, and there is no cost-sharing for preventive services and immunizations. Annual limits on coverage must meet standards set by the Department of Health and Human Services and will be eliminated altogether in 2014.

Health Insurance Exchanges

An HIE will be a state agency or nonprofit corporation that offers health coverage through qualified health plans. HIEs will prequalify health plans that offer standard benefit packages and provide educational materials to consumers, and will offer numerous health insurers and plans to consumers (the Connecticut Exchange currently offers 48 different health insurers and plans). HIEs must coordinate enrollment with Medicaid and the State Children's Health Insurance Plan (SCHIP).

By January 1, 2014, states must establish HIEs for individuals (American Health Benefit Exchanges) and for small businesses (Small Business Health Options Program Exchange).

HIEs will offer four benefit levels:

- Bronze, which covers 60% of the cost of benefits with out-of-pockets limits based on Health Savings Account limits and income.
- Silver, which covers 70% of the cost of benefits with out-of-pockets limits based on Health Savings Account limits and income.
- Gold, which covers 80% of the costs of benefits with out-of-pockets limits based on Health Savings Account limits and income.
- Platinum, which covers 90% of the cost of benefits with out-of-pockets limits based on Health Savings Account limits and income.

Medicaid Expansion

Effective January 1, 2014, states must cover all individuals (except undocumented aliens) under age 65 years with adjusted gross incomes below 133% of the federal poverty level (currently $29,327 for a family of 4). In addition, states must cover foster care children to age 26 years. This will result in a very large increase in the number of individuals who will be covered by Medicaid. Each State must fund the state match for these individuals.

Accountable Care Organizations

Health care reform legislation allows demonstration of pediatric Accountable Care Organizations (ACOs) to share in savings they achieve for the Medicaid program. ACOs must be accountable for the overall care of their covered beneficiaries, have adequate primary care physicians, define a process to promote evidence-based medicine, report on quality and costs, and coordinate care. The ability to capture, share, and analyze data will be an important aspect of ACOs. The legislation also allows Medicare ACO demonstrations. ACOs may be the model for other payers and future reorganizations of the health care delivery system.

IMPACT OF HEALTH CARE REFORM ON SCHOOL-BASED HEALTH CARE

The impact of health care reform is that a larger portion of children will be covered by some form of health coverage. This will mean less reliance on grants and other funding sources and greater reliance on billing insurers and health plans. If Connecticut's experience holds true, SBHCs will have to be able to deal with a number of insurers and health plans and be recognized by them as a source of care. Medicaid eligibility will be simplified so it will be easier for SBHCs to assist families in gaining eligibility. For managed care providers and ACOs, SBHCs will have to become a part of an ACO or potentially lose the right to treat portions of the school population.

One important section of the PPACA mandates the creation of a patient-centered medical home. This is defined as a mode of care that includes personal physicians; whole person orientation; coordinated and integrated care; safe and high-quality care through evidence-informed medicine, appropriate use of health information technology, and continuous quality improvements; expanded access to care; and payment that recognizes added value from additional components of patient-centered care. This may pose problems for SBHCs if they cannot link to the child's primary care provider.

Medicaid payments to primary care physicians for primary care services will be increased to 100% of Medicare rates in January 2013. The difference between current rates and the new primary care rates will be covered with 100% federal financing in 2013 and 2014.

Health Information Technology

The health care industry lags most others in the use of information technology for its core business (clinical care), although HIT is extensively used in some aspects (such as billing and claims submission). Even though health information may be created and stored electronically, it is often not shared electronically across or even within organizations.

Medicaid Incentive Payment

As an incentive for providers to adopt HIT, the HITECH Act (enacted as part of ARRA) authorized financial incentive payments through Medicare and Medicaid to eligible medical professionals and hospitals for efforts to adopt, implement, upgrade, and meaningfully use certified electronic health record (EHR) technology. The purpose of EHRs and meaningful use is to improve quality, safety, efficiency, and reduction of health disparities; engage patients and families in their health care; improve care coordination; improve population and public health; and ensure adequate privacy and security protections for personal health information.

The ARRA amended the Social Security Administration to authorize a 100% federal match for a portion of payments to encourage the adoption of EHRs (including support services and maintenance) to certain Medicaid providers who meet certain requirements. Allowable costs are paid directly to the health care provider without any deduction or rebate, the provider is responsible for payment of the EHR technology costs, the user certifies "meaningful use," and the technology is compatible with federal administrative management systems.

Eligible providers would include physicians, nurse midwives, pediatricians, and nurse practitioners who are not hospital-based and who have patient volume of at least 30% attributable to Medicaid patients. In order to be eligible, the provider would be required to waive any right to Medicare EHR incentive payments.

This provider group would be eligible for payments of up to 85% of their net allowable technology costs. However, the allowable costs of the purchase and initial implementation of EHR technology cannot exceed $25,000 or include costs over a period of five years. Annual allowable costs not associated with the initial implementation or purchase of the EHR technology may not exceed $10,000 per year or be made over a period of five years. Aggregate allowable costs, after application of the 85% adjustment, may not exceed $63,750.

Rural health care clinics, physician assistant-led rural clinics, and federally qualified health centers with at least 30% patient volume attributable to Medicaid patients would also be eligible for Medicaid incentive payments at amounts to be determined by the Secretary of Health and Human Services.

Detailed information regarding provider criteria and determination of Medicaid patient volume may be found at: https://www.cms.gov/EHRIncentivePrograms/15_Eligibility.asp. Additional information on meaningful use may be found at: http://healthit.hhs.gov/portal/server.pt?open=512&objID=2996&mode=2. Certified technology information may be found at: https://www.cms.gov/EHRIncentivePrograms/25_Certification.asp.

Regional Extension Centers

Regional Extension Centers (RECs) are federally designated entities dedicated to helping providers navigate the complex EHR marketplace by providing neutral, unbiased information and support. Their role is to assist providers throughout the entire adoption process from selecting and adopting an EHR to meaningfully using it to improve the quality of care delivered to their patients.

RECs will help the provider in vendor selection and group purchasing, implementation and project management, practice and workflow redesign, functional interoperability and health information exchange, and privacy and security best practices. Supporting meaningful use includes education on Stage 1 meaningful use objectives, oversight on vendor compliance on meeting meaningful use criteria, assisting practices in data capture for quality reporting, conducting post-implementation review, evaluating practices meeting meaningful use criteria, and monitoring meaningful use reporting.

Health Information Exchange

The HITECH Act provides requirements for the State HIE Cooperative Agreement Program. The State HIE Cooperative Agreement Program is a federal program that funds states' efforts to rapidly build capacity for exchanging health information across the health care system both within and across states. The State HIE Cooperative Agreement Program awards funding to states to develop and advance mechanisms for information sharing across the health care system, including establishing health information exchange capacity among health care providers and hospitals in their jurisdiction, ultimately enabling exchange across states.

Participating states will also be expected to use their authority and resources to:

- Develop and implement up-to-date privacy and security requirements for HIE with and across state borders.
- Develop state-level directories and technical services to enable interoperability within and across states.
- Coordinate with Medicaid and state public health programs to enable information exchange and support monitoring of provider participation in the HIE.
- Remove barriers that may hinder effective HIE, particularly those related to interoperability across laboratories, hospitals, clinician offices, health plans, and other HIE partners.
- Ensure an effective model for HIE governance and accountability is in place.
- Convene health care stakeholders to build trust in and support for a statewide approach to HIE.[4]

Additional information is available at http://healthit.hhs.gov/programs/stateHIE.

IMPACT OF HEALTH INFORMATION TECHNOLOGY ON SCHOOL-BASED HEALTH CENTERS

The SBHC's role in preventive and primary care becomes very complicated when other collaborating providers are involved. The sharing of information is either very slow or nonexistent. Once the SBHC becomes enrolled in the HIE, the ability to coordinate an individual's care will be greatly enhanced. Safety and efficiency are the obvious end results of this coordination. SBHCs are strongly encouraged to work with their sponsors on HIT. Given the size of most SBHCs, the financial and personnel status of the SBHC does not readily lend itself to implementing its own certified HIT program that meets meaningful use criteria. Most sponsors (e.g., hospitals, federally qualified health centers) may already be in the process of adopting, implementing, or upgrading their existing technology.

The accumulated database from the SBHC will enable the providers (both SBHC and other care providers) to provide a long-term positive impact on students ranging from better health to greater academic performance. SBHCs will be able to reaffirm their contributions to the students' health and educational efforts through analysis of this data. Many decried the critical shortage of data that has meaning to policymakers and purseholders and show the value of important medical and non-medical functions of school-based health care. How do SBHCs demonstrate that they are keeping kids out of emergency rooms and other inappropriate health care settings? That compared to traditional pediatric and adolescent health care practices, SBHCs do a better job of achieving primary care goals? How can school-based health care data incorporate national medical and public health quality assurance yardsticks and goals such as the Healthcare Effectiveness Data Information Set and Healthy People 2010? How can these yardsticks be augmented to include preventive services, such as the American Medical Association's Guidelines for Adolescent Preventive Services? Advocates suggested that data from the New York SBHC Medicaid carve out will be very valuable. How will the extensive billing of more than 100 SBHCs inform a national audience about normative access and utilization for school-age Medicaid enrollees?[5]

Many SBHCs lack staffing, software, and administrative structures to support billing third-party payers, such as Medicaid, for their services. SBHCs are adopting HIT to enhance their work with more than half (56%) using electronic billing systems, and 53% with a management information system. A smaller number use an electronic medical record (32%) and electronic prescribing (22%) and 7% of SHBCs have a telemedicine system.[2]

RECOMMENDATIONS

The SBHCs in the school and community can be a vital access point for health services for the student population. The following recommendations will allow the SBHCs to continue to provide these needed services effectively and efficiently.

- The SBHCs must strengthen their ability and capacity to bill Medicaid and commercial insurances for the eligible services. The SBHCs must not solely rely on the schools and community to fund these clinics. With the expansion of Medicaid eligibility, more students will likely be seen by these clinics, resulting in more demand on the financial status of the clinics. Billing Medicaid and commercial insurances will be a necessity.

- Medicaid eligibility requirements will become easier. Staff at the SBHC should become familiar with Medicaid eligibility requirements so they may assist families to enroll in Medicaid. SBHCs should develop a relationship with the local Department of Human Services to facilitate these enrollments.
- The eligible providers within the SBHCs must become meaningful users of HIT. This will strengthen the quality of the services they render and greatly enhance the communications between the primary providers and other ancillary providers for this population. Stronger communications between primary providers will help create the patient-centered family home.
- Analyze the service history to identify new coverage rules. There may be new opportunities for billing previously uncovered services, such as immunizations and other preventive care. Mental health services are provided by many of the SBHCs. These services may now be billable to Medicaid and/or commercial insurers.
- Connect to resources that can support the development of meaningful use for HIT, including RECs and HIEs. These connections will assist the SBHC to obtain certified HIT and attain meaningful use. The RECs and HIEs are there to help eligible providers.
- Participate in the larger service delivery organizations, such as ACOs or MCOs, as part of their provider panel. The SBHCs may be rendering services that may be duplicative of the ACO or MCO. Being part of the ACO or MCO will also assist in the continuous flow of information and patient-centered family home.
- Take advantage of the SBHC organizational capacity to build expertise across the network. Let the associations work for the SBHCs. The associations can collectively analyze the importance, capabilities, and abilities of the SBHCs to enhance the physical and mental health of the student population thereby enhancing their academic health. The strength of the associations can assist with the legislative opportunities to recognize and fund SBHCs nationally and statewide.

REFERENCES

1. Texas Department of aState Health Services. School-based health centers. Available at: http://www.dshs.state.tx.us/schoolhealth/healctr.shtm#2. Accessed October 4, 2010.

2. Strozer J, Juszczak L, Ammerman A. *2007–2008 National School-Based Health Care Census*. Washington, DC: National Assembly on School-Based Health Care; 2010.

3. Ammerman A. School-based health care: how it is funded. 2010. Available at: http://www.seenmagazine.us/Sections/ArticleDetail/tabid/79/ArticleID/864/smid/403/reftab/326/Default.aspx. Accessed October 20, 2010.

4. US Department of Health and Human Services, The Office of the National Coordinator for Health Information Technology. Get the facts about state health information exchange program. 2010. Available at: http://healthit.hhs.gov/portal/server.pt?open=512&mode=2&objID=1834. Accessed October 25, 2010.

5. National Assembly on School-Based Health Care. Issue brief: critical issues in school-based health care financing: a report of the National Assembly on School-Based Health Care, September 1999. 1999. Available at: http://ww2.nasbhc.org/RoadMap/Public/Funding_IB_CriticalIssues.pdf. Accessed October 26, 2010.

About the Author

Denise Holmes–is Associate Dean for Government Relations and Outreach at Michigan State University's (MSU's) College of Human Medicine and Director of the Institute for Health Care Studies, an organization providing research, policy analysis, education, and quality improvement assistance to Michigan government and health care organizations. Prior to joining MSU in 2002, Denise was the Director of the Michigan Department of Community Health's Bureau of Medicaid Policy and Federal Affairs, responsible for development and promulgation of Medicaid and State Children's Health Insurance Plan policies. Over her 32-year career with the State of Michigan, she was the Bureau Chief, Health Plan Development and Medicaid Policy; Chief, Office of Policy, Planning, and Evaluation; and Chief, Bureau of Community Services.

Center for School, Health, and Education of the American Public Health Association

Terri D. Wright

The preceding chapters of this book demonstrate the substantial advances of school-based health care over the last two decades. From models that focused on the school nurse assuring that every student was in compliance with their schedule of immunizations to the provision of comprehensive physical, mental, oral, and preventive health care services and education, school-based health care has been established as a viable source of health care delivery in urban and rural communities that responds to the needs of school-age children and adolescents. And with regard to adolescents whose health and social risks are heavily driven by their behaviors, the school-based health care model for service delivery is highly desired by them. Additionally we now have several years of practice and empirical evidence that suggest that there is an opportunity for school-based health care and school-based health centers (SBHCs) to adopt a future direction that is both strategic and proactive. They have the opportunity to leverage the trust they have earned and the reputation they have established to be a catalyst and a champion for the health and educational equity of our nation's most vulnerable children and adolescents.

The social environment of the school-age population holds many challenges and potential obstacles to their educational success and school graduation. Students today are confronted with social circumstances that include homelessness, food insecurity, substance abuse, pregnancy, traumatic stress, mental distress, and violence. They don't feel safe at school or in their communities, and they lack access to the resources that contribute to their success and well-being. The best teachers and schools cannot compensate for illness, fear, and distress.

As a result, nearly one third of all students in the United States do not graduate from high school on time. For Black, Latino, and American Indian students, that number jumps to 50%.[1] Young people who do not graduate suffer a wide range of negative social, economic, political, health, and criminal justice outcomes, with effects that last over generations.[2] Research indicates that education is the strongest predictor of long-term health. Poor health is largely found in those with less education, less income, and low-status occupations and employment.[3(p1)] Furthermore, the consequences of low educational attainment are found in adults who are more likely to die from cardiovascular disease, cancer, infection, lung disease, and diabetes.[3(p2)] These findings support the position that school dropout is a public health issue that requires urgent attention.

SBHCs have the power to eliminate or reduce the barriers to graduation and prevent school dropout. SBHCs should expand their influence beyond the clinic walls and student-patient into the school population as a community of focus for public health. They have the capacity to impact the obstacles that derail students from educational success through schoolwide programs and policies that benefit every student. This is the impetus for the creation of the Center for School, Health, and Education (CSHE) within the American Public Health Association (APHA).

CSHE was established in 2010 to emphasize the inextricable relationship between health and educational attainment particularly of the K–12 population and to recognize that school dropout is a public health priority. Its focus is on the health and social factors that determine educational success and therefore prevent school dropout. Many if not most of the social obstacles to school graduation (violence, food insecurity, poverty, drug use, teen pregnancy) are the same obstacles to health. The CSHE advances school-based health care as a comprehensive strategy for improving graduation rates for the K–12 population. SBHCs can identify and address social barriers to learning in two ways:

1. They are catalysts for developing comprehensive strategies, including prevention programs that can create a healthy school climate and improve the well-being and educational success of all students. For example, SBHCs can examine the data, design, implement, and evaluate the schoolwide policies and programs that prevent bullying, increase access to healthier food in the cafeteria, address depression and distress to prevent suicide, prevent teen pregnancy, reduce school violence, help students deal with the aftermath of violence, and whatever else students need to stay in school, learn, and graduate.

2. By serving as a doctor's office in the school, they provide physical and mental health care and services to students who may not have access to such services. Research shows that students who use the centers have improvements in their grade point average and attendance.[4]

The Center's location within the APHA underscores the fact that high school completion is a public health priority and is poised to champion this new and expanded direction for school-based health care. Educational success starts with healthy students, and individuals who complete high school are more likely to have a lifetime of better health and economic opportunities. Through partnerships, policies, and advocacy, the CSHE is a catalyst for collaborative initiatives between the educational and public health communities to ensure that all students, particularly those facing social inequities, are supported to graduate.

REFERENCES

1. Freudenberg N, Ruglis J. Reframing school dropout as a public health issue. *Prev Chronic Dis.* 2007;4(4):A107.

2. Freudenberg N, Ruglis J. Toward a healthy high schools movement: strategies for mobilizing public health for educational reform. *Am J Public Health.* 2010;100(9):1565–1571.

3. Alliance For Excellent Education. Healthier and wealthier: decreasing health care costs by increasing educational attainment. *Issue Brief.* 2006. http://www.all4ed.org/publication_material/healthier_wealthier. Accessed January 23, 2011.

4. Walker SC, Kerns SE, Lyon AR, Bruns EJ, Cosgrove TJ. Impact of school-based health center use on academic outcomes. *J Adolesc Health.* 2010;46(3):251–257.

About the Author

Terri D. Wright, MPH, ABD – is the Director of the newly established Center for School, Health, and Education at the American Public Health Association. She provides leadership to the strategic development of school-based health programming and policy to avert school dropout. Formerly, she served for 12 years as a Program Director for Health Policy at the W. K. Kellogg Foundation and provided leadership for Foundation's school-based health care policy program. Terri was Maternal and Child Health Director and Bureau Chief for Child and Family Services at the Michigan Department of Community Health where she managed policy, programs, and resources with the goal of reducing preventable maternal, infant, and child morbidity and mortality. She has her Bachelor's Degree in Community and School Health and Master's of Public Health. She is currently a doctoral candidate in Public Health at the University of Michigan. Terri takes an active leadership role in several professional and community organizations including the Institute of Medicine Roundtable on the Promotion of Health Equity and the Elimination of Health Disparities.

Appendix

For information about School-Based Health Centers see the links below[a]:

National Assembly on School-Based Health Care (NASBHC)

http://www.nasbhc.org

"The National Assembly on School-Based Health Care (NASBHC) was founded in 1995 and is the national voice for school-based health centers (SBHCs). Built from the grassroots up by individuals from state and federal government agencies, national and regional foundations, child health and education organizations, and SBHCs, we are a true reflection of the field we support. NASBHC advocates for national policies, programs, and funding to expand and strengthen SBHCs, while also supporting the movement with training and technical assistance."

Center for School, Health and Education (CSHE)

http://www.schoolbasedhealthcare.org

"The Center advances the well-being and educational success of the school-age population through partnerships, policy and advocacy. The Center promotes school-based health centers as uniquely positioned to create learning-friendly environments, increase access to physical and mental health care, and promote lifelong healthy behaviors for children and teens."

American School Health Association

http://www.ashaweb.org

"The American School Health Association (ASHA) is the leading membership organization for school health professionals. It is concerned with all health factors that are necessary for students to be ready to learn, including optimum nutrition, physical fitness, emotional well-being, and a safe and clean environment. This broad spectrum of topics makes ASHA unique among health and education organizations and sets the stage for collaboration among its membership and partners."

---

[a] Descriptions are verbatim from each website.

Centers for Disease Control and Health Promotion (CDC)

http://www.cdc.gov/HealthyYouth/index.htm

"CDC's mission is to collaborate to create the expertise, information, and tools that people and communities need to protect their health—through health promotion, prevention of disease, injury and disability, and preparedness for new health threats."

US Department of Education National Center for Education Statistics

http://nces.ed.gov/

"The National Center for Education Statistics (NCES) is the primary federal entity for collecting and analyzing data related to education in the U.S. and other nations. NCES is located within the US Department of Education and the Institute of Education Sciences."

US Government Accountability Office

School-Based Health Centers: Available Information On Federal Funding

http://www.gao.gov/products/GAO-11-18R

"The US Government Accountability Office (GAO) is an independent, non-partisan agency that works for Congress. Often called the 'congressional watchdog,' GAO investigates how the federal government spends taxpayer dollars. Our mission is to support the Congress in meeting its constitutional responsibilities and to help improve the performance and ensure the accountability of the federal government for the benefit of the American people. We provide Congress with timely information that is objective, fact-based, nonpartisan, nonideological, fair, and balanced."

The Center For Health and Healthcare in Schools

http://www.healthinschools.org

"The Center for Health and Health Care in Schools (CHHCS) is a non-partisan policy and program resource center at George Washington University's School of Public Health and Health Services. The Center's mission is to strengthen the well-being of children and youth through effective health programs and health care services in schools."

Index

Note: The italicized *f* and *t* following page numbers refer to figures and tables, respectively. The italicized *n* refers to footnotes.

racial/ethnic disparities, 397
  SBHC status and, 109*t*
  socioeconomic status and, 164
Opposition messages, in poll, 218–219, 219*t*
Oral health. *See* Dental and oral health care
Oral Health Executive Committee, 20
Orleans Parish public school study
  conclusions, 112
  limitations, 112
  methodology, 103–105
  participant demographics, 105, 105*t*
  participating schools, 104, 104*t*
  purpose, 103
  results, 106–112, 106*t*, 109*t*, 110*t*, 307
Orleans Parish SBHCs, 305
Orleans Parish Youth Risk Behavioral
      Survey (YRBS), 102
Orleans Recovery School District, 304, 307
Overweight. *See* Obesity and overweight

P
Parental consent. *See also* Minor consent
      health rights
  in New York SBHCs, 350
  public opinion, 216–217, 218, 221–222
  service decisions and, 311
Parent education, 66
Parent productivity losses, 218, 282,
      406–407, 410
Partnership for Child Development, 338
Partnerships. *See also* Education and health
      partnerships
  from funder's perspective, 317
  with private sector, 429
Patient-Centered Medical Home, 364–365,
      364*t*. *See also* Medical home
Patient population, 3, 31*t*, 436–437
Patient Protection and Affordable Care Act
      (PPACA)
  impact on SBHCs, 4, 440–443
  insurance mandates and provisions,
      438–440

SBHC funding in, 161, 354, 425
SBHCPP impact on, 133–134
Patient satisfaction, 39, 103
Patrick, Deval, 292
Pediatric health care shortfalls, 15
Personal level of change, 183, 194
Philanthropy
  investment risks, 134–135
  leadership from, 136
  relationship building through, 137
Physical discomfort, 52*t*, 53*t*, 55, 56–57*t*, 59
Physical activity, 15–23, *passim*
  obesity prevention program, 17
  results of studies, 37, 51, 52*t*, 53*t*, 54,
      56–57*t*, 58, 60
  SBHC status and, 109*t*, 110*t*, 111
  weight management intervention, 119,
      120
Physical health. *See* Health outcomes;
      Medical services
Plaquemines Parish schools, 304
Playground initiative, 263–265
Policy advocacy. *See also* National Assem-
      bly on School-Based Health Care
  communication, 138, 139–140, 201–203,
      220–223
  community engagement, 136, 138–139
  eight-step process, 264*f*, 265*f*
  guidelines for progress, 140–142
  in Indian Country, 195–198
  integrated approaches, 170–173, 171*f*,
      180
  leadership, 135–136, 139
  lobbying, 147–151
  multicultural lens, 179–180, 181*f*,
      185–188, 188*t*, 193–195
  organizational capacity, 135
  philanthropic support, 134–137
  SBHCPP impact on, 133–134, 143
  variations in progress, 138
  youth advocacy, 136–137, 143, 261–265,
      265*f*